HEAD AND NECK CANCER

Cancer Treatment and Research
Steven T. Rosen, M.D., *Series Editor*

Goldstein, L.J., Ozols, R. F. (eds): *Anticancer Drug Resistance. Advances in Molecular and Clinical Research.* 1994. ISBN 0-7923-2836-1.

Hong, W.K., Weber, R.S. (eds): *Head and Neck Cancer. Basic and Clinical Aspects.* 1994. ISBN 0-7923-3015-3.

Thall, P.F. (ed): *Recent Advances in Clinical Trial Design and Analysis.* 1995. ISBN 0-7923-3235-0.

Buckner, C. D. (ed): *Technical and Biological Components of Marrow Transplantation.* 1995. ISBN 0-7923-3394-2.

Winter, J.N. (ed.): *Blood Stem Cell Transplantation.* 1997. ISBN 0-7923-4260-7.

Muggia, F.M. (ed): *Concepts, Mechanisms, and New Targets for Chemotherapy.* 1995. ISBN 0-7923-3525-2.

Klastersky, J. (ed): *Infectious Complications of Cancer.* 1995. ISBN 0-7923-3598-8.

Kurzrock, R., Talpaz, M. (eds): *Cytokines: Interleukins and Their Receptors.* 1995. ISBN 0-7923-3636-4.

Sugarbaker, P. (ed): *Peritoneal Carcinomatosis: Drugs and Diseases.* 1995. ISBN 0-7923-3726-3.

Sugarbaker, P. (ed): *Peritoneal Carcinomatosis: Principles of Management.* 1995. ISBN 0-7923-3727-1.

Dickson, R.B., Lippman, M.E. (eds.): *Mammary Tumor Cell Cycle, Differentiation and Metastasis.* 1995. ISBN 0-7923-3905-3.

Freireich, E.J, Kantarjian, H. (eds): *Molecular Genetics and Therapy of Leukemia.* 1995. ISBN 0-7923-3912-6.

Cabanillas, F., Rodriguez, M.A. (eds): *Advances in Lymphoma Research.* 1996. ISBN 0-7923-3929-0.

Miller, A.B. (ed.): *Advances in Cancer Screening.* 1996. ISBN 0-7923-4019-1.

Hait , W.N. (ed.): *Drug Resistance.* 1996. ISBN 0-7923-4022-1.

Pienta, K.J. (ed.): *Diagnosis and Treatment of Genitourinary Malignancies.* 1996. ISBN 0-7923-4164-3.

Arnold, A.J. (ed.): *Endocrine Neoplasms.* 1997. ISBN 0-7923-4354-9.

Pollock, R.E. (ed.): *Surgical Oncology.* 1997. ISBN 0-7923-9900-5.

Verweij, J., Pinedo, H.M., Suit, H.D. (eds): *Soft Tissue Sarcomas: Present Achievements and Future Prospects.* 1997. ISBN 0-7923-9913-7.

Walterhouse, D.O., Cohn, S. L. (eds.): *Diagnostic and Therapeutic Advances in Pediatric Oncology.* 1997. ISBN 0-7923-9978-1.

Mittal, B.B., Purdy, J.A., Ang, K.K. (eds): *Radiation Therapy.* 1998. ISBN 0-7923-9981-1.

Foon, K.A., Muss, H.B. (eds): *Biological and Hormonal Therapies of Cancer.* 1998. ISBN 0-7923-9997-8.

Ozols, R.F. (ed.): *Gynecologic Oncology.* 1998. ISBN 0-7923-8070-3.

Noskin, G. A. (ed.): *Management of Infectious Complications in Cancer Patients.* 1998. ISBN 0-7923-8150-5

Bennett, C. L. (ed): *Cancer Policy.* 1998. ISBN 0-7923-8203-X

Benson, A. B. (ed): *Gastrointestinal Oncology.* 1998. ISBN 0-7923-8205-6

Tallman, M.S. , Gordon, L.I. (eds): *Diagnostic and Therapeutic Advances in Hematologic Malignancies.* 1998. ISBN 0-7923-8206-4

von Gunten, C.F. (ed): *Palliative Care and Rehabilitation of Cancer Patients.* 1999. ISBN 0-7923-8525-X

Burt, R.K., Brush, M.M. (eds): *Advances in Allogeneic Hematopoietic Stem Cell Transplantation.* 1999. ISBN 0-7923-7714-1

Angelos, P. (ed): *Ethical Issues in Cancer Patient Care* 2000. ISBN 0-7923-7726-5

Gradishar, W.J., Wood, W.C. (eds): *Advances in Breast Cancer Management.* 2000. ISBN 0-7923-7890-3

Sparano, Joseph A. (ed): *HIV & HTLV-I Associated Malignancies.* 2001. ISBN 0-7923-7220-4.

Ettinger, David S. (ed): *Thoracic Oncology.* 2001. ISBN 0-7923-7248-4.

Bergan, Raymond C. (ed): *Cancer Chemoprevention.* 2001. ISBN 0-7923-7259-X.

Raza, A., Mundle, S.D. (eds): *Myelodysplastic Syndromes & Secondary Acute Myelogenous Leukemia* 2001. ISBN: 0-7923-7396.

Talamonti, Mark S. (ed): *Liver Directed Therapy for Primary and Metastatic Liver Tumors.* 2001. ISBN 0-7923-7523-8.

Stack, M.S., Fishman, D.A. (eds): *Ovarian Cancer.* 2001. ISBN 0-7923-7530-0.

Bashey, A., Ball, E.D. (eds): *Non-Myeloablative Allogeneic Transplantation.* 2002. ISBN 0-7923-7646-3

Leong, Stanley P.L. (ed): *Atlas of Selective Sentinel Lymphadenectomy for Melanoma, Breast Cancer and Colon Cancer.* 2002. ISBN 1-4020-7013-6

Andersson , B., Murray D. (eds): *Clinically Relevant Resistance in Cancer Chemotherapy.* 2002. ISBN 1-4020-7200-7.

Beam, C. (ed.): *Biostatistical Applications in Cancer Research.* 2002. ISBN 1-4020-7226-0.

Brockstein, B., Masters, G. (eds): *Head and Neck Cancer.* 2002. ISBN 1-4020-7336-4.

HEAD AND NECK CANCER

edited by

Bruce Brockstein, M.D.
Evanston Northwestern Healthcare, Evanston, IL
Robert H. Lurie Cancer Center of Northwestern University,
Feinberg School of Medicine, Chicago IL

Gregory Masters, M.D.
Evanston Northwestern Healthcare, Evanston, IL
Robert H. Lurie Cancer Center of Northwestern University,
Feinberg School of Medicine, Chicago IL

KLUWER ACADEMIC PUBLISHERS
Boston / Dordrecht / London

Distributors for North, Central and South America:
Kluwer Academic Publishers
101 Philip Drive
Assinippi Park
Norwell, Massachusetts 02061 USA
Telephone (781) 871-6600
Fax (781) 681-9045
E-Mail: kluwer@wkap.com

Distributors for all other countries:
Kluwer Academic Publishers Group
Post Office Box 322
3300 AH Dordrecht, THE NETHERLANDS
Telephone 31 786 576 000
Fax 31 786 576 474
E-Mail: services@wkap.nl

Electronic Services < http://www.wkap.nl >

Library of Congress Cataloging-in-Publication Data

A C.I.P. Catalogue record for this book is available
from the Library of Congress.

Printed on acid-free paper.

Printed in the United States of America.

The Publisher offers discounts on this book for course use and bulk purchases.
For further information, send email to laura.walsh@wkap.com.

TABLE OF CONTENTS

Preface vii
List of Contributors ix

Chapter 1   **Overview of Head and Neck Cancer**
             Gregory Masters, M.D.,
             Bruce Brockstein, M.D. 1

Chapter 2   **Epidemiology, Staging, and Screening of Head and Neck
             Cancer**
             Athanassios Argiris, M.D. and
             Cathy Eng, M.D..15

Chapter 3   **Oral Preneoplasia and Chemoprevention of Squamous
             Cell Carcinoma of the Head and Neck**
             Omer Kucuk, M.D., FACN 61

Chapter 4   **Early Stage Head and Neck Cancer – Surgery**
             Steven J. Charous, M.D. 85

Chapter 5   **Radiation Therapy in the Management of Early-Stage
             Head and Neck Cancer**
             Russell W. Hinerman, M.D.,
             William M. Mendenhall, M.D. and
             Robert J. Amdur, M.D. 115

Chapter 6   **Advanced Head and Neck Cancer-Surgery and
             Reconstruction**
             Brandon G. Bentz, M.D. and
             Dennis H. Kraus, M.D. 145

Chapter 7   **Modified Fractionated Radiotherapy in Head and Neck
             Squamous Cell Carcinoma (HNSCC) & Re-irradiation in
             Recurrent Head and Neck Carcinomas**
             R. De Crevoisier, M.D. and
             J. Bourhis M.D., PhD and
             F. Eschwège, M.D..199

Chapter 8   **Organ preservation-Induction Chemotherapy**
             A. Dimitrios Colevas, M.D. 213

Chapter 9   **Organ Preservation for Advanced Head and Neck
               Cancer, Concomitant Chemoradiation**
               Bruce Brockstein, M.D. 235

Chapter 10   **Unresectable, Locoregionally Advanced Head and Neck
               Cancer**
               Fred Rosen, M.D...249

Chapter 11   **Nasopharyngeal Cancer**
               Anthony TC Chan, M.D.,
               Peter ML Teo, M.D. and
               Philip J. Johnson, M.D..275

Chapter 12   **Treatment of Metastatic Head and Neck Cancer:
               Chemotherapy and Novel Agents**
               Edward S. Kim, M.D. and
               Bonnie S. Glisson, M.D..295

Chapter 13   **New Therapies for Locoregionally Advanced and
               Locoregionally Recurrent Head and Neck Cancer**
               Barry L. Wenig, M.D., M.P.H...................................315

Chapter 14   **Quality of Life and Late Toxicities in Head and Neck
               Cancer**
               Marcy A. List, PhD and
               John Stracks, BA..331

Chapter 15   **Oral, Dental, and Supportive Care in the Cancer Patient**
               Harry Staffileno, Jr. DDS, MS and
               Leslie Reeder, DDS..353

Index 371

PREFACE

Bruce Brockstein, M.D., Gregory Masters, M.D.
Evanston Northwestern Healthcare, Evanston IL and Robert Lurie Cancer Center of Northwestern University, Feinberg School of Medicine, Chicago IL.

Squamous cell carcinoma of the head and neck affects more than 40,000 people each year in the U.S., and at least 13,000 people each year die of this disease. In many countries, oral cancers are one of the leading causes of cancer incidence, and a major cause of morbidity and mortality. Sadly, these statistics have not improved despite clear delineation of tobacco and alcohol as contributory or etiologic in at least 80% of cases.

Exciting advances are occurring in the understanding of the molecular pathogenesis of squamous head and neck cancers. This progress may allow for earlier detection using molecular markers in blood, saliva, or tissue. Molecular diagnostic tools to distinguish between second primary upper aerodigestive tract tumors and metastases may be routinely used clinically in the near future. Understanding the significance of molecular markers such as p53 mutations improves our ability to use these as both prognostic markers of outcome, and predictive markers of response to our therapies.

For early stage head and neck cancer, surgery and radiotherapy remain standard therapies, with cure achieved in 60-90% of such patients. Although there is still room for improvement in these numbers, a significant need for these patients is effective chemoprevention of second primary malignancies. These occur in the head and neck, lung, and esophagus at the rate of 5% per year in those who continue to smoke, and slightly less in those who have quit. Eagerly awaited data from large randomized trials of chemoprevention agents will emerge in the next few years, and preclinical and early clinical work promise further advances in the near future.

Locoregionally advanced head and neck cancer, the most common presentation, and metastatic head and neck cancer are both considered stage IV disease. This reflects the unique biology of HNC in which the majority of patients die of locoregional, not metastatic, disease. Traditional treatment with surgery and postoperative radiotherapy has led to cure in 30-35% of patients, and less in unresectable patients treated with radiotherapy alone. In the last decade, a clear role for chemotherapy has emerged in the multimodality treatment of head and neck cancer. This has led to improved outcome in virtually all categories for which it has been used. Larynx preservation is demonstrated to be feasible for two-thirds or more of larynx and hypopharyx cancer patients treated with induction chemotherapy and radiation. Even higher rates of larynx preservation are possible with concomitant chemotherapy and radiation. Concomitant chemoradiation has clearly improved survival in unresectabele HNC when compared to RT alone, and this modality continues to be studied in resectable HNC. In the postoperative setting chemoradiation shows promise for improving survival versus radiation alone. This approach can allow organ preservation while preserving or improving cure rates when used as a substitute for surgery. Advances in reconstruction for patients requiring extensive surgeries have allowed for improved cosmesis and function.

Despite our best efforts, any treatment for HNC has the potential to lead to anatomic, functional or cosmetic sequelae, and altered quality of life. Many efforts are currently underway to describe, quantify and compare these adverse outcomes in the various treatments used for HNC. Understanding and improving these outcomes is a fertile arena for ongoing investigation.

Notwithstanding all of the advances in the multidisciplinary treatment of head and neck cancer, we continue to hope that through primary prevention we can eliminate more head and neck cancer cases and deaths than we can with all of the diagnostic and therapeutic measures discussed in this book.

LIST OF CONTRIBUTORS

Robert J. Amdur, M.D. Department of Radiation Oncology, University of Florida College of Medicine, Gainesville, Florida

Athanassios Argiris, M.D. Assistant Professor of Medicine, Division of Hematology/Oncology, Department of Medicine, Northwestern University, Feinberg School of Medicine and the Robert H. Lurie Comprehensive Cancer Center Chicago, Illinois

Brandon G. Bentz, M.D. Division of Head & Neck Surgery, Department of Surgery, Memorial Sloan-Kettering Cancer Center

J. Bourhis, M.D. PhD. Institut Gustave-Roussy, 39 rue Camille Desmoulins 94805 Villejuif Cédex, France

Bruce Brockstein, M.D. Evanston Northwestern Healthcare, Evanston, IL and Robert H. Lurie Cancer Center of Northwestern University, Feinberg School of Medicine, Chicago IL

Anthony TC Chan, M.D. Chinese University of Hong Kong, HKSAR, China

Steven J. Charous, M.D. Assistant Professor, Rush-Presbyterian-St. Luke's Medical Center & Evanston Northwestern Healthcare Hospitals

A. Dimitrios Colevas, M.D. Senior Investigator, Investigational Drug Branch, NCI/CTEP, 6130 Executive Blvd. EPN 7130, Rockville MD 20852

R. De Crevoisier, M.D. Institut Gustave-Roussy, 39 rue Camille Desmoulins 94805 Villejuif Cédex, France

Cathy Eng, M.D. Fellow, Division of Hematology/Oncology, The University of Chicago, Chicago, Illinois

F. Eschwège, M.D. Institut Gustave-Roussy - 39 Rue Camille Desmoulins - 94805 VILLEJUIF Cedex, France

Bonnie S. Glisson, M.D. Professor of Medicine, Chief, Section of Head and Neck Medical Oncology, Department of Thoracic/Head and Neck Medical Oncology, University of Texas M. D. Anderson Cancer Center, 1515 Holcombe Blvd. Box 432, Houston, TX 77030

Russell W. Hinerman, M.D. Department of Radiation Oncology, University of Florida College of Medicine, Gainesville, Florida

Philip J Johnson, M.D. Chinese University of Hong Kong, HKSAR, China

Barbara Ann Karmanos Cancer Institute, Wayne State University, Detroit, Michigan

Edward S. Kim, M.D. Assistant Professor of Medicine, Department of Thoracic/Head and Neck Medical Oncology, University of Texas M. D. Anderson Cancer Center, 1515 Holcombe Blvd. Box 432, Houston, TX 77030

Dennis H. Kraus, M.D., Division of Head & Neck Surgery, Department of Surgery, Memorial Sloan-Kettering Cancer Center

Omer Kucuk, M.D., FACN Professor of Medicine, Oncology and Nutrition (adjunct), Leader, Prevention Program, Barbara Ann Karmanos Cancer Institute, Wayne State University, 3990 John R, 5 Hudson, Detroit, MI 48201

Marcy A. List, Ph.D. University of Chicago Cancer Research Center, Chicago, IL 60637

Gregory Masters, M.D. Evanston Northwestern Healthcare, Evanston, IL and Robert H. Lurie Cancer Center of Northwestern University, Feinberg School of Medicine, Chicago IL

William M. Mendenhall, M.D. Department of Radiation Oncology, University of Florida College of Medicine, Gainesville, Florida

Leslie Reeder, DDS , Northwestern University, Feinberg School of Medicine, Chicago,IL 60611, Evanston Northwestern Healthcare, Evanston, IL 60201

Fred Rosen, M.D. University of Illinois at Chicago, Department of Medicine, Section of Hematology/Oncology, Chicago, Illinois 60612

Harry Staffileno, Jr. DDS, MS , Northwestern University, Feinberg School of Medicine, Chicago,IL 60611, Evanston Northwestern Healthcare, Evanston, IL 60201

John Stracks, B.A. University of Chicago Cancer Research Center, Chicago, IL 60637

Peter ML Teo, M.D. Chinese University of Hong Kong, HKSAR, China

Barry L. Wenig, M.D., M.P.H. Professor of Otolaryngology – Head and Neck Surgery, Feinberg School of Medicine, Northwestern University, Director, Division of Otolaryngology - Head and Neck Surgery, Evanston Northwestern Healthcare

Chapter 1

OVERVIEW OF HEAD AND NECK CANCER

Gregory Masters, M.D., Bruce Brockstein, M.D.
Evanston Northwestern Healthcare, Evanston, IL and
Robert H. Lurie Cancer Center of Northwestern University, Feinberg School of Medicine, Chicago IL

HEAD AND NECK CANCER – RISK FACTORS

Head and neck cancer is a significant health problem for high-risk populations. This chapter briefly outlines the most important aspects of this disease, which are described in detail in subsequent chapters.

Head and neck cancer (HNC) accounts for approximately 3% of all malignancies in the United States. Approximately 40,000 individuals were diagnosed with HNC in 2001 leading to nearly 12,000 deaths. This disease preferentially affects men with a three to five times higher incidence in males compared to females. The majority of patients have an extensive history of cigarette, cigar or pipe smoking, chewing tobacco use, and/or alcohol abuse. There appears to be a multiplicative carcinogenic affect of tobacco and alcohol in this population with an approximately 38-fold increased risk of HNC in patients with heavy tobacco and alcohol use. This malignancy more commonly affects patients with a lower socioeconomic status, and has a higher incidence in African-Americans compared to whites (18.7 versus 13.4 cases per 100,000) (1). The median age of diagnosis of HNC 62 years.

Additional risk factors for HNC include exposure to various carcinogenic viruses including the Human Papillomavirus, which is found in approximately 35% of HNCs and to an even greater extent in tonsillar carcinoma. The HPV-16 subtype is most commonly associated with this malignancy (2). Other viruses associated with an increase risk of HNC include the Epstein-Barr virus (EBV), which has been strongly associated with nasopharyngeal carcinoma. The herpes simplex virus has also been described in malignancies of the head and neck.

HNC often is predated by premalignant lesions in the oral cavity and pharynx with oral leukoplakia being the most common premalignant lesion observed. This is observed most often in smokers. Malignant transformation of these precancerous changes can occur in up to 44% of patients (3).

A genetic predisposition may also be relevant in the development of these cancers. There may be some association with familial cancer syndromes and an increased risk for HNC, although this is a relatively underdeveloped field in hereditary carcinogeneses (4).

There is a sequence of genetic changes that occur in the development and progression of HNC from the premalignant lesion to overt invasive cancer. Loss of the chromosomal region 9p21 is the most common genetic change observed in this malignant transformation. This genetic abnormality leads to the inactivation of the p16 gene, which appears to be important in cell cycle regulation. Therefore, loss of this can lead to malignant degeneration (5). Approximately 50 % of tumors in the head and neck region contain a mutation of the p53 gene located at chromosome region 17 p13. Loss of p53 function seems to be important in development of invasive cancer from premalignant lesions (6).

Testing for the genetic alternations occurring in the malignant transformation of HNC may help identify patients at increased risk, and direct the screening of high-risk patients, potentially leading to a higher overall cure rate by earlier diagnosis.

Patients with HNC often develop multiple primary tumors and remain at increased risk for further malignancies after successful treatment of an initial cancer. Second primary tumors develop at a rate as high as 5% per year following treatment of an initial cancer (7). This development of multiple primary lesions appears to relate to a field cancerization effect, which can occur throughout the entire aerodigestive tract.

The prognosis for patients with HNC depends on the stage of the disease at the time of diagnosis. Early stage (I and II) patients have an 60% to 95% chance of cure with local treatment alone, but patients with more advanced disease have a greater than 50% risk of recurrence or development of distant metastatic disease. Lymph node metastases and distant metastases are the most important predictors of prognosis. Traditional staging has included computed tomography (CT) and magnetic resonance imaging (MRI) to optimally evaluate the tumor, lymph nodes, and regional structures in this disease. Improvements in our ability to diagnose, evaluate, and stage these patients can improve individualization of treatment. New imaging modalities, such as positron emission tomography (PET), may improve our ability to optimally stage tumors in the head and neck region.

Molecular analysis with molecular staging using the increasing knowledge of genetic alterations occurring in these patients may also contribute to our ability to evaluate these patients (8). These techniques improve our understanding of the behavior of HNC in order to predict the likelihood of local tumor recurrence and/or development of distant metastatic disease. Ultimately, they may also be helpful in determining whether a second tumor represents a recurrence of the original malignancy or a second primary cancer.

Although HNC preferentially affects a distinct population based on socioeconomic status, alcohol, and tobacco abuse, no definite screening guidelines have been developed. Nonetheless, there is a general recommendation for oral examination by a qualified professional such as a dentist or primary care health professional in an attempt to detect these cancers or premalignant lesions earlier. A randomized trial in India in which patients received either an intensive screening examination versus routine care has yet to demonstrate a decrease in oral cancer mortality (9).

TREATMENT OF HEAD AND NECK CANCERS

Early Stage Head and Neck Cancer

Early stage HNC (stage I and II) is curable in 60% to 95% of patients. Specific cure rates dependent on the size and location of the tumor and the ability to deliver the necessary treatment. Virtually all of these tumors are technically resectable, and surgical resection and radiotherapy (RT) are equivalent in terms of cure. For some subtypes surgery may have a higher chance of one-time local control than radiotherapy. Thus the choice of RT versus surgery for stage I and stage II HNC is dependent upon a number of factors. These include the site of the tumor, the potential for long-term morbidity due to treatment, the expertise of the treating physician, patient preference, comorbidities, and prior history of radiation or anticipated need for future radiation.

Within the glottic or supraglottic larynx, surgery and RT are essentially equivalent in terms of likelihood of curing the cancer. All patients should meet with a surgeon and radiation oncologist and have a detailed explanation of the differences between treatment modalities and expected outcomes and participate whenever possible in the treatment choice. For T1 glottic tumors, initial locoregional control with larynx preservation surgery, such as vertical hemilaryngectomy, is 90% to 100%. With radiotherapy it is 75% to 95%. For T2 glottic tumors, conservation therapy results in initial locoregional control of 75% to 95% and radiotherapy is 75% to 80%. The slightly lower chance of locoregional control with radiotherapy may be solely a function of selection bias (10). With salvage for RT failures, locoregional control with either modality is approximately equivalent. For supraglottic tumors, T1 tumors are controlled 90% to 100% of time with supraglottic laryngectomy and 80% to 100% of the time with radiotherapy. Initial locoregional control of T2 tumors is 85% to 100% with conservation surgery and 65% to 90% with radiotherapy. This does not appear to be a difference attributable to selection bias (10). In all the above cases, however, survival is equivalent with either treatment (11). Notably, after five years, death from intercurrent disease and new primaries are more common than death from the primary cancer. Voice quality appears to be somewhat better long-term with radiotherapy than with partial laryngectomy, but recurrences with radiotherapy requiring salvage surgery generally require total laryngectomy and total loss of voice. Major complications are higher in the surgical group.

Oral cavity tumors can be treated with radiotherapy or surgery. There is a however a tendency to treat oral cavity tumors with surgery, with generally low morbidity, due to the side effects of radiotherapy within the oral cavity. These include acute mucositis and long-term xerostomia or tongue discomfort, dental decay and possible long-term changes in diet. Most patients recover relatively uneventfully from surgery for oral cavity tumors with relatively good function. In the oropharynx, however, early stage tumors are more frequently treated with radiation. Although there exists a risk of xerostomia and some mild to moderate swallowing dysfunction, surgery generally causes more morbidity when used to treat oropharyngeal tumors than radiation therapy. As with larynx cancers, in both the oral cavity and oropharynx, outcome in terms of tumor control is approximately equivalent with 50% to 90% of patients achieving cure depending on factors such as size, stage, location, and functional status of the patient.

Most tumors of the nasopharynx are not easily resectable. Therefore radiation therapy is almost always utilized for nasopharyngeal tumors. Although chemotherapy has been definitively integrated into the treatment of most nasopharyngeal tumors, the relatively uncommon stage I or II nasopharyngeal carcinoma is usually treated with radiotherapy alone. In those patients with endemic ("lymphoepithelioma") nasopharyngeal cancers, greater than 80% with early stage tumors will be cured with radiotherapy alone.

These cure rates are somewhat lower with early stage squamous cell nasopharyngeal cancers.

Locoregionally Advanced Head and Neck Cancers

Locoregionally advanced HNC generally refers to stage III or stage IV cancers. These patients include those with large or locally progressive T3 or T4 tumors or those with involvement of lymph nodes within the neck. Notably, a large number of patients present with stage IV (stage IVA) tumors. Although in most other carcinomas the designation of stage IV is reserved for patients with metastatic disease, stage IV tumors of the head and neck include those that are locoregionally advanced, reflecting the morbidity and mortality of locoregionally advanced HNC. Nonetheless, it is very important to note that non-metastatic stage IV HNC is curable. This contrasts with metastatic HNC and local regionally recurrent advanced HNC, both of which are generally not curable and carry a median survival of only about six months.

The treatment of local regionally advanced HNC is somewhat controversial. Treatment options differ for patients with resectable versus those with unresectable disease. A great difficulty however exists within the reproducibility of the definition of resectability. This definition is somewhat dependent upon surgeon, institution, and the willingness of a patient to lose essential organs such as the tongue, mandible, pharynx and larynx. For most subsites within the head and neck there are no good randomized studies assessing survival or organ preservation endpoints for surgery versus radiotherapy or chemoradiotherapy. Overall survival outcomes for patients undergoing primary surgery of stage III and IV tumors, often involving postoperative radiation, appears to be better than that for patients receiving radiotherapy only. There is, however, a clear bias in that those receiving radiotherapy only frequently have more advanced or unresectable disease than those who have resectable tumors. Patients who undergo successful surgery by definition have resectable disease.

Very good evidence exists for the use of sequential or concomitant chemotherapy and radiation in lieu of surgery for stage III or IV larynx or hypopharynx cancer. Outside of the larynx, the utility of organ preservation strategies has not been established in randomized trials. There is however an abundance of nonrandomized data which suggests that surgery may be safely eliminated in many patients with HNC without sacrificing the chance of cure and with allowance for organ preservation. Ultimately this decision on surgery versus radiation or combined modality therapy for an individual patient should be based on a multidisciplinary approach and a decision that involves patient discussion with radiation oncologist, medical oncologist and surgeon and a group discussion between the involved physicians. The likelihood of cure, the patient's performance status and the likelihood of morbidity or mortality from treatment will affect this decision. A major current focus of ongoing studies of advanced HNC includes short-term and long-term functional sequelae and quality of life measures.

Surgery for "resectable" locoregionally advanced HNC has not been directly compared to RT or chemotherapy with RT except in the larynx. A number of trials however have reported outcome data from which some indirect comparisons can be made. Large multi-institutional trials of surgery, usually with post-operative RT, generally comprise approximately 60% stage IV and 40% stage III patients. Five-year survival after primary surgery plus radiation is approximately 30% in these multi-institutional trials (12-14). Some single institution studies have reported higher survival figures. For patients with unresectable HNC, five-year survival figures are in the range of 20% with RT alone (15,16). Almost all of these unresectable patients have stage IV disease. Again, single institution studies have reported slightly higher numbers. There are a few large-scale studies that have looked at radiotherapy for resectable disease. The few studies that have assessed this have suggested five-year survival rates of approximately 30%. These patients have a demographic distribution resembling that of surgical patients more than radiation patients who receive RT for unresectable disease.

Altered fraction radiation implies methodologies such as hyperfractionation (dividing the daily doses in smaller fractions but not shortening the duration of treatment) and accelerated radiation therapy (delivering a course of radiation in a shorter period of time with higher daily doses). A number of randomized studies have assessed the utility of both of these modalities. In general, hyperfractionated radiotherapy, in particular within the oropharynx, has been shown to improve locoregional control and survival versus standard fraction radiation. In general, however, the side effects are greater. Accelerated RT has not consistently shown the benefit that hyperfractionated radiotherapy has shown. A large randomized trial of four different radiation schedules (RTOG 9003) showed that hyperfractionated RT or accelerated RT with a "concomitant boost" yield superior 2 year locoregional control compared to standard fraction RT or accelerated split course RT (17).

Combined modality therapy, utilizing chemotherapy and radiotherapy, began being assessed in earnest in the late 1970s to early 1980s. It was recognized that presurgical ("neoadjuvant or induction") chemotherapy almost always led to dramatic tumor responses. This led to a number of studies that compared chemotherapy given prior to RT or surgery in a randomized fashion versus the same locoregional therapy alone. Although primary tumor responses were very high, survival in general was not improved with neoadjuvant chemotherapy. There is a small survival benefit that has been demonstrated for induction cisplatin and 5-FU versus the same locoregional therapy alone (18). The focus of combined modality therapy then turned towards the goal of organ preservation with survival as a secondary endpoint. At least two large studies in larynx cancer, one in United States (19) and one in Europe (20), randomized patients to: 1) two or three cycles of induction chemotherapy with cisplatin and 5-FU followed by RT in responders, or 2) surgery plus RT. Short and long-term follow-up of these studies have demonstrated that survival is approximately equivalent and that two-thirds of patients can have larynx preservation when treated with induction chemotherapy plus RT for tumors of the larynx or hypopharynx. Preliminary results of a subsequent study however, RTOG 9111, showed that concomitant chemoradiation appears to be better than induction chemotherapy followed by RT, at least in terms of locoregional control (21). No large randomized trial has tested induction chemotherapy as a tool for organ preservation outside of the larynx or hypopharynx.

In a similar fashion, investigations began in the 1980's for concomitant, or simultaneous, delivery of chemotherapy and RT (concomitant chemoradiotherapy- CRT) as a means of overcoming radiation resistance in HNC. Patients were randomized to RT alone, in general for unresectable HNC, versus the same RT plus chemotherapy. Initial studies generally utilized single agent chemotherapy but in some, mostly later, studies multi-agent chemotherapy was utilized. Individual studies as well as a large individual patient data meta-analyses (18) have demonstrated a clear improvement of survival for CRT therapy versus RT alone. Multi-agent chemotherapy leads to even greater overall survival benefit than single agent chemotherapy (18). Unfortunately, no trial has yet randomized "resectable" patients to concomitant CRT versus surgery plus RT. There are, however, a large number of small to medium sized phase II studies that have assessed outcome of CRT in resectable patients (22,23). These have included patients with resectable or both resectable and unresectable disease, and have shown cure rates of 30% to 50%- as high or higher than those traditionally seen in patients who received surgery. The possible implication is that without sacrificing survival, CRT can be used with elimination of surgery or with its use as a salvage tool only.

For patients who have locoregional relapses of HNC after primary treatment, the outcome in general is fairly poor. Some patients who undergo primary RT will have potential for cure with salvage surgery. Likewise, a small number of patients, especially those with early stage HNC who had surgery only, will be salvaged with RT or combined radiotherapy and chemotherapy. For patients with unresectable relapses who have already had radiation therapy, re-irradiation, generally with chemotherapy, can lead to long-term locoregional control in up to 20% of very carefully selected patients (24).

Metastatic Disease

Patients who develop locoregionally recurrent, incurable or metastatic HNC have a poor prognosis. Median survival is approximately three to four months without chemotherapy and approximately five to six months with chemotherapy. A number of single agent chemotherapy drugs result in response rates of 15% to 25%. These drugs include cisplatin, carboplatin, paclitaxel, docetaxel, 5-fluorouracil and methotrexate. Combination chemotherapy results in higher response rates of 30% to 35%. These combination therapies generally include cisplatin or carboplatin and paclitaxel or docetaxel, or 5FU. Unfortunately survival remains the same whether single agent or multi-agent chemotherapy is given (25).

A number of new treatment modalities are under evaluation for HNC. Included are a variety of biologically targeted therapies. Epidermal growth factor receptor (EGFR) is over-expressed in the majority of head neck cancers. EGFR thus can be made a target for the treatment of HNC either with monoclonal antibodies directed against EGFR or downstream targets of EGFR. A majority of HNC patients either over-express p53 or express mutated p53. As a result, p53 has become a target or focus of "gene therapy" or "gene transfer". These therapies utilize a vector such as an adenovirus, which can be made replication competent or deficient, to deliver a mutant or wild type p53. Phase I and phase II studies have shown that gene transfer utilizing p53 is feasible and efficacious. Large scale phase III trials are now in progress testing the efficacy of gene transfer therapy when added to standard chemotherapy for locoregionally advanced head neck cancer.

In summary, for patients with stage I to stage IVA cancer, the goal of therapy is cure. Stage I and II patients are cured 60% to 95% of the time with surgery or radiation. The treatment modality of choice is dependent upon the size and site of the primary tumor, patient co-morbidities, expertise of the treating physician, and patient preferences. For patients with locally advanced disease, treatment options include surgery plus radiation, concomitant chemotherapy and radiation, or RT alone for patients with poor functional status. For advanced nasopharyngeal cancer, concomitant chemoradiation is considered as standard (26). For stage III and IV larynx cancer patients who do not have vocal cord destruction, concomitant chemoradiation (21), or perhaps induction chemotherapy followed by radiation is one standard treatment option, though surgery plus RT is an equivalent option if preferred by patients. For patients with resectable advanced tumors at other sites, combined modality treatment can be offered as a means of organ preservation and/or improved outcome, but no randomized studies have yet definitively shown CRT to be equivalent to surgery plus radiation in terms of survival. Patients with metastatic disease or locoregionally recurrent, unresectable disease already irradiated generally are treated for palliation.

SUPPORTIVE CARE AND QUALITY OF LIFE

The successful management of HNC patients lies not only in choosing the proper treatment but also in successfully shepherding the patient through the acute and chronic side effects of therapy. Patients who undergo surgery or radiation generally have a prolonged period of difficulty eating and frequently will require non-oral nutrition via gastric, jejunal, or intravenous feedings. Pain management, management of mucositis, skin breakdown, infection and depression require skilled multi-specialty support. Long-term attention to xerostomia, swallowing dysfunction, aspiration, dental issues and psychosocial issues are also necessary.

Oral Hygiene

The importance of adequate oral care is crucial in management of patients undergoing therapy for HNC. Each of the treatment modalities for this disease contributes to oral problems. The oral mucosa has a high-metabolic index and rapid cell turnover. Therefore, chemotherapy can preferentially affect these tissues. There is also a complex bacterial flora observed in the oral cavity. Interruption of the oral mucous membranes can lead to pathogenesis of these normal bacteria. Therapy for HNC can also affect saliva quality and quantity, and this can lead to further difficulties in oral health. Finally the normal function of the mouth including breathing, chewing, eating, swallowing, and drinking are affected by the tumor and associated therapies. Tissue injury in this region can interrupt normal function. All patients undergoing therapy for HNC should undergo dental examination due to the high-risk of concurrent dental or oral pathology and the risk for further problems developing as patients go through treatment. This is particularly true for patients undergoing multimodality therapy with chemotherapy and radiation. As described above, each of these modalities can lead to oral problems and prophylaxis, early identification and treatment may reduce the intensity of oral complications. This may include dental extraction for carious teeth, dental cleaning, and prophylaxis and treatment of invasive infections and mucositis.

A comprehensive education of patients undergoing such treatment is crucial to reduce complications such as mucositis, fungal overgrowth (such as candidiasis), xerostomia, loss of taste sensation, trismus, dental caries, and osteoradionecrosis. Education regarding diet, oral hygiene, and avoidance of exacerbating factors such as alcohol, tobacco, and peroxide, and other typical mouth care products is important for this population and requires an integrated multimodality approach. Specific guidelines have been developed as described later in this book regarding the management of each of these potential complications whether due to the primary tumor or the toxicities of therapy.

Given the broad range of effects that HNC can have, improving our understanding of quality of life as patients are diagnosed and receive therapy for this disease becomes increasingly important. Formal quality of life analysis is crucial in understanding the entire impact this malignancy has on the patient's well being. The study of quality of life has been refined over recent years, with improved science in this field. Quality of life must reflect the patient's own perception of the impact of his or her illness and associated therapy for this disease. This extends beyond the more traditional evaluation of symptoms of the cancer itself or toxicities of therapy and incorporates the beneficial effect of therapy on a patients' well being and how these affect a patients sense of well being. This may include the physical symptoms as well as social, emotional, and psychological factors and their impact on functional independence. New strategies for the study and analysis of quality of life are developing including the Functional Assessment of Cancer Theory (FACT) and the European Organization for Research and Treatment of Cancer Quality of Life Questionnaire (EORTCQLQ-30) (27).

It is clear that treatment interventions do have an impact on quality of life. Surgical resection can often lead to disfigurement, voice loss, and difficulty with swallowing. Radiation therapy can lead to difficulties with eating, swallowing and dry mouth as well as alterations in sensation such as taste and smell. Ultimately, long-term effects of radiation can lead to pharyngeal or esophageal stricture and osteoradionecrosis and early dental decay. Chemotherapy can exacerbate the effects of radiation with an increased level of mucositis and dermatitis. Chemotherapy also leads to fatigue, nausea, hair loss, and other systemic side effects.

Quality of life research can improve our ability to manage this disease by identifying specific areas of the overall quality of life that may need further attention (28). This could include the above-mentioned toxicities of therapy as well as the pain associated with malignancy and its therapy, and alternation of mood such as depression, anxiety, and fatigue. Ultimately the impact of a patient's own social behaviors including alcohol and tobacco abuse must be integrated in assessment of quality of life. Patients often have extreme difficulty in giving up these addictions due to physical and psychological components of addiction.

Overall, however, there is evidence that the toxicities of therapy we administer for these malignancies diminish over time, and that overall quality of life does benefit from treatment of the disease. By 12 months following treatment, most studies have shown that full or nearly complete recovery has occurred in overall symptoms and quality of life. It remains to be seen how quality of life measurements and analysis will affect an individual patient, as these instruments are being integrated into research efforts on population-based samples (29).

In summary, the multimodality treatment of head and cancer requires that a comprehensive understanding of the disease and therapies as well as their potential toxicities and effect on quality of life are taken into account by all of the members of the treatment team. This book will address each of these specific components and is aimed at developing an optimal strategy for the multimodality evaluation and care of this patient population.

REFERENCES

1.   Ries LAG, Eisner MP, Kosary CL, et al. SEER Cancer Statistics Review, 1973-1998, National Cancer Institute. Bethesda, MD, http://seer.cancer.gov/publications/CSR1973_1998/,2001.
2.   McKaig RG, Baric RS, Olshan AF. Human papillomavirus and head and neck cancer: epidemiology and molecular biology. Head Neck 1998; 20:250-65.
3.   Silverman S. Oral Cancer. In: Silverman S, ed. Atlanta: The American Cancer Society, 1990.
4.   Copper MP, Jovanovic A, Nauta JJ, et al. Role of genetic factors in the etiology of squamous cell carcinoma of the head and neck. Arch Otolaryngol Head Neck Surg 1995;121:157-60.

5.   Van der Riet P, Nawroz H, Hruban RH, et al. Frequent loss of chromosome 9p21-22
        early in head and neck cancer progression. Cancer Res 1996; 56:2488-92.
6.   Somers K, Merrick MA, Lopez ME, Incognito LS, Schechter GL, Casey G. Frequent
        p53 mutations in head and neck cancer. Cancer Res 1992; 52:5997-6000.
7.   Cooper JS, Pajak TF, Rubin P, et al. Second malignancies in patients who have head
        and neck cancer: incidence, effect on survival and implications based on the RTOG
        experience. Int J Radiat Oncol Biol Phys 1989; 17:449-56.
8.   Forastiere A, Koch W, Trotti A, and Sidransky D. Head and neck cancer. N Engl J
        Med 2001; 345:1890.
9.   Sankaranarayanan R, Mathew B, Jacob BJ, et al. Early findings from a community-
        based, cluster-randomized, controlled oral cancer screening trial in Kerala, India.
        The Trivandrum Oral Cancer Screening Study Group. Cancer 2000; 88:664-73.
10.   Dickens WJ, Cassisi NJ, Million RR, et al. Treatment results of early vocal cord
        carcinoma: A comparison of apples and oranges. Laryngoscope 1983; 93:216-219.
11.   Mendenhall MM, Hinerman RW, Stringer Sp, et al. Management of Early and
        Advanced Laryngeal Cancer: Current status of larynx preservation. Updates in Head
        and Neck Cancer 2001; 1:1-14.
12.   Laramore GB, Scott CB, Al-Sarraf M, et al. Adjuvant chemotherapy for resectable
        squamous cell carcinomas of the head and neck: report on Intergroup study 0034. Int
        J Radiat Oncol Biol Phys 1992; 23:705-713.
13.   Head and Neck Contracts Program. Adjuvant chemotherapy for advanced head and
        neck squamous carcinoma. Final report of the head and neck contracts program.
        Cancer 1987; 60:301-311
14.   Paccagnella A, Orlando A, Marchiori C, et al. Phase III trial of initial chemotherapy
        in stage III or IV head and neck cancers: a study by the Gruppodidi Studio SUI
        Tumori Della Testa E Del Collo. J Natl Cancer Inst 1994;86:265-272.
15.   Sanchiz F, Milla A, Torner J, et al. Single fraction per day versus two fractions per
        day versus radiochemotherapy in the treatment of head and neck cancer. Int J
        Radiation Oncol Biol Phys 1990; 19:1347-1350
16.   Merlano M, Vitale V, Rosso R, et al. Treatment of Advanced squamous cell
        carcinoma of the head and neck with alternating chemotherapy and radiotherapy. N
        Engl J Med 1992; 327:1115-1121
17.   Fu KK, Pajak TF, Trotti A, et al. A radiation therapy oncology group (RTOG) phase
        III randomized study to compare hyperfractionated and two variants of accelerated
        fractionation to standard fractionated radiotherapy for head and neck squamous cell
        carcinomas: First report of RTOG 9003. Int J Radiation Oncology Biol Phys 2000;
        48:7-16.
18.   Pignon JP, Bourhis J, Domenge C, Designe L. Chemotherapy added to locoregional
        treatment for head and neck squamous cell carcinoma: three meta-analyses of
        updated
19.   Induction chemotherapy plus radiation compared with surgery plus radiation in
        patients with advanced laryngeal cancer. The Department of Veterans Affairs Cancer
        Study Group. N Engl J Med 1991; 324:1685-1690.
20.   Lefebvre, JL, Chevalier, D, Luboinski B, et al. Larynx preservation in pyriform sinus
        cancer: Preliminary results of a European Organization for research of cancer phase
        II trial. J Natl Cancer Inst 1996; 88:890-899.
21.   Forastiere AA, Berkey B, Maor M, et al. Phase III trial to preserve the larynx:
        Induction chemotherapy and radiotherapy versus concomitant chemoradiotherapy
        versus radiotherapy alone, Intergroup trial R91-11. Proc ASCO 2001; 20:abstract 4.
22.   Kies MS, Haraf DJ, Rosen F, et al. Concomitant infusional paclitaxel and
        fluorouracil, oral hydroxyurea, and hyperfractionated radiation for locally advanced
        squamous head and neck cancer. J Clin Oncol 2001; 19:1961-1969.

23.   Adelstein DJ, Lavertu P, Saxton JP et al. Mature results of a phase III randomized trial comparing concurrent chemoradiotherapy with radiation therapy alone in patients with stage III and IV squamous cell carcinoma of the head and neck. Cancer 2000;88:876-883.

24.   Brockstein B, Haraf DJ, Stenson K, et al. A phase I-II study of concomitant chemoradiotherapy with paclitaxel (one-hour infusion), 5-fluorouracil and hydroxyurea with gcsf support for patients with poor prognosis head and neck cancer. Annals of Oncology 2000;11:721-728

25.   Brockstein BE, Vokes EE. Principles of Chemotherapy in the management of head and neck cancer. In: Bailey BJ, ed. Head and Neck Surgery-Otolaryngology, 3rd ed. Lippincott Williams and Wilkins. Philadelphia, 2001.

26.   Al-Sarraf M, LeBlanc M, Shanker Giri PG, et al. Chemoradiotherapy versus radiotherapy in patients with advanced nasopharyngeal cancer: Phase III randomized intergroup study 0099. J Clin Oncol 1998; 16:1310-1317.

27.   Cella DF, Tulsky DS, Gray G, et al. The functional assessment of cancer therapy scale: development and validation of the general measure. J Clin Oncol 1993; 11:570-9.

28.   Aaronson NK, Ahmedzai S, Bergman B, et al. The European Organization for Research and Treatment of Cancer QLQ-C30: a quality-of-life instrument for use in international clinical trials in oncology. J Natl Cancer Inst 1993; 85:365-76.

29.   List MA, Siston A, Haraf D, et al. Quality of life and performance in advanced head and neck cancer patients on concomitant chemoradiotherapy: a prospective examination. J Clin Oncol 1999; 17:1020-8.

Chapter 2

EPIDEMIOLOGY, STAGING, AND SCREENING OF HEAD AND NECK CANCER

Athanassios Argiris, M.D.
Northwestern University Medical School and the
Robert H. Lurie Comprehensive Cancer Center
Chicago, Illinois

Cathy Eng, M.D.
Fellow, Division of Hematology/Oncology
The University of Chicago
Chicago, Illinois

Head and neck cancer accounts for 3% of all malignancies in the United States, and 10% of all malignancies worldwide [1,2]. Cancers of the head and neck cancer are a heterogeneous group of diseases with differences in natural history, treatment, and prognosis. A unifying feature, besides their location, is that approximately 95% of head and neck tumors are squamous cell carcinomas [3], which invariably arise from the upper aerodigestive epithelium and are strongly associated with tobacco and/or alcohol use. Salivary gland and thyroid tumors as well as melanomas, sarcomas and other rare tumors, such as esthesioneuroblastomas and paragangliomas, are usually examined separately. Nasopharyngeal carcinomas, even though they are of squamous cell histology, are distinct in their epidemiology, etiology, and clinical behavior [4]. Despite the fact that approximately three-quarters of head and neck cancers are attributable to tobacco and/or alcohol consumption, only a minority of smokers and drinkers eventually develop head and neck cancer. It is assumed that there is a continuous interaction between carcinogens and the individual's susceptible genetic makeup, the details of which remain to be unveiled, that leads to a succession of molecular alterations and eventually to invasive cancer.

EPIDEMIOLOGY AND ETIOLOGY

Incidence and Mortality

Worldwide

Globally, it is estimated that head and neck cancer affected approximately 634,000 men (14% of all new cancer cases in males), and 227,000 women (6% of all new cancer cases in females) in the year 1999, i.e. approximately 10% in both sexes combined, and resulted in 9% of all cancer-related deaths in both sexes in the same year (Table 1) [2]. Head and neck cancer ranks as the fifth most common malignancy in men, after lung, stomach, prostate, and colorectal cancers, and the eighth most common cancer in women, after breast, uterine cervix, colorectal, stomach, lung, ovarian, and uterine corpus cancers [2]. Cancer of the oral cavity/pharynx is 2.5 times more common in males, whereas laryngeal cancer is 7 times more common in males compared to females [2]. In men, the incidence of oral cavity/pharyngeal cancer is highest in Melanesia, Northern France, Southern India, Central and Eastern Europe, and Latin America and lowest in China and Japan [2, 5]. Amongst women, the highest incidence is observed in India and the Philippines with a preponderance of cancer of the oral cavity, where chewing betel quid is common. The age-standardized incidence rates of oral cavity/pharynx cancer are 13.5 versus 11.5 per 100,000 persons for males and 3.0 versus 5.1 per 100,000 persons for females in developed and developing countries, respectively [2]. The incidence of oral cancer is decreasing in developing countries but an increase in the incidence of oral cavity/pharyngeal cancer has been noted in many developed countries, such as in countries of the Southern and Eastern Europe [5]. In Melanesia, where tobacco chewing is popular, 95% of the mouth/pharynx cancers occur in the mouth compared to 56% in Western Europe [2]. Laryngeal cancer is more common in Europe, South America, and Western Asia. An increase in the incidence of oral cavity cancer, especially of tongue cancer, has been noted in individuals below the age of 40 [6]. In the United States (U.S.), the incidence in this age group has risen from 3% of oral cavity/pharyngeal cancers in 1973 to 6% in 1993, whereas in India 16-28% of oral cancers occur in people younger than 40 years of age [6].

Table 1.**Estimates age-standardized incidence and mortality rates per 100,000 worldwide**[2].

SITE	INCIDENCE		MORTALITY	
	Male	Female	Male	Female
Mouth	6.6	2.9	3.1	1.4
Nasopharynx	1.8	0.7	1.1	0.4
Mouth/Pharynx	12.1	4.4	6.6	2.3
Other Pharynx	3.6	0.7	2.4	0.5
Larynx	5.7	0.7	3.1	0.4

United States

In the U.S., an estimated 40,100 individuals were diagnosed with head and neck cancer in 2001, with 11,800 deaths [1]. The incidence is 3-5 fold higher in males than females (see Table 2), and it varies by tumor site. The male to female ratio has been decreasing over time presumably as a result of the growing number of women smokers.

Table 2. **Age-adjusted Incidence, Mortality, and Survival of Patients with Head and Neck Cancer in the United States (SEER DATABASE 1994-98)** [1]

Site	Annual Incidence per 100,000	% of all head and neck sites	Incidence Ratio in males/females	Mortality per 100,000	5-year relative survival (1992-97)
Lip	1.0	7	1.8/0.3 6.0	0.0	94%
Tongue	2.2	16	3.2/1.4 2.3	0.6	51.5%
Salivary gland	1.0	7	1.3/0.8 1.6	0.2	72.4%
Floor of mouth	0.9	7	1.3/0.5 2.6	0.1	52%
Nasopharynx	0.6	4	0.9/0.4 2.2	0.2	57%
Tonsil	1.1	8	1.8/0.5 3.6	0.2	52.5%
Oropharynx	0.3	2	0.4/0.1 4.0	0.2	33%
Hypopharynx	0.9	7	1.5/0.4 3.7	0.1	32%
All oral cavity/pharynx	9.9	73	14.8/5.8 2.6	2.6	56%
Larynx	3.7	27	6.5/1.4 4.6	1.3	64.5%

Surveillance, Epidemiology, and Surveillance Program (SEER) Database.

The SEER program collects data from 11 geographic areas in the U.S. that represent approximately 15% of the population. Head and neck malignancies are grouped in two major categories: oral cavity/pharyngeal cancers, and laryngeal cancers. Head and neck cancer is the sixth most common solid malignancy in males, and the tenth commonest malignancy in females [7]. In the years 1973 to 1998, the age-adjusted incidence of head and neck cancer was 13.6 per 100,000 and the mortality 3.9 per 100,000 [7]. The incidence was higher in African-Americans (18.7 per 100,000) in comparison to whites (13.4/100,000). The lifetime risk of oral cavity/pharyngeal cancer was 1.45% in males and 0.71% in females, and of laryngeal cancer 0.67% in males and 0.17% in females [7].

In the past two decades, the incidence and mortality from head and neck malignancies in the U.S. have been declining. From 1973 to 1998 there has been a 14.7% decrease in the incidence of oral cavity/pharyngeal cancer (0.7% per year) and a 23% decrease in the incidence of laryngeal cancer (1%/year), with a corresponding decrease in mortality of 31.4% (1.6%/year) for oral cavity/pharyngeal cancer and 14.7% (0.6%/year) for laryngeal cancer (Figures 1 and 2). These changes primarily reflect a major decrease in the incidence of head and neck cancer in white males, which is apparently due to declining rates of tobacco consumption in this population. In white males, the incidence of oral cavity and pharyngeal cancer decreased from 17.6 in 1973 to 14.4 in 1997; a smaller decrease was seen in white females (6.1 to 5.8 per 100,000). However, an increase in the incidence of cancer of the oral cavity and pharynx was observed in black males that peaked in the 1980's with a recent decline in 1997. Nevertheless, in 1997, the incidence of laryngeal cancer in black males was almost two-fold higher in comparison to that of white males (11.6 vs. 6.2 per 100,000), and the incidence of oral cavity/pharyngeal cancers was approximately 20% higher than that of white males (17.1 vs. 14.4/100,000).

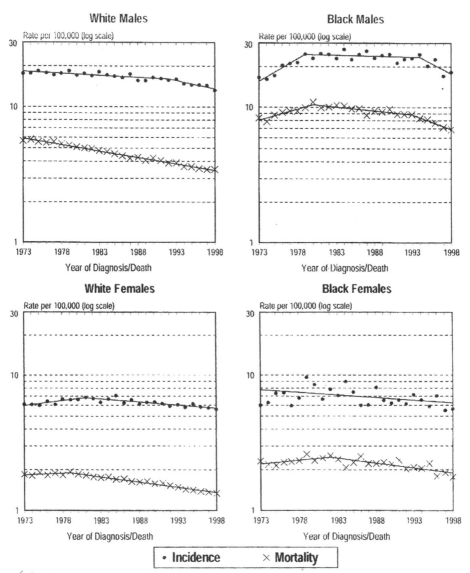

Figure 1 .

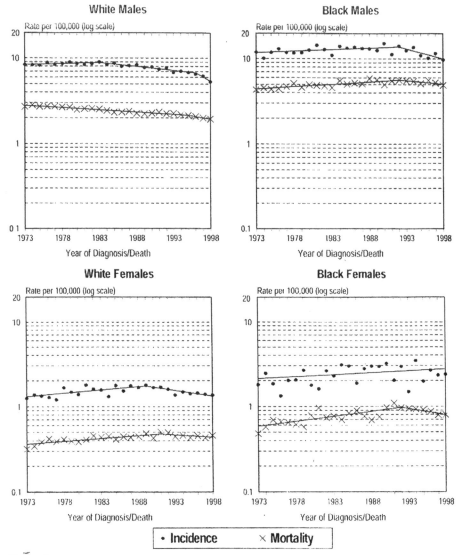

Figure 2.

AGE

According to SEER data, over the years 1994-98, the median age of diagnosis of head and neck malignancies for all sexes and races was 59-69 years, with the exception of patients with nasopharyngeal carcinoma who were diagnosed at a younger median age of 55. The incidence of oral cavity/pharyngeal cancer for people of 65 years of age or older is 43.6 versus 6.3/100,000 for younger individuals, whereas the incidence of laryngeal cancer is 18.5 versus 2.1/100,000, respectively. Laryngeal cancer is exceptionally rare below the age of 35; its age-specific incidence peaks at ages 70-74. On the other hand, oral cavity/pharyngeal cancer has an age-specific incidence of 0.3 between the ages 10-14 that gradually increases with advancing age with a peak between the ages of 80-84. Other studies have also reported a higher percentage of younger age groups among patients with oral cavity cancer compared to other sites [8].

RACE AND SOCIOECONOMIC FACTORS

Head and neck cancer is more common in blacks in comparison to whites with more pronounced differences in laryngeal cancer and in males. Higher rates of tobacco and alcohol consumption in blacks primarily account for these differences [9]. Moreover, data from the SEER database show that between 1989-1996 blacks were diagnosed with a higher incidence of distant disease at presentation when compared to whites for both laryngeal and oral cavity/pharyngeal cancers. The majority of patients with nasopharyngeal carcinoma are of Asian descent.

Social and socioeconomic parameters have been linked to the development of head and neck cancer [10-14]. However, differences in smoking and alcohol habits as well as other risk factors that may correlate with education or occupational status are strong potential confounding factors. Mackillop et al reviewed data from the U.S. and Canada and reported that in both countries there were strong inverse relationships between income and the incidence of head and neck cancer [12]. Elwood et al demonstrated an association between low socioeconomic status, based on occupation, and marital status and head and neck cancer [13]. After adjusting for other risk factors, a relative risk of 1.6 (95% CI=1-2.5) was observed. In a case-control study and after adjustment for other risk factors, Greenberg et al found that a lower percentage of years worked, but not the level of education or occupational status, was associated with an increased risk for oral/pharyngeal cancer [14].

RISK FACTORS

Tobacco and Alcohol Exposure

Tobacco and alcohol have long been recognized as the leading causes of head and neck cancer [15]. Although tobacco and alcohol are independent risk factors, it is often difficult to separate their contribution since they usually coexist. In the U.S., Blot et al calculated an attributable population risk for oral cavity/pharyngeal cancer due to tobacco and /or alcohol of 74% (80% for males, 61% for females) [16]. These two carcinogens result in a multiplicative rather than an additive effect. An approximately 38-fold increased risk for oral cavity/pharyngeal cancer in subjects who smoked more than 2 packs of cigarettes per day and drank more than 30 alcoholic drinks per week has been reported (see Table 3)[16]. Accordingly, Tuyns et al found a 43-fold increased risk for cancer of the larynx for smokers of more than 26 cigarettes a day and heavy drinkers (Table 4) [17]. Another case-control study found a 80-fold increased risk for oral cavity/pharyngeal cancer and a 12-fold increased risk for laryngeal cancer with heavy cigarette and alcohol consumption [18]. Similar results have been reported in other case-control and cohort studies in the U.S. and other countries [19-26]. Religious denominations such as the Seventh-Day Adventists and Mormons who generally abstain from tobacco and alcohol use have a multiple times less lower risk of head and neck cancer in comparison to the general population [27-29]. Different habits of tobacco use increase the risk of cancer in specific sites of the upper aerodigestive epithelium. For example, chewing tobacco has been particularly associated with an increased incidence of cancer of the oral cavity and pharynx, and reverse smoking increases the risk of hard palate cancer.

Table 3. **Relative risks for oral cavity/pharyngeal cancer among males according to amount of smoking and alcohol use (modified from Blot et al [16]).**

Cigarettes/day (for 20+ years)	Alcohol drinks per week					Total (for smoking). with 95% CI
	<1	1-4	5-14	15-29	30+	
Nonsmokers	1	1.3	1.6	1.4	5.8	1.0
1-19	1.7	1.5	2.7	5.4	7.9	1.6 (0.9-2.7)
20-39	1.9	2.4	4.4	7.2	23.8	2.8 (1.8-4.3)
40+	7.4	0.7	4.4	20.2	37.7	4.4 (2.7-7.2)
Total (for alcohol), with 95% CI	1.0	1.2 (0.7-2.0)	1.7 (1-2.7)	3.3 (2-5.4)	8.8 (5.4-14.3)	

Table 4. **Relative risks for laryngeal cancer among males according to amount of smoking and alcohol use (modified from Tuyns et al [17]).**

Cigarettes/day	Alcohol grams per day				Total (for smoking)
	0-40	41-80	81-120	121+	
0-7	1	1.6	2 3	3.8	1.0
8-15	6.7	5.9	10.7	12.2	4.5
16-25	12.7	10.7	21.0	31.5	9.3
26+	11.5	12.2	23.5	43.2	11 1
Total (for alcohol)	1.0	1.1	1.8	2.7	

Cigarette Smoking

Smoking is a major health problem in the U.S. and worldwide. In the U.S., an estimated 24.4% of male and 21.2% of female adults were active smokers in 2000 [30]. More than 50 carcinogens are found in the tobacco smoke, the major categories of which are the polycyclic aromatic hydrocarbons (PAHs), nitrosamines, and aromatic amines [31]. The relative risk for head and neck cancer increases with the intensity (cigarettes per day) as well as the duration of smoking. A higher risk of head and neck cancer has been documented in females compared to males when exposed to the same degree of tobacco [16, 22, 32, 33]. Smoking cessation gradually reduces the risk for head and neck cancer. After 10 years of abstinence from smoking, the risk for head and neck cancer approaches that of nonsmokers [16, 17, 34]

The deleterious effects of smoking persist beyond the diagnosis of a first tobacco-related primary malignancy. Patients with head and neck cancer carry a high-risk for a second-tobacco-related tumor, especially if they continue to smoke [35, 36]. The prevalence of continued tobacco use in patients with head and neck cancer ranges from 26-61% [37]. Potential predictors of continued tobacco use include an oral cavity primary, earlier stage of disease, surgical management alone [37], and heavy smoking [38]. Continued tobacco smoking during radiation therapy has been associated with decreased overall survival and inferior response to treatment [39].

Alcohol

Ethanol metabolites, such as acetaldehyde [40], but not pure ethanol, have been shown to be carcinogenic in animal studies. In addition, alcohol may facilitate the carcinogenic effect of other known carcinogens, especially those present in tobacco. After eliminating the profound effect of smoking, alcohol becomes the predominant etiologic factor for head and neck cancer [17, 41]. However, mild-moderate alcohol use, which has been defined as less than 20 grams per day [25] (usually 10-15 g of alcohol equals one drink), up to 1-6 oz of alcohol/day [34], or 1-14 drinks per week [16], results in minimal or not significantly increased risk for head and neck cancer in nonsmokers. All types of alcoholic beverages have been associated with an increased risk for the development of head and neck cancer. However, contradictory results have been reported between studies regarding the magnitude of the risk associated with wine intake [16, 18, 22, 24, 42], which can be attributed to the arduous task of the controlling for consumption of other types of alcoholic beverages. It can be concluded that the most commonly consumed alcoholic beverages in the population, i.e. wine for Italian and French studies [18, 24, 42], hard liquor/beer for many studies in the U.S. [16, 43], and beer alone for other studies (e.g. in Norway [26], Denmark [23]), have demonstrated the strongest association with head and neck cancer. Certain head and neck cancer sites, such as the lip and glottis, are less strongly associated with alcohol consumption [8, 17].

Cigar and Pipe Smoking

Although cigar and pipe smoking has been generally been misperceived by the public as safer than cigarettes, its use has been conclusively shown to increase the risk of head and neck cancer. Cigar sales were noted to have risen by nearly 50% between the years of 1993 and 1998 [44]. Blot et al conducted a subset analysis of 52 males with oral/pharyngeal cancer who exclusively smoked cigars and/or pipes in comparison to 56 healthy controls [16]. After adjusting for alcohol consumption, the risk for oral/pharyngeal cancer was almost 2-fold but increased to 16.9 with heavy cigar use. Mashberg et al reported a relative risk of 2.6 for cigar smoking and 3.2 for pipe smoking for the development of oral cavity/oropharyngeal cancer [19]. Furthermore, in a cohort study by Iribarren et al, cigar smokers had a two-fold increased relative risk for cancers of the upper aerodigestive tract (95% CI=1.01-4.06) [45]. A dose response relationship as well as a synergistic effect between cigar smoking and alcohol intake was demonstrated. A common practice amongst some Indian women is smoking homemade "chuttas" or cigars [29]. This custom results in squamous cell carcinoma of the hard palate as a consequence of the burning end of the chutta being held in the mouth while puffing continuously. This smoking habit is also seen in certain parts of Italy, the Caribbean, and South America [29].

Smokeless tobacco

Smokeless tobacco is a strong risk factor for cancers of the oral cavity/pharynx [29]. A weak association has been made between smokeless tobacco and cancers of the larynx, nasal cavity, and paranasal sinuses [46]. After a decline in the use of smokeless tobacco with a concomitant increase in cigarette consumption, a resurgence of this habit was noted in the 1970s and 1980s, with high rates of usage among high school and college students [46]. Women in Southeastern U.S. have a higher than expected incidence of oral cancer that is attributed to the use of snuff.

Snuff dipping involves placing a small amount of chewing tobacco between the buccal mucosa and gum for prolonged periods, a habit that is prevalent in the Southern and Western U.S. [46]. Oral cavity malignancies usually occur at the sites where tobacco is in contact with oral mucosa. Oral leukoplakia, a premalignant lesion, develops in 18-64% of smokeless tobacco users. [46] In a case-control study of 255 women with oral cavity/pharyngeal cancer in North Carolina, Winn et al reported a relative risk of 4.2 (95% CI=2.6-6.7) associated with snuff dipping [47]. Chronic snuff use for 50 years or more increased the risk of developing gum and buccal mucosa cancer by approximately 50 times. The vast majority of epidemiological studies have reported similar results [46]. The carcinogens that are present in snuff include [210] Po, an α-particle emitting metal, benzo(a)pyrene, a polycyclic aromatic hydrocarbon, and various nitrosamines [29, 46]. Approximately 15% of adult males in Sweden have used "Swedish" oral snuff, a moist, non-fermented tobacco product that is rarely used outside Scandinavia [25]. In contrast to the studies conducted in the U.S., the use of Swedish snuff did not confer an increased risk for squamous cell carcinoma [25]

A popular custom in South Asia is chewing betel-nut quid, also known as pan. Various ingredients, including tobacco, lime, spices, and areca (betel) nut are placed in a betel leaf which is folded and held in the mouth for hours or even days [48]. Oral cavity cancers, especially of the buccal mucosa and gingiva, are the most common head and neck malignancies in India as a result of these habits. The risk of developing a carcinoma is almost 8-fold higher in pan chewers, and relates to the duration of the mucosal exposure to the quid [49]. Chronic premalignant lesions are usually seen in the oral mucosa. Tobacco is not the only carcinogen found in betel-nut quid. In Malaysia and Papua, New Guinea the incidence of oral cavity/pharyngeal cancers is high despite the fact that tobacco is not an ingredient of their version of betel-nut quid.

Nonsmokers

Studies of head and neck cancer in nonsmokers have reported a higher proportion of women and that the tumors develop preferentially in the oral cavity as compared to smokers [50, 51]. Koch and colleagues identified 46 nonsmokers, who rarely used alcohol, if at all, and reported a larger proportion of females, oral tongue tumors, and a wider age range in this sub-group as compared to smokers with head and neck cancer [52]. A case-control study found a lower rate of smokers among young adults (40 years or younger) with head and neck cancer versus older patients (30% versus 9%) [53].

At a molecular level, the rate of p53 mutations [52, 54] and chromosome abnormalities [52] is lower in nonsmokers as compared to smokers with head and neck cancer. The role of viruses, such as HPV, for the development of head and neck cancer in nonsmokers requires further investigation.

Marijuana

The tar phase of marijuana contains common elements to cigarette smoke including phenols and polycyclic aromatic hydrocarbons. Benzo(a)pyrene has a 50% higher concentration in marijuana tar than in an unfiltered cigarette [55]. Smoking marijuana results in a 3-fold increase in inhaled tar and a nearly 5-fold greater increase in blood carboxyhemoglobin level compared to smoking tobacco [56]. In a case control study, Zhang and colleagues reported that the use of marijuana increased the risk of squamous cell carcinoma of the head and neck by 2.6 times (95% CI= 1.1-6.6) [57]. In this study, laryngeal and tongue cancers were the two leading cancers associated with marijuana use. A dose-response relationship was found to correlate with years of marijuana use (1-5 years vs. greater than 5 years, p=0.03) and frequency (once vs. more than once a day, p=0.036) [57]. Although this study can be criticized for bias in the selection of control group and the possibility of underreporting the use of an illicit drug, it demonstrates that smoking marijuana should be recognized as a potential risk factor for head and neck cancer.

Environmental and Other Risk Factors

Possible environmental carcinogens that have been implicated in head and neck carcinogenesis include polycyclic aromatic hydrocarbons, asbestos, wood dust, welding fumes, industrial heat, formaldehyde, nickel, and chromium. Asbestos exposure has been reported to increase the risk of laryngeal cancer by 1.4- to 15-fold [58-60]. Gustavvson and colleagues reported an approximately 2-fold increased risk of pharyngeal and laryngeal cancer following a more than 8 years of exposure to welding fumes. Formaldehyde has been classified as a probable carcinogen (group 2A) by the International Agency for Research on Cancer (IARC) based on animal studies [61]. Formaldehyde exposure has often been linked to nasopharyngeal cancer [62-66], but this association has been disputed [67]. Wood dust has been strongly associated with adenocarcinoma of the nasal cavity and paranasal sinuses [68-71]. The contribution of exposure to environmental tobacco smoke to the development of head and neck cancer was suggested by a case control study [72]. The etiologic role of dietary factors is controversial. However, a high intake of fruits has been consistently shown to have a protective effect [26, 73-75]. The association between salted fish intake and nasopharyngeal cancer is discussed below. Other established risk factors include sunlight exposure for cancer of the lip and ionizing radiation for carcinomas of the salivary and thyroid glands [29, 76]. Parameters that relate to poor dentition and/or poor dental hygiene [77, 78] as well as the frequent use of mouthwashes with high alcohol content [79] have been implicated as risk factors for head and neck cancer but a causative relationship cannot be firmly established [20, 80-82] due to the presence of multiple confounding variables. Finally, solid organ transplantation and immunosuppression has been recognized as a risk factor for cancer of the lip [83], and may also increase the risk for other squamous cell carcinomas of the head and neck.

PREMALIGNANT LESIONS

Oral leukoplakia (a white mucosal patch or plaque) is the commonest premalignant lesion of the oral cavity, and is a marker of an increased risk of cancer anywhere in the oral cavity [84]. The prevalence of oral leukoplakia varies between studies from 1.1-11.7%, probably as a result of variability in definition, with a mean of 2.9% [85]. The vast majority of patients with oral leukoplakia (25-97%) are smokers; prevalence rates of 0.03-3.8% have been reported in non-smokers and 4-60% in smokers [85]. Although approximately 15% of patients with oral and oropharyngeal cancers have leukoplakic mucosal changes [48], the risk of malignant tranformation of oral leukoplakia is relatively low and unpredictable. Up to 44% of leukoplakia lesions will spontaneously regress. Smoking cessation results in resolution of leukoplakia in 43-60% of cases [85]. The rate of malignant transformation of oral leukoplakia lesions is estimated to be approximately 5% [86], but it ranges between series from 0.3-17.5%, and it occurs at a mean period of 3.5-10 years [48]. The degree of dysplasia and continued use of tobacco are risk factors for the development of invasive cancer in patients with leukoplakia [86]. Erythroplakia is a red discoloration of the mucosa that has a higher risk of up to 15% for the development of head and neck cancer [87]. It is important to note that the vast majority of patients with head and neck cancer do not have an identifiable preexisting premalignant lesion. Therefore, the identification and treatment of oral premalignant lesions may not have a significant impact on the morbidity and mortality from head and neck cancer.

VIRAL EXPOSURE

Human Papillomavirus

Human papillomavirus (HPV) is a DNA virus with oncogenic potential that has been associated with anogenital and cervical carcinomas. Some HPV subtypes, such as HPV 16 and 18, result in high-risk infections for malignant transformation. HPV encodes two major oncogenes E6 and E7, which are involved in the regulation of the cell cycle. The E6 and E7 proteins are believed to promote tumor growth by inactivating the p53 and retinoblastoma tumor suppressor gene products, respectively. The preponderance of evidence from epidemiologic and molecular biology studies support an association between HPV with head and neck cancer, especially with oropharyngeal tumors [88, 89]. A sexual mode of transmission has been suggested but has yet to be proven. Patients with other HPV-associated neoplasms or premalignant conditions may be at a higher risk for the development of head and neck cancer. An increased risk for oropharyngeal cancer among spouses of women with a history of cervical dysplasia attributed to HPV has been reported [90]. Another study showed a higher risk of tonsillar cancer in patients with history of anogenital cancer [91]. Moreover, an increased incidence of tonsillar carcinoma amongst HIV positive men (relative risk of 2.6) was reported in a study of HPV-associated cancers in over 300,000 HIV positive subjects. [92]

Approximately 35% of all head and neck cancers and 77% of tonsillar cancers harbor HPV, with greater than 60% of cases being the HPV 16 subtype, as shown by polymerase chain reaction (PCR) analysis [89]. A recent study of 253 tumor specimens of patients with newly diagnosed or recurrent head and neck cancers reported that HPV was identified by PCR in 25% of cases, with the high risk HPV 16 type being present in 90% of positive samples [93]. Oropharyngeal tumors were 6 times more likely to demonstrate HPV positivity than other sites. HIV-positive oropharyngeal tumors were more likely to have wild-type p53, basaloid morphology, and to occur in nonsmokers or nondrinkers [93]. In addition, these and other investigators have reported that patients with HPV-positive tumors have a favorable outcome in comparison with patients with HPV-negative tumors [94], which contradicts results of previous smaller studies [89].

A number of case-control studies have investigated the association between HPV and head and neck cancer. Brandsma et al reported a very low prevalence of approximately 5% of HPV expression by Southern blot analysis in squamous cell carcinoma samples when compared to normal tissue samples obtained from control subjects, and failed to establish an association between the presence of HPV and head and neck cancer [95]. Maden et al performed PCR for HPV on exfoliated oral cavity cells from male subjects with oral squamous cell cancers and healthy controls. They found a higher risk of oral cancer in subjects with HPV 6 and HPV 16 infection, which was statistically significant only for the former [96]. Smith et al reported that the presence of HPV in exfoliated oral cavity cells conferred an increased risk of oral cavity/pharyngeal cancer of 3.7 (95% CI= 1.5-9.3), after adjusting for tobacco and alcohol use [97]. Two case-control studies have documented an association between the presence of HPV antibodies in the serum and head and neck cancer [98, 99]. Schwartz et al reported a relative risk of 2.3 (95% CI=1.6-3.3) for individuals with HPV 16 seropositivity versus controls [98]. The risk of developing a squamous cell cancer positive for HPV 16 DNA was 7 times higher in subjects seropositive for HPV 16 compared to seronegative subjects. Among males, the risk of oral cancer increased with younger age at first intercourse, increasing number of sex partners, and a history of genital warts. On the other hand, HPV expression in exfoliated oral tissues was not a significant risk factor. More recently, Mork and colleagues reported a case-control study of 292 squamous cell head and neck patients in comparison to 1568 matched controls [99]. The prevalence of seropositivity for HPV-16 was higher in patients with head and neck cancer versus controls (12 versus 7%), whereas it was similar for other HPV types. After adjusting for smoking history by the use of serum cotinine levels, seropositivity for HPV-16 was associated with an increased odds ratio for squamous cell carcinoma of the head and neck of 2.2 (p<0.001). As in the study by Gillison et al, the adjusted odds ratio was highest for oropharyngeal cancer (14.4) and base of the tongue tumors (20.7).

Nasopharyngeal Carcinoma

Nasopharyngeal carcinoma (NPC) is an epithelial tumor with multifactorial etiology and distinct geographic distribution. The worldwide annual incidence of NPC is 1.8 per 100,000 persons in males and 0.7 per 100,000 in females [2]. NPC is rare in the U.S. with an incidence of 0.4/100,000, which represents 4.4% of squamous cell cancers of the upper aerodigestive tract in the SEER database [3]. However, NPC is a very common malignancy in Cantonese in Southern China and Malaysians in Southeast Asia; its incidence in males is approximately 26/100,000 in Hong Kong [100]. NPC has an intermediate incidence in Alaskan Eskimos and North African Arabs [100, 101]. The possible causes include genetic and environmental factors, which may be viral and/or dietary [101, 102]. The increased risk of NPC is maintained in first-generation Chinese immigrants to the U.S. [100, 103]. In the U.S., the keratinizing (WHO I) type of NPC accounts for more than two-thirds of NPC cases, whereas in Asians as well as in Asians immigrant to the US the non-keratinizing (WHO type II) and the undifferentiated squamous cell carcinoma types (WHO type III) predominate [104]. Many case-control studies have determined a strong association between NPC and salted fish and other preserved food ingestion, especially during childhood, in Chinese populations [105-112]. In addition, certain HLA loci, such as HLA-A2a, have been linked to NPC [113, 114]. Finally, an association between tobacco use and NPC has been documented in the U.S., where the keratinizing type of NPC is prevalent [115-117], but the association is weak or controversial in Asia [105, 118, 119]. A case-control study conducted in the U.S. demonstrated a 3-fold increased risk of nasopharyngeal cancer associated with heavy tobacco and alcohol use [117]. Furthermore, a cohort study of U.S. Veterans found a 3.9 times increased risk (95% CI=1.5-10.3) of mortality from nasopharyngeal cancer in smokers compared to nonsmokers, with a pronounced risk of 6.4 amongst smokers of 2 or more packs per day [116]. Vaughan et al observed a strong dose-response relationship between cigarette smoking and risk for the WHO type 1 NPC but no association with WHO type II or WHO type III [120]. Moreover, heavy alcohol use (21 or more drinks/week) resulted in a 2.9 times (CI 95% CI, 1.2-6.9) higher risk for the development of WHO type 1 NPC [120]. Finally, certain genetic pleomorphisms in the CYP2E1 [121] and Glutathione S-transferase M1 (GSTM1) [122] enzymes which are involved in the metabolism of carcinogens may increase the risk for NPC.

Epstein-Barr Virus

Epstein-Barr virus (EBV) is a human herpesvirus that has been strongly linked with NPC. The association between EBV and NPC was first suggested by serological studies [123]. Subsequently, this association was demonstrated by identification of EBV viral genome in tumor biopsy samples of NPC [124]. Expression of the viral genes and proteins that are associated with the latent phase of EBV infection, such as the latency membrane proteins (LMPs) and the EBV nuclear antigen (EBNA), is commonly found in NPC, but it varies according to the histological type of NPC. The frequency of EBV positivity approaches 100% in WHO types II and III NPC, whereas it is relatively low in WHO type 1 NPC [125-128]. Although multiple studies have reported that EBV testing by PCR is highly specific for EBV. other investigators have reported false positive results with this method that has been attributed to the presence of contaminating EBV-positive lymphocytes. It has been suggested that in situ hybridization of the EBV encoded RNAs (EBERs) is a more specific method for detecting EBV in NPC than PCR [128].

EBER1 signal by in situ hybridization has been identified in nuclei of malignant epithelial cells in the primary tumor, lymph node metastasis, and distant metastasis of NPC [128, 129]. EBER1 in situ hybridization has been used to examine fine needle aspiration specimens from 10 NPC tumors and 19 squamous cell carcinomas from other sites of the head and neck [130]. EBER1 signal was detected in all NPC tumors but in none of the other squamous cell carcinomas. Finally, EBV DNA levels in serum/plasma or blood cells has been shown to correlate with the extent of NPC and may prove to be a useful prognostic parameter as well as a diagnostic tool for monitoring patients with NPC after treatment [131-134].

High-titers of IgA antibodies against EBV are found in the serum of patients with NPC, especially with WHO types 2 and 3 NPC, but also in the general population [135-137]. In a prospective study in the U.S., elevated antibody titers directed against viral capsid antigen and early antigen were observed in 85% of the patients with WHO types II and III tumors but in only 16% of patients with WHO type I NPC [136, 137]. Serology for EBV may identify subjects at high risk for the development of NPC. A recent prospective cohort study of almost 10,000 Taiwanese men reported an adjusted relative risk of NPC of 32.8 (95% CI=7.3-147.2) for subjects with history of a positive serology for two EBV markers (IgA antibodies against capsid antigen and neutralizing antibodies against EBV DNase) and a relative risk of 4.0 (95% CI= 1.6-10.2) when one of the two markers was positive, as compared with subjects with neither marker positive [138]. The overall prevalence of positivity for IgA against EBV capsid antigen was 1.2% and for anti-EBV DNase 12%. A total of 22 cases of NPC were diagnosed from 1 to 15 years after recruitment, 9 of which in the 1173 seropositive patients, for an overall annual incidence of 16.7/100,000. These results suggest a potential role for population screening with serology for NPC in endemic areas. Previous serological screening studies from China have also supported the usefulness of EBV serology in the early diagnosis of NPC [139, 140]. However, no randomized study has evaluated the impact of screening on NPC-related mortality.

Herpes Simplex Virus

Limited data exist regarding a potential association between head and neck cancer and herpes simplex virus (HSV). In a case-control study, Maden et al reported a non-statistically significant increased risk of oral cancer in males with serologically detected HSV infection [96]. Kassim and colleagues reported that 42% of patients were HSV-1 seropositive in comparison to 0%

in controls [141]. Finally, an association between HSV-1 serology and survival of patients with oral cancer has been reported [142].

GENETIC SUSCEPTIBILITY

Genetic predisposition may play an important role for the development of cancer of the head and neck that is not fully understood at the present time. A model of molecular progression for head and neck cancer that spans from benign hyperplasia and dysplasia to invasive cancer has been proposed [143]. Environmental factors may interact with the host's genetic material resulting in an accumulation of a series of detrimental genetic alterations that lead to invasive cancer. A 3-4-fold higher risk of developing head and neck cancer has been reported in individuals with a first-degree relative with head and neck cancer [144, 145]. Patients with Hereditary Nonpolyposis Colorectal Cancer (HNPCC) and Li Fraumeni syndrome have been described to develop laryngeal cancer [146]. Hereditary chromosomal instability syndromes, such as Fanconi's anemia and ataxia-telangiectasia, have also been associated with the development head and neck malignancies [146].

GENETIC DIFFERENCES IN CARCINOGEN METABOLISM

Major tobacco carcinogens, i.e. polycyclic aromatic hydrocarbons, nitrosamines, and aromatic amines, are being activated by the so-called phase I enzymes of the cytochrome P-450 (CYP) metabolic pathway, such as CYP1A1, to DNA-reactive metabolites that are carcinogenic [31, 147]. Subsequently, epoxide intermediates are formed, for example benzo(a)pyrene diol epoxide (BPDE), which release free radicals and may bind and modify DNA. Phase II enzymes, such as glutathione S-tranferases (GSTs), act to detoxify these free radicals. Thus, imbalances between these two types of enzymes are postulated to account for a genetic predisposition to head and neck cancer. In recent years, multiple molecular epidemiological studies have examined the role of genetic susceptibility due to polymorphisms in CYP and GSTs in the development of head and neck cancer. These studies have reported conflicting results, whereas even in studies that documented an association between common gene polymorphisms and head and neck cancer the magnitude of the risk was small or moderate. Finally, these results should be examined in the context of underlying ethnic variations in the prevalence of gene polymorphisms [148, 149].

Cytochrome P-450

Multiple genetic polymorphisms of the CYP1A1 gene due to point mutations (m1-m4) have been described [150]. A number of case-control studies have investigated the role of polymorphism in CYP1A1 in increasing the risk for head and neck cancer with mixed results: four studies produced negative results [151-154], whereas four other were positive [155-158], with reported odds ratios for CYP1A1 m2 homozygotes that ranged from 2.3 to 3.6. The significance of mutations in other CYP enzymes has also been investigated. Whereas all 5 case-control studies of CYP2E1 were negative [152, 153, 155, 159, 160] one positive study has been reported for CYP1B1 [161]. Finally, one positive [162] and two negative studies [153, 160] were reported for the association between CYP2D6 and head and neck cancer.

Glutathione S-Transferase

Glutathione S-transferases (GSTs) conjugate glutathione to DNA-damaging electrophiles which renders them hydrophilic and nontoxic [147]. Five different groups of GSTs have been described within the GST superfamily: Alpha (A), Mu (M), Theta (T), Pi (P), and Z [147]. Genetic polymorphisms relevant to altered GST expression have been demonstrated in GSTM1, GSTM3, GSTT1, and GSTP1 genes. Approximately 50% of Caucasians (range 38-67%) lack a functional GSTM1 allele (GSTM1 null genotype) [148]. It is hypothesized that individuals with the GSTM1 null genotype have an impaired ability to detoxify carcinogens resulting in a high risk for the development of head and neck cancer. A link between GSTM1-null and laryngeal cancer was first suggested by Lafuente et al [163]. Positive associations between GSTM1-null and head and neck cancer have also been reported in subsequent case-control studies, the majority of which were conducted in Japan [154, 158, 164-167]. Moderate relative risks that ranged from 1.5-3.0 over healthy controls were observed in the above studies. In contrast, multiple other studies, primarily in Caucasians, have failed to demonstrate an association between GSTM1 and head and neck cancer [151, 153, 155-157, 160, 168, 169]. Racial differences appear to play an important role in determining the contribution of certain genotypes in genetic susceptibility for head and neck cancer. A relationship between GSTM1-null and oral cancer was described in African-Americans but not in Caucasians in one study [170].

Polymorphisms in GSTP1 have been linked predominantly to the development of oral/pharyngeal cancers [169, 171-173] but not to laryngeal cancers. [155, 174] Moreover, controversial results have been reported for the association between head and neck cancer and polymorphisms in GSTM3 and GSTT1 [147]. Finally, the combination of CYP1A1 mutations and GSTM1 null genotype may result in a synergistic risk for carcinogenesis [150, 175]. However, this remains to be proven in large molecular epidemiological studies.

Alcohol metabolism enzymes

Alcohol dehydrogenases (ADHs) are enzymes involved in the first-pass metabolism of ethanol to acetaldehyde, a proven animal carcinogen. Aldehyde dehydrogenases (ALDH) are also important enzymes for alcohol metabolism that convert acetaldehyde to acetic acid. Polymorphisms in genes for ADH2, ADH3, and ALDH2 have been characterized [176]. The ADH3*1 allele is associated with a 2-3-fold increased conversion rate of ethanol to acetaldehyde compared to the ADH3*2 allele [176]. A study conducted in Puerto Rico and a smaller French study [177] showed that homozygosity for ADH3*1 increases the risk for oral cancer in alcoholics [178]. In the French study, the combination of GSTM1 deficient genotype and ADH3*1 homozygosity resulted in the highest risk for head and neck cancer [177]. Conflicting results were reported in a case-control study in the U.S. that showed that the risk for oral cancer associated with alcohol was potentiated in homozygotes for ADH3*2 [179]. Additional studies in Europe and the U.S. have failed to show an association between ADH3 polymorphism and head and neck cancer [180-182]. The mutant allele for ALDH2 (ALDH2*2) is prevalent in Asians, but is not seen in Caucasian or African-Americans [149]. Finally, a Japanese case-control study showed that ADH2 genotypes may be important for carcinogenesis [183]. After adjusting for other risk factors, including alcohol, homozygosity for ADH2*1 or heterozygosity for ALDH2*1/2*2 significantly increased the risk for head and neck cancer [183].

Mutagen sensitivity as evident by quantifying bleomycin-induced chromosomal breaks within peripheral blood lymphocytes in vitro has also been associated with an increased risk for head and neck cancer [184, 185]. The significance of polymorphisms in cyclin D1 [186] and DNA repair enzymes [187] is under investigation.

SECOND PRIMARY TUMORS

Patients with head and neck cancer are at high risk for a second primary tumor (SPT), which is often fatal [86]. The term "field cancerization" was introduced by Slaughter in the early 1950s to denote that the entire aerodigestive epithelium has been exposed to chronic carcinogenic insults and is predisposed to develop multiple foci of premalignant and malignant lesions [188]. Second primary tumors are considered to be synchronous if diagnosed within 6 months of the primary tumor, and metachronous, if developed more than 6 months after the diagnosis of primary tumor. Routine screening may reveal a synchronous tumor in 9-14% of patients, of which 42-70% are in the head and neck, 5-26% in the lung, 15-43% in the esophagus [189]. Metachronous malignancies develop in approximately 10-20% of patients with head and neck cancer at a median interval of 31 to 43 months [190-195]. More than 60% of SPTs affect the aerodigestive tract; usually the lung or head and neck is affected, and less frequently the esophagus. The annual rate of SPTs is estimated to be 3-5%, and it remains constant over time.[193] However, the reported risk varies according to the site of the original tumor, continued tobacco exposure, curability of the primary tumor, and the length and quality of follow-up [86]. The risk of SPTs is relatively low among patients with nasopharyngeal cancer compared to other head and neck cancer sites [196], but it may be higher than the expected risk in the general population, at least in Asian countries [197].

The patient's age and the amount of tobacco use have been found to correlate with the risk of a second primary tumor [198]. The risk decreases after 5 years of smoking cessation after the diagnosis of the first primary [199] but it is considerably higher in patients who continue to smoke. In a study by Moore et al, amongst 203 patients who were disease-free for 3 years or more, and therefore, presumed cured from their primary head and neck cancer, 40% of patients who continued to smoke developed a SPT versus 6% of patients who quit smoking (p<0.001) [35]. The largest prospective study of SPTs up to date has been a randomized placebo-controlled chemoprevention trial with cis-retinoic acid that enrolled a total of 1191 eligible patients with stage I-II head and neck cancer [200]. SPTs developed in 172 patients (14%), at an annual rate of 5.1%. Sixty-six percent of SPTs developed in the aerodigestive tract, of which 50% developed in the lung, 44% in head and neck, and 5% in the esophagus. Smoking-related SPT developed at an annual rate of 4.2%, 3.2%, and 1.9% in current, former, and never smokers, respectively (p= 0.034) [200]. However, the distinction between a SPT, which is usually of squamous cell histology, and a recurrence of the primary malignancy is often difficult. The distance between the location of the primary and the subsequent lesion (>2 cm of clinically normal epithelium) as well as the length of the interval between diagnosis of the original tumor and the subsequent tumor (>3 years) have been used as criteria for the definition of a SPT in randomized trials [200]. Molecular techniques may be useful for this differentiation by demonstrating clonality [201]. SPTs along with cardiovascular diseases are the major causes of death for patients with early stage head and neck cancer. Vikram et al showed that after 3 years, the leading cause of cancer-related mortality is SPTs[202]. Smoking cessation and screening and chemopreventive strategies are important goals for improving the outcome of patients with potentially curable head and neck cancer.

EVALUATION AND DIAGNOSIS

The initial patient evaluation should include a thorough history and physical examination. Frequently, the signs and symptoms of head and neck cancer are subtle and overlooked by the patient and/or the examiner, whereas early stage tumors are often asymptomatic. The time interval from the onset of symptoms to diagnosis may exceed 3 months in 34-55% of cases and one year in 7-10% of cases [203]. Although the oral cavity is readily accessible to physical examination, delays from the first professional visit to diagnosis have been reported from a minimum of 2 weeks to a maximum of 1 year, with a mean of 20 weeks [203]. Subtle signs as facial pain, mild trismus, earaches, and headaches can herald the presentation of nasopharyngeal carcinoma and may be confused with benign disorders [204]. Specific symptoms should be elicited from the patient, including the presence of neck masses, throat pain, dysphagia, epistaxis, diplopia, unilateral hearing deficit, and nasal obstruction. Therefore, education of primary care physicians, dentists, and patients is paramount. Physical examination should not only include inspection but also bimanual palpation of the oral cavity. The mouth should be examined with the dentures removed. Application of topical anesthetic may optimize examination for patients with an overactive gag reflex. Careful examination of the neck lymph nodes should be performed. A tumor map or diagram will provide much needed information when evaluating the patient's response. Clinical examination including the use of a nasolaryngoscope by an otolaryngologist is essential for the diagnosis and staging of head and neck cancer.

All patients should have a histological diagnosis. Tumors that are evident during examination of the oral cavity and oropharyngeal cavity may be biopsied in the office setting. Fine needle aspiration (FNA) is a useful diagnostic tool when evaluating neck masses. Needle or excisional biopsies of neck lymph nodes should be generally avoided, unless the other work-up is unrevealing, because they can potentially alter the lymphatics and compromise the outcome of a subsequent node dissection. In the setting of an unknown primary malignancy, a panendoscopy with random biopsies of the nasopharynx, tonsil, and base of tongue and piriform sinus, which are common sites of silent primaries, may reveal the primary malignancy.

Computed tomography (CT) and magnetic resonance imaging (MRI) of the neck provide invaluable information about invasion of adjacent structures and lymph node involvement. MRI provides multiplanar imaging and can detect subtle differences in the soft tissues. MRI is superior to CT scanning for evaluation of the nasopharynx, paranasal sinuses, salivary glands, retropharyngeal and prevertebral space, and the oropharynx. CT scanning is faster and less costly than MRI, and it is as least as good for assessing neck lymphadenopathy, whereas it has improved accuracy for the evaluation of bony erosions (e.g. invasion of the mandible or base of skull) and areas that may produce motion artifact, such as the larynx. Angiography is rarely indicated, but it is particularly useful in the assessment of invasion of the carotid artery, when surgical management is contemplated, and when the diagnosis of paraganglioma is entertained.

Distant metastases are diagnosed at presentation in 12-17% of patients with locoregionally advanced disease [205-208], whereas 20-36% of patients develop clinically detected distant metastases after primary therapy [202, 209-212]. The risk for developing distant metastases is higher for more advanced stage at presentation, especially with advanced N stage, and for nasopharyngeal and hypopharyngeal primaries. The lungs, bone, liver, and mediastinal lymph nodes are common sites of spread in head and neck cancer [213]. It is recommended that all patients undergo evaluation with chest radiographs [214]. However, chest radiographs have a low sensitivity for metastases and fail to demonstrate lung lesions in more than two-thirds of patients with lung metastases [206, 215]. With the use of CT scan of the chest, infraclavicular malignant lesions, including synchronous primary lung tumors, are detected in approximately 10-20% of patients with locoregionally advanced head and neck cancer [206, 215-217]. Therefore, patients with considerable risk for distant metastasis should be evaluated with CT scan of the chest, including the upper abdomen. A bone scan should also be considered, but its yield may be low [218]. The need for additional imaging studies for staging work-up is determined by the presence of clinical or laboratory abnormalities.

Lymph node metastases are frequently seen (70-90%) with nasopharyngeal, tonsillar, base of tongue, and nasopharyngeal primaries, even with small primary tumors [219]. The identification of occult neck lymphadenopathy, not detected by clinical examination, is of major importance, and usually modifies the treatment plan. Anatomical imaging usually relies on size criteria, which are not highly accurate for diagnosing malignant lymphadenopathy. Therefore, newer imaging modalities, such as positron emission tomography (PET) scan and ultrasound-guided-FNA have been utilized for the optimal staging of the neck.

PET scanning with [¹⁸F] fluoro-2-deoxy-D-glucose (FDG) may be helpful in the assessment of neck lymphadenopathy as well as of distant metastases. Multiple studies have shown the superiority of PET scan over CT scan and MRI in detecting lymph node involvement by cancer [220, 221]. Adams et al conducted a prospective comparison of PET scan, CT, MRI, and ultrasonography of the neck [221]. Based on histopathological findings, FDG-PET correctly identified lymph node metastases with a sensitivity of 90% and a specificity of 94%, which were statistically higher than the sensitivity and specificity of CT scan (82% and 85%), MRI (80% and 79%), and ultrasonography (72% and 70%). PET scan may provide useful information for the management of clinical N0 neck [222] but further investigation is needed. A recent prospective study showed that imaging modalities, including PET scan, US, CT, and MRI, were suboptimal in predicting histological lymph node involvement from oral cavity squamous cell carcinoma [223]. PET scan showed the highest specificity of 82% and ultrasonography the highest sensitivity of 84% compared to the other modalities. Nevertheless, PET scan resulted in the diagnosis of unexpected second primary tumors or distant metastases in 10% of patients [223]. PET scan may also be helpful in the diagnostic work-up of metastatic cervical lymphadenopathy from an occult primary. In 21-38% of these cases, PET scan will detect an occult primary tumor of the head and neck [224-228], which usually leads to modifications of the treatment plan. However, a high rate of false-positive findings and a limited added value to other imaging modalities has been reported in some studies [224, 229, 230]. PET scan may be particularly useful in the post-treatment evaluation of the patient in order to assess response and detect tumor recurrence [228, 231-235]. Due to its ability to differentiate active tumor from fibrotic changes, PET scan has a higher sensitivity and specificity than anatomical imaging with CT scan and MRI in detecting recurrent head and neck cancer [231, 235]. However, imaging within the first 3 months post irradiation should be interpreted with caution since it may produce false positive results [231]. Overall, the optimal use of PET scan in the management of patients with head and neck cancer remains to be defined, especially as PET scanners are becoming widely available. Currently, PET scanning should be considered as a complementary diagnostic modality that is particularly useful in the evaluation of a patient with ambiguous disease involvement. Of great promise is its potential role in response assessment post chemoradiotherapy as well as in the early diagnosis of disease recurrence. Correlation with more detailed anatomical imaging with CT scan or MRI findings is always required in the interpretation of PET scan findings. Dual PET/CT scanners that produce fused PET and CT images are being evaluated [236].

Ultrasonography-guided FNA improves the accuracy of clinical examination in assessing for neck lymphadenopathy [237, 238], and may be superior to other imaging modalities for this purpose [239]. In subsequent studies, ultrasonography-guided FNA has produced equal [238] or inferior results [240-242] when compared to CT scan and/or MRI for the evaluation of clinical N0 neck. Some lymph node areas, e.g. retropharyngeal, cannot be assessed by ultrasonography due to their deep-seated location, whereas aspirating small sized lymph nodes is technically demanding [243]. On the other hand, ultrasonography-guided FNA may detect malignancy in normal-appearing lymph nodes by CT scan [242], and it may be a valuable adjunct diagnostic tool for the evaluation of the neck. Its role in the routine management of patients with head and neck cancer has yet to be determined.

AJCC STAGING SYSTEM

The American Joint Committee on Cancer (AJCC) has established a staging system that incorporates three aspects of tumor growth: extent of the primary tumor (T), involvement of regional lymph nodes (N), and distant metastasis (M). The TNM staging system is based primarily on clinical examination and describes the anatomic extent of the tumor. Information from clinical staging guides the initial treatment decisions. The TNM staging systems does incorporate imaging techniques i.e., cortical involvement upgrades a patient to T4. Information for pathological staging is derived from operative findings and histopathological review and it should be recorded separately. In general, the T stage is relatively similar for each subdivision of head and neck cancer but varies on anatomical considerations. The N stage is unique in nasopharyngeal and thyroid cancer. The M stage is uniform throughout. At presentation, approximately two-thirds of patients with head and neck cancer are diagnosed with advanced disease (AJCC stage III or IV) and one-third with early-stage disease (AJCC stage I or II). The last revision of the AJCC system was in 1997. Major revisions were undertaken in the staging of nasopharyngeal cancer.

AJCC STAGING SYSTEM CLASSIFICATION, HEAD AND NECK CANCERS

TUMOR (T) STAGE

Lip and Oral Cavity

Tx	Primary tumor cannot be assessed
T0	No evidence of primary tumor
T1	Tumor < 2 cm in greatest dimension
T2	Tumor not more than 2 cm but less than 4 cm in greatest dimension
T3	Tumor more than 4 cm in greatest dimension
T4 (lip)	Tumor invades adjacent structures (i.e., through cortical bone, inferior alveolar nerve, floor of mouth, skin of face)
T4 (oral cavity)	Tumor invades adjacent structures (i.e., through cortical bone, deep muscle of tongue, maxillary sinus, and skin.

PHARYNX, SUBSITES

Tx-T$_1$ (All)

Tx	Primary tumor cannot be assessed
T0	No evidence of primary tumor
Tis	Carcinoma in situ

Nasopharynx

T1	Tumor confined to the nasopharynx
T2	Tumor extends to the soft tissue of oropharynx and/or nasal fossa
T2a	Without parapharyngeal extension
T2b	With parapharyngeal extension
T3	Tumor invades bony structures and/or paranasal sinuses
T4	Tumor with intracranial extension and/or involvement of cranial nerves, infratemporal fossa, hypopharynx, or orbit

Oropharynx

T1	Tumor 2 cm or less in greatest dimension
T2	Tumor more than 2 cm but not more than 4 cm in greatest dimension
T3	Tumor more than 4 cm in greatest dimension
T4	Tumor invades adjacent structures (e.g., pterygoid muscle[s], mandible, hard palate, deep muscle of the tongue. larynx)

Hypopharynx

T1	Tumor limited to one subsite of hypopharynx and 2 cm or less in greatest dimension
T2	Tumor involves more than one subsite of hypopharynx or an adjacent site, or measures more than 2 cm but not more than 4 cm in greatest diameter without fixation of hemilarynx
T3	Tumor measures more than 4 cm in greatest dimension or with fixation of hemilarynx
T4	Tumor invades adjacent structures (e.g., thyroid/cricoid cartilage, carotid artery, soft tissues of the neck, prevertebral fascia/muscles, thyroid and/or esophagus)

Larynx

Tx	Primary tumor cannot be assessed
T0	No evidence of primary tumor
Tis	Carcinoma in situ

Supraglottic

T1	Tumor limited to one subsite of supraglottic with normal cord mobility
T2	Tumor invades mucosa of more than one adjacent subsite of supraglottis or glottis or region outside the supraglottis (e.g., mucosa of the base of tongue, vallecula, medial wall of pyriform sinus) without fixation of the larynx
T3	Tumor limited to the larynx with vocal cord fixation and/or invades any of the following: postcricoid area, pre-epiglottic tissues, deep base of tongue
T4	Tumor invades through the thyroid cartilage, and/or extends into soft tissues of the neck, thyroid and/or esophagus

Glottis

T1		Tumor limited to the vocal cord(s) (may involve anterior or posterior commissure) with normal mobility
	T1a	Tumor limited to one vocal cord
	T1b	Tumor involves both vocal cords
T2		Tumor extends to supraglottis and/or subglottis, and or with impaired vocal cord mobility
T3		Tumor limited to the larynx with vocal cord fixation
T4		Tumor invades through the thyroid cartilage and/or to other tissues beyond the larynx (e.g., trachea, soft tissue of the neck, including thyroid, esophagus)

Subglottis

T1	Tumor limited to the subglottis
T2	Tumor extends to vocal cord(s) with normal or impaired mobility
T3	Tumor limited to larynx with vocal cord fixation
T4	Tumor invades through cricoid or thyroid cartilage and/or extends to other tissues beyond the larynx (e.g., trachea, soft tissues of neck, including thyroid, esophagus)

Paranasal Sinus

Maxillary Sinus:

Tx	Primary tumor cannot be assessed
T0	No evidence of primary tumor
T1	Tumor limited to the antral mucosa with no erosion or destruction of bone
T2	Tumor causing bone erosion or destruction, except for the posterior antral wall, including extension into the hard palate and/or middle nasal meatus
T3	Tumor invades any of the following: bone of the posterior wall of maxillary sinus, subcutaneous tissues, skin of cheek, floor or medial wall of orbit, infratemporal fossa, pterygoid plates, ethmoid sinuses
T4	Tumor invades orbital contents beyond the floor or medial wall including any of the following: the orbital apex, cribiform plate, base of skull, nasopharynx, sphenoid, frontal sinuses

Ethmoid Sinus

T1	Tumor confined to the ethmoid with or without bone erosion
T2	Tumor extends into the nasal cavity
T3	Tumor extends to the anterior orbit, and/or maxillary sinus
T4	Tumor with intracranial extension, orbital extension including apex, involving sphenoid, and/or frontal sinus and/or skin of external nose

Major Salivary Glands (parotid, submandibular, sublingual)

Tx	Primary tumor cannot be assessed
T0	No evidence of primary tumor
T1	Tumor 2 cm or less in greatest dimension without extraparenchymal extension
T2	Tumor more than 2 cm but not more than 4 cm in greatest dimension without extraparenchymal extension
T3	Tumor having extraparenchymal extension without seventh nerve involvement and/or more than 4 cm but not more than 6 cm in greatest dimension
T4	Tumor invades the skull base, seventh nerve, and/or exceeds 6 cm in greatest dimension

REGIONAL LYMPH NODES (N) STAGE

Nasopharynx

Nx		Regional lymph nodes cannot be assessed
N1		Unilateral metastasis in lymph node(s), 6 cm or less in greatest dimension, above the supraclavicular fossa
N2		Bilateral metastasis in lymph nodes(s), 6 cm or less in greatest dimension, above the supraclavicular fossa
N3		Metastasis in a lymph node(s)
	N3a	Greater than 6 cm in greatest dimension
	N3b	Extension to the supraclavicular fossa

Oropharynx . Hypopharynx, Larynx, Oral Cavity, Paranasal Sinuses, Salivary Glands

Nx		Regional lymph nodes cannot be assessed
N0		No regional lymph nodes metastasis
N1		Metastasis in a single ipsilateral lymph node, 3 cm or less in greatest dimension
N2		Metastasis in a single ipsilateral lymph node, more than 3 cm but not more than 6 cm in greatest dimension; or in multiple ipsilateral lymph nodes, none more than 6 cm in greatest dimension; or in bilateral or contralateral lymph nodes. none more than 6 cm in greatest dimension
	N2a	Metastasis in single ipsilateral lymph node more than 3 cm but not more than 6 cm in greatest dimension
	N2b	Metastasis in multiple ipsilateral lymph nodes. none more than 6 cm in greatest dimension
	N2c	Metastasis in bilateral or contralateral lymph nodes. none more than 6 cm in greatest dimension
N3		Metastasis in a lymph node more than 6 cm in greatest dimension

DISTANT METASTASIS (M): ALL SITES

Mx	Distant metastasis cannot be assessed
M0	No distant metastasis
M1	Distant metastasis

STAGE GROUPINGS:

NASOPHARYNX

Stage	T	N	M
Stage 0	Tis	N0	M0
Stage I	T1	N0	M0
Stage IIA	T2a	N0	M0
Stage IIB	T1	N1	M0
	T2a	N1	M0
	T2b	N0-1	M0
Stage III	T1	N2	M0
	T2a,b	N2	M0
	T3	N0-2	M0
Stage IVA	T4	N0-2	M0
Stage IVB	Any T	N3	M0
Stage IVC	Any T	Any N	M1

SALIVARY GLANDS

Stage	T	N	M
Stage I	T1	N0	M0
	T2	N0	M0
Stage II	T3	N0	M0
Stage III	T1	N1	M0
	T2	N1	M0
Stage IV	T4	N0	M0
	T3	N1	M0
	T4	N1	M0
	Any T	N2	M0
	Any T	N3	M0
	Any T	Any N	M1

ALL OTHERS (oral cavity, oropharynx, hypopharynx, larynx,,paranasal sinuses)

Stage	T	N	M
Stage 0	Tis	N0	M0
Stage I	T1	N0	M0
Stage II	T2	N0	M0
Stage III	T3	N0	M0
	T1	N1	M0
	T2	N1	M0
	T3	N1	M0
Stage IVA	T4	N0	M0
	T4	N1	M0
	Any T	N2	M0
Stage IVB	Any T	N3	M0
Stage IVC	Any T	Any N	M1

SCREENING

Ways to contribute to head and neck cancer control include education about the risks of tobacco and alcohol, screening, and chemopreventive agents. Oral cavity and oropharyngeal cancer (i.e. oral cancer) usually occurs in sites that are accessible to the examiner by inspection and/or palpation. Therefore, a large number of screening studies for oral cancer, but not for laryngeal cancer [244], have been conducted, especially in Asian countries. However, the benefit of screening asymptomatic subjects for head and neck cancer has yet to be proven in randomized studies.

Population screening studies for oral cancer and/or premalignant lesions, excluding serological studies for NPC, have been conducted in India [245, 246], Sri Lanka [247], Japan [248-250], U.K. [251-253], Italy [254], Hungary [255], Sweden [256], U.S. [257], and Cuba [258]. Great variability in the examiners is noted in these studies from basic health care workers to dentists and otolaryngologists. In general, a discouraging number of subjects would fail to comply with referral recommendations.

A major problem for the implementation of population screening is the relative low prevalence of head and neck cancer in most countries. The yield of biopsy-confirmed cancerous lesions in screening studies has been very low (0.05% or less in most studies), whereas the rate of false-positive referrals may be unacceptably high [259]. As a result, the vast majority of individuals will be subjected to unnecessary testing associated with potential risks and discomfort.

Cuba has implemented the only national oral cancer screening program that requires annual oral examination by dentists [258]. From 1983 to 1990 a total of 10 million people were screened. The annual participation was 12-26% of the eligible population; only 27% of the 30,478 subjects with suspicious lesions (0.3% of screened population) complied with referral recommendations [258, 260]. The program identified 28.8% of the oral cancers reported by the Cuban National Registry of Cancer during 1983-1990 [260]. Despite an observed increase in the diagnosis of stage I head and neck malignancies after the introduction of the screening program in Cuba, from 23% in 1982 to 43% in 1988, no improvement in oral cancer-specific mortality has been observed over the last decade in this country [258, 260]. In the United States, a screening program in Minnesota consisting of 23,616 participants was completed between the years of 1957-1972 [257]. More than 10% of patients were diagnosed with leukoplakia, and 12.2% were found to be invasive squamous cell carcinomas. The use of staining with toluidine blue as an adjunct to clinical examination by specialized physicians may increase the accuracy of screening, but the yield remains low due to the low prevalence of head and neck cancer [261]

The only randomized population screening study is currently underway in Kerala, India, a high-risk region for oral cancer. Subjects were randomized by virtue of their residence in a total of 13 geographic areas, and as a result, some imbalances in risk factors between groups were observed. The intervention group consisted of 59,894 patients, of whom 49,179 were screened, and the control group was comprised of 54,707 subjects [245]. Screening examinations were performed by visiting health care workers who had undergone a 3-month training program, and included mouth examination. Follow-up was achieved mainly through the regional tumor registry. After the first screening session, and despite an approximately 50% compliance with referral recommendations, a total of 47 oral cancers were diagnosed in the screened population (25% were cancers of the tongue and 55% of the buccal mucosa), of whom 36 as a result of screening, and 16 in the control group (44% of the cases involved the tongue and 31% the buccal mucosa). The sensitivity and specificity of the screening method was 76.6% and 76.2%, respectively, however, the positive predictive value was only 1%. An increase in the diagnosis of early stage I/II cancers (72.3%) versus that of the control group (12.5%) was observed. Moreover, the 3-year fatality rate of patients with oral cancer was increased in the control versus the intervention arm (56% vs. 15 %). Nevertheless, a significant difference in mortality from oral cancer, a widely accepted endpoint to assess the impact of a cancer screening program, has yet to be demonstrated. In the above study, 7 deaths have occurred in the screened and 9 in the control population [245].

Targeting high-risk groups for head and neck cancer may increase the yield and the cost-effectiveness of screening. However, certain high-risk groups, such as the alcoholics, may not be sufficiently compliant with screening procedures. Another target population for screening is patients who have already been diagnosed with a primary head and neck cancer and who carry a significant risk for a second aerodigestive malignancy. Synchronous tumors are found in 2-16% of these patients [262]. Screening procedures in this group of patients have not been thoroughly evaluated. The use of CT scan of the chest or PET scan in this setting warrants investigation. The use of staining with toluidine blue may also be helpful for detection of a local recurrence or a new lesion but requires specialized training [263].

Screening Recommendations and Guidelines

Given the lack of proof from randomized studies, significant variability exists between screening recommendations from various organizations. Consensus reports have advised against screening for oral cancer, whereas the need for randomized studies has also been questioned [264]. Limited data are available for screening for laryngeal cancer [244, 264], and no recommendations can be generated for this head and neck site. The American Cancer Society advocates an oral examination every 3 years for patients over the age of 20 and annually for those over the age of 40, as part of a cancer-related check-up [265]. The guidelines of the Canadian Task Force advise against population screening for oral cancer, however, they state that opportunistic screening may be considered during annual examinations for high-risk individuals, such as those with history of tobacco smoking and/or excessive alcohol consumption [259]. The U.S. Preventive Task Force recognizes the insufficient data to recommend for or against routine screening of asymptomatic subjects for oral cancer [266]. Finally, there is universal agreement in that smoking cessation is beneficial and that smoking cessation counseling should be implemented during office visits. National health policies should pursue tobacco use cessation as the best preventive measure for head and neck cancer.

REFERENCES

1.   Greenlee RT, Hill-Harmon MB, Murray T, Thun M. Cancer statistics, 2001. CA Cancer J Clin 2001; 51:15-36.
2.   Parkin DM, Pisani P, Ferlay J. Global cancer statistics. CA Cancer J Clin 1999; 49:33-64, 1.
3.   Skarsgard DP, Groome PA, Mackillop WJ, et al. Cancers of the upper aerodigestive tract in Ontario, Canada, and the United States. Cancer 2000; 88:1728-38.
4.   Vokes EE, Liebowitz DN, Weichselbaum RR. Nasopharyngeal carcinoma. Lancet 1997; 350:1087-91.
5.   Franceschi S, Bidoli E, Herrero R, Munoz N. Comparison of cancers of the oral cavity and pharynx worldwide: etiological clues. Oral Oncol 2000; 36:106-15.
6.   Llewellyn CD, Johnson NW, Warnakulasuriya KA. Risk factors for squamous cell carcinoma of the oral cavity in young people--a comprehensive literature review. Oral Oncol 2001; 37:401-18.
7.   Ries LAG, Eisner MP, Kosary CL, et al. SEER Cancer Statistics Review, 1973-1998, National Cancer Institute. Bethesda, MD, http://seer.cancer.gov/publications/CSR1973_1998/,2001.
8.   Brugere J, Guenel P, Leclerc A, Rodriguez J. Differential effects of tobacco and alcohol in cancer of the larynx, pharynx, and mouth. Cancer 1986; 57:391-5.
9.   Day GL, Blot WJ, Austin DF, et al. Racial differences in risk of oral and pharyngeal cancer: alcohol, tobacco, and other determinants. J Natl Cancer Inst 1993; 85:465-73.
10.   Thorne P, Etherington D, Birchall MA. Head and neck cancer in the South West of England: influence of socio- economic status on incidence and second primary tumours. Eur J Surg Oncol 1997; 23:503-8.
11.   Williams RR, Horm JW. Association of cancer sites with tobacco and alcohol consumption and socioeconomic status of patients: interview study from the Third National Cancer Survey. J Natl Cancer Inst 1977; 58:525-47.
12.   Mackillop WJ, Zhang-Salomons J, Boyd CJ, Groome PA. Associations between community income and cancer incidence in Canada and the United States. Cancer 2000; 89:901-12.

13. Elwood JM, Pearson JC, Skippen DH, Jackson SM. Alcohol, smoking, social and occupational factors in the aetiology of cancer of the oral cavity, pharynx and larynx. Int J Cancer 1984; 34:603-12.
14. Greenberg RS, Haber MJ, Clark WS, et al. The relation of socioeconomic status to oral and pharyngeal cancer. Epidemiology 1991; 2:194-200.
15. Wynder EL, Bross IJ, Feldman RM. A study of etiological factors in cancer of the mouth. Cancer 1957; 10:1300-23.
16. Blot WJ, McLaughlin JK, Winn DM, et al. Smoking and drinking in relation to oral and pharyngeal cancer. Cancer Res 1988; 48:3282-7.
17. Tuyns AJ, Esteve J, Raymond L, et al. Cancer of the larynx/hypopharynx, tobacco and alcohol: IARC international case-control study in Turin and Varese (Italy), Zaragoza and Navarra (Spain), Geneva (Switzerland) and Calvados (France). Int J Cancer 1988; 41:483-91.
18. Franceschi S, Talamini R, Barra S, et al. Smoking and drinking in relation to cancers of the oral cavity, pharynx, larynx, and esophagus in northern Italy. Cancer Res 1990; 50:6502-7.
19. Mashberg A, Boffetta P, Winkelman R, Garfinkel L. Tobacco smoking, alcohol drinking, and cancer of the oral cavity and oropharynx among U.S. veterans. Cancer 1993; 72:1369-75.
20. Franco EL, Kowalski LP, Oliveira BV, et al. Risk factors for oral cancer in Brazil: a case-control study. Int J Cancer 1989; 43:992-1000.
21. Zheng TZ, Boyle P, Hu HF, et al. Tobacco smoking, alcohol consumption, and risk of oral cancer: a case- control study in Beijing, People's Republic of China. Cancer Causes Control 1990; 1:173-9.
22. Macfarlane GJ, Zheng T, Marshall JR, et al. Alcohol, tobacco, diet and the risk of oral cancer: a pooled analysis of three case-control studies. Eur J Cancer B Oral Oncol 1995; 31B:181-7.
23. Bundgaard T, Wildt J, Frydenberg M, Elbrond O, Nielsen JE. Case-control study of squamous cell cancer of the oral cavity in Denmark. Cancer Causes Control 1995; 6:57-67.
24. Andre K, Schraub S, Mercier M, Bontemps P. Role of alcohol and tobacco in the aetiology of head and neck cancer: a case-control study in the Doubs region of France. Eur J Cancer B Oral Oncol 1995; 31B:301-9.
25. Lewin F, Norell SE, Johansson H, et al. Smoking tobacco, oral snuff, and alcohol in the etiology of squamous cell carcinoma of the head and neck: a population-based case-referent study in Sweden. Cancer 1998; 82:1367-75.
26. Kjaerheim K, Gaard M, Andersen A. The role of alcohol, tobacco, and dietary factors in upper aerogastric tract cancers: a prospective study of 10,900 Norwegian men. Cancer Causes Control 1998; 9:99-108.
27. Enstrom JE. Cancer mortality among Mormons. Cancer 1975; 36:825-41.
28. Phillips RL, Garfinkel L, Kuzma JW, Beeson WL, Lotz T, Brin B. Mortality among California Seventh-Day Adventists for selected cancer sites. J Natl Cancer Inst 1980; 65:1097-1107.
29. Baden E. Prevention of cancer of the oral cavity and pharynx. CA Cancer J Clin 1987; 37:49-62.
30. State-specific prevalence of current cigarette smoking among adults, and policies and attitudes about secondhand smoke-united States, 2000. MMWR 2001; 50:1101-6.
31. Hecht SS. Tobacco smoke carcinogens and lung cancer. J Natl Cancer Inst 1999; 91:1194-210.
32. Spitz MR, Fueger JJ, Goepfert H, Hong WK, Newell GR. Squamous cell carcinoma of the upper aerodigestive tract. A case comparison analysis. Cancer 1988; 61:203-8.

33.   Wynder EL, Stellman SD. Impact of long-term filter cigarette usage on lung and larynx cancer risk: a case-control study. J Natl Cancer Inst 1979; 62:471-7.
34.   Wynder EL, Stellman SD. Comparative epidemiology of tobacco-related cancers. Cancer Res 1977; 37:4608-22.
35.   Moore C. Cigarette smoking and cancer of the mouth, pharynx, and larynx. A continuing study. Jama 1971; 218:553-8.
36.   Silverman S, Jr., Griffith M. Smoking characteristics of patients with oral carcinoma and the risk for second oral primary carcinoma. J Am Dent Assoc 1972; 85:637-40.
37.   Ostroff JS, Jacobsen PB, Moadel AB, et al. Prevalence and predictors of continued tobacco use after treatment of patients with head and neck cancer. Cancer 1995; 75:569-76.
38.   Gritz ER, Carr CR, Rapkin D, et al. Predictors of long-term smoking cessation in head and neck cancer patients. Cancer Epidemiol Biomarkers Prev 1993; 2:261-70.
39.   Browman GP, Wong G, Hodson I, et al. Influence of cigarette smoking on the efficacy of radiation therapy in head and neck cancer. N Engl J Med 1993; 328:159-63.
40.   Acetaldehyde. IARC Monogr Eval Carcinog Risk Chem Hum 1985; 36:101-32.
41.   Fioretti F, Bosetti C, Tavani A, Franceschi S, La Vecchia C. Risk factors for oral and pharyngeal cancer in never smokers. Oral Oncol 1999; 35:375-8.
42.   Barra S, Franceschi S, Negri E, Talamini R, La Vecchia C. Type of alcoholic beverage and cancer of the oral cavity, pharynx and oesophagus in an Italian area with high wine consumption. Int J Cancer 1990; 46:1017-20.
43.   Kabat GC, Wynder EL. Type of alcoholic beverage and oral cancer. Int J Cancer 1989; 43:190-4.
44.   Satcher D. Cigars and public health. N Engl J Med 1999; 340:1829-31.
45.   Iribarren C, Tekawa IS, Sidney S, Friedman GD. Effect of cigar smoking on the risk of cardiovascular disease, chronic obstructive pulmonary disease, and cancer in men. N Engl J Med 1999; 340:1773-80.
46.   Connolly GN, Winn DM, Hecht SS, Henningfield JE, Walker B, Jr., Hoffmann D. The reemergence of smokeless tobacco. N Engl J Med 1986; 314:1020-7.
47.   Winn DM, Blot WJ, Shy CM, Pickle LW, Toledo A, Fraumeni JF, Jr. Snuff dipping and oral cancer among women in the southern United States. N Engl J Med 1981; 304:745-9.
48.   Silverman S. Oral Cancer. In: Silverman S, ed. Atlanta: The American Cancer Society, 1990.
49.   Jussawalla DJ, Deshpande VA. Evaluation of cancer risk in tobacco chewers and smokers: an epidemiologic assessment. Cancer 1971; 28:244-52.
50.   Hodge KM, Flynn MB, Drury T. Squamous cell carcinoma of the upper aerodigestive tract in nonusers of tobacco. Cancer 1985; 55:1232-5.
51.   Ng SK, Kabat GC, Wynder EL. Oral cavity cancer in non-users of tobacco. J Natl Cancer Inst 1993; 85:743-5.
52.   Koch WM, Lango M, Sewell D, Zahurak M, Sidransky D. Head and neck cancer in nonsmokers: a distinct clinical and molecular entity. Laryngoscope 1999; 109:1544-51.
53.   Schantz SP, Byers RM, Goepfert H, Shallenberger RC, Beddingfield N. The implication of tobacco use in the young adult with head and neck cancer. Cancer 1988; 62:1374-80.
54.   Brennan JA, Boyle JO, Koch WM, et al. Association between cigarette smoking and mutation of the p53 gene in squamous-cell carcinoma of the head and neck. N Engl J Med 1995; 332:712-7.
55.   Hoffman D, Brunnemann DX, Gori GB, Wynder EL. On the carcinogenicity of marijuana smoke. Recent Adv. Phytochem., 1975; 9:63-81.
56.   Wu TC, Tashkin DP, Djahed B, Rose JE. Pulmonary hazards of smoking marijuana as compared with tobacco. N Engl J Med 1988; 318:347-51.

57.   Zhang ZF, Morgenstern H, Spitz MR, et al. Marijuana use and increased risk of squamous cell carcinoma of the head and neck. Cancer Epidemiol Biomarkers Prev 1999; 8:1071-8.
58.   Burch JD, Howe GR, Miller AB, Semenciw R. Tobacco, alcohol, asbestos, and nickel in the etiology of cancer of the larynx: a case-control study. J Natl Cancer Inst 1981; 67:1219-24.
59.   Rothman KJ, Cann CI, Flanders D, Fried MP. Epidemiology of laryngeal cancer. Epidemiol Rev 1980; 2:195-209.
60.   Gustavsson P, Jakobsson R, Johansson H, Lewin F, Norell S, Rutkvist LE. Occupational exposures and squamous cell carcinoma of the oral cavity, pharynx, larynx, and oesophagus: a case-control study in Sweden. Occup Environ Med 1998; 55:393-400.
61.   IARC monographs on the evaluation of the carcinogenic risk of chemicals to humans, International Agency for Research on Cancer Working Group. Wood dust and formaldehyde, Lyon, France, 1995.
62.   Blair A, Stewart P, O'Berg M, et al. Mortality among industrial workers exposed to formaldehyde. J Natl Cancer Inst 1986; 76:1071-84.
63.   Blair A, Saracci R, Stewart PA, Hayes RB, Shy C. Epidemiologic evidence on the relationship between formaldehyde exposure and cancer. Scand J Work Environ Health 1990; 16:381-93.
64.   Roush GC, Walrath J, Stayner LT, Kaplan SA, Flannery JT, Blair A. Nasopharyngeal cancer, sinonasal cancer, and occupations related to formaldehyde: a case-control study. J Natl Cancer Inst 1987; 79:1221-4.
65.   West S, Hildesheim A, Dosemeci M. Non-viral risk factors for nasopharyngeal carcinoma in the Philippines: results from a case-control study. Int J Cancer 1993; 55:722-7.
66.   Vaughan TL, Strader C, Davis S, Daling JR. Formaldehyde and cancers of the pharynx, sinus and nasal cavity: II. Residential exposures. Int J Cancer 1986; 38:685-8.
67.   Armstrong RW, Imrey PB, Lye MS, Armstrong MJ, Yu MC, Sani S. Nasopharyngeal carcinoma in Malaysian Chinese: occupational exposures to particles, formaldehyde and heat. Int J Epidemiol 2000; 29:991-8.
68.   Demers PA, Kogevinas M, Boffetta P, et al. Wood dust and sino-nasal cancer: pooled reanalysis of twelve case- control studies. Am J Ind Med 1995; 28:151-66.
69.   Cecchi F, Buiatti E, Kriebel D, Nastasi L, Santucci M. Adenocarcinoma of the nose and paranasal sinuses in shoemakers and woodworkers in the province of Florence, Italy (1963-77). Br J Ind Med 1980; 37:222-5.
70.   Hayes RB, Gerin M, Raatgever JW, de Bruyn A. Wood-related occupations, wood dust exposure, and sinonasal cancer. Am J Epidemiol 1986; 124:569-77.
71.   Brinton LA, Blot WJ, Becker JA, et al. A case-control study of cancers of the nasal cavity and paranasal sinuses. Am J Epidemiol 1984; 119:896-906.
72.   Zhang ZF, Morgenstern H, Spitz MR, et al. Environmental tobacco smoking, mutagen sensitivity, and head and neck squamous cell carcinoma. Cancer Epidemiol Biomarkers Prev 2000; 9:1043-9.
73.   McLaughlin JK, Gridley G, Block G, et al. Dietary factors in oral and pharyngeal cancer. J Natl Cancer Inst 1988; 80:1237-43.
74.   Zheng W, Blot WJ, Shu XO, et al. Risk factors for oral and pharyngeal cancer in Shanghai, with emphasis on diet. Cancer Epidemiol Biomarkers Prev 1992; 1:441-8.
75.   Riboli E, Kaaks R, Esteve J. Nutrition and laryngeal cancer. Cancer Causes Control 1996; 7:147-56.

76.   de Visscher JG, van der Waal I. Etiology of cancer of the lip. A review. Int J Oral Maxillofac Surg 1998; 27:199-203.

77.   Maier H, Zoller J, Herrmann A, Kreiss M, Heller WD. Dental status and oral hygiene in patients with head and neck cancer. Otolaryngol Head Neck Surg 1993; 108:655-61.

78.   Marshall JR, Graham S, Haughey BP, et al. Smoking, alcohol, dentition and diet in the epidemiology of oral cancer. Eur J Cancer B Oral Oncol 1992; 28B:9-15.

79.   Winn DM, Blot WJ, McLaughlin JK, et al. Mouthwash use and oral conditions in the risk of oral and pharyngeal cancer. Cancer Res 1991; 51:3044-7.

80.   Velly AM, Franco EL, Schlecht N, et al. Relationship between dental factors and risk of upper aerodigestive tract cancer. Oral Oncol 1998; 34:284-91.

81.   Mashberg A, Barsa P, Grossman ML. A study of the relationship between mouthwash use and oral and pharyngeal cancer. J Am Dent Assoc 1985; 110:731-4.

82.   Young TB, Ford CN, Brandenburg JH. An epidemiologic study of oral cancer in a statewide network. Am J Otolaryngol 1986; 7:200-8.

83.   Seymour RA, Thomason JM, Nolan A. Oral lesions in organ transplant patients. J Oral Pathol Med 1997; 26:297-304.

84.   Lippman SM, Hong WK. Molecular markers of the risk of oral cancer. N Engl J Med 2001; 344:1323-6.

85.   Banoczy J, Gintner Z, Dombi C. Tobacco use and oral leukoplakia. J Dent Educ 2001; 65:322-7.

86.   Lippman SM, Hong WK. Second malignant tumors in head and neck squamous cell carcinoma: the overshadowing threat for patients with early-stage disease. Int J Radiat Oncol Biol Phys 1989; 17:691-4.

87.   Mashberg A, Morrissey JB, Garfinkel L. A study of the appearance of early asymptomatic oral squamous cell carcinoma. Cancer 1973; 32:1436-45.

88.   Franceschi S, Munoz N, Bosch XF, Snijders PJ, Walboomers JM. Human papillomavirus and cancers of the upper aerodigestive tract: a review of epidemiological and experimental evidence. Cancer Epidemiol Biomarkers Prev 1996; 5:567-75.

89.   McKaig RG, Baric RS, Olshan AF. Human papillomavirus and head and neck cancer: epidemiology and molecular biology. Head Neck 1998; 20:250-65.

90.   Hemminski K, Dong C, Frisch M. Tonsillar and other upper aerodigestive tract cancers among cervical cancer patients and their husbands. Eur J Cancer Prev 2000; 9:433-437.

91.   Frisch M, Biggar RJ. Aetiological parallel between tonsillar and anogenital squamous-cell carcinomas. Lancet 1999; 354:1442-3.

92.   Frisch M, Biggar RJ, Goedert JJ. Human papillomavirus-associated cancers in patients with human immunodeficiency virus infection and acquired immunodeficiency syndrome. J Natl Cancer Inst 2000; 92:1500-10.

93.   Gillison ML, Koch WM, Capone RB, et al. Evidence for a causal association between human papillomavirus and a subset of head and neck cancers. J Natl Cancer Inst 2000; 92:709-20.

94.   Mellin H, Friesland S, Lewensohn R, Dalianis T, Munck-Wikland E. Human papillomavirus (HPV) DNA in tonsillar cancer: clinical correlates, risk of relapse, and survival. Int J Cancer 2000; 89:300-4.

95.   Brandsma JL, Abramson AL. Association of papillomavirus with cancers of the head and neck. Arch Otolaryngol Head Neck Surg 1989; 115:621-5.

96.   Maden C, Beckmann AM, Thomas DB, et al. Human papillomaviruses, herpes simplex viruses, and the risk of oral cancer in men. Am J Epidemiol 1992; 135:1093-102.

97.   Smith EM, Hoffman HT, Summersgill KS, Kirchner HL, Turek LP, Haugen TH. Human papillomavirus and risk of oral cancer. Laryngoscope 1998; 108:1098-103.
98.   Schwartz SM, Daling JR, Doody DR, et al. Oral cancer risk in relation to sexual history and evidence of human papillomavirus infection. J Natl Cancer Inst 1998; 90:1626-36.
99.   Mork J, Lie AK, Glattre E, et al. Human papillomavirus infection as a risk factor for squamous-cell carcinoma of the head and neck. N Engl J Med 2001; 344:1125-31.
100.   Ho JH. An epidemiologic and clinical study of nasopharyngeal carcinoma. Int J Radiat Oncol Biol Phys 1978; 4:182-98.
101.   Liebowitz D. Nasopharyngeal carcinoma: the Epstein-Barr virus association. Semin Oncol 1994; 21:376-81.
102.   Yu MC. Diet and nasopharyngeal carcinoma. Prog Clin Biol Res 1990; 346.93-105.
103.   Buell P. The effect of migration on the risk of nasopharyngeal cancer among Chinese. Cancer Res 1974; 34:1189-91.
104.   Fremgen AM, Bland KI, McGinnis LS, Jr., et al. Clinical highlights from the National Cancer Data Base, 1999. CA Cancer J Clin 1999; 49:145-58.
105.   Armstrong RW, Armstrong MJ, Yu MC, Henderson BE. Salted fish and inhalants as risk factors for nasopharyngeal carcinoma in Malaysian Chinese. Cancer Res 1983; 43:2967-70.
106.   Yu MC, Ho JH, Henderson BE, Armstrong RW. Epidemiology of nasopharyngeal carcinoma in Malaysia and Hong Kong. Natl Cancer Inst Monogr 1985; 69:203-7.
107.   Yu MC, Ho JH, Lai SH, Henderson BE. Cantonese-style salted fish as a cause of nasopharyngeal carcinoma: report of a case-control study in Hong Kong. Cancer Res 1986; 46:956-61.
108.   Yu MC, Huang TB, Henderson BE. Diet and nasopharyngeal carcinoma: a case-control study in Guangzhou, China. Int J Cancer 1989; 43:1077-82.
109.   Yu MC, Mo CC, Chong WX, Yeh FS, Henderson BE. Preserved foods and nasopharyngeal carcinoma: a case-control study in Guangxi, China. Cancer Res 1988; 48:1954-9.
110.   Zheng YM, Tuppin P, Hubert A, et al. Environmental and dietary risk factors for nasopharyngeal carcinoma: a case-control study in Zangwu County, Guangxi, China. Br J Cancer 1994; 69:508-14.
111.   Ning JP, Yu MC, Wang QS, Henderson BE. Consumption of salted fish and other risk factors for nasopharyngeal carcinoma (NPC) in Tianjin, a low-risk region for NPC in the People's Republic of China. J Natl Cancer Inst 1990; 82:291-6.
112.   Lee HP, Gourley L, Duffy SW, Esteve J, Lee J, Day NE. Preserved foods and nasopharyngeal carcinoma: a case-control study among Singapore Chinese. Int J Cancer 1994; 59:585-90.
113.   Simons MJ, Wee GB, Goh EH, et al. Immunogenetic aspects of nasopharyngeal carcinoma. IV. Increased risk in Chinese of nasopharyngeal carcinoma associated with a Chinese- related HLA profile (A2, Singapore 2). J Natl Cancer Inst 1976; 57:977-80.
114.   Lu SJ, Day NE, Degos L, et al. Linkage of a nasopharyngeal carcinoma susceptibility locus to the HLA region. Nature 1990; 346:470-1.
115.   Henderson BE, Louie E, SooHoo Jing J, Buell P, Gardner MB. Risk factors associated with nasopharyngeal carcinoma. N Engl J Med 1976; 295:1101-6.
116.   Chow WH, McLaughlin JK, Hrubec Z, Nam JM, Blot WJ. Tobacco use and nasopharyngeal carcinoma in a cohort of US veterans. Int J Cancer 1993; 55:538-40.
117.   Nam JM, McLaughlin JK, Blot WJ. Cigarette smoking, alcohol, and nasopharyngeal carcinoma: a case- control study among U.S. whites. J Natl Cancer Inst 1992; 84:619-22.

118.   Lin TM, Chang HJ, Chen CJ, et al. Risk factors for nasopharyngeal carcinoma. Anticancer Res 1986; 6:791-6.

119.   Yu MC, Garabrant DH, Huang TB, Henderson BE. Occupational and other non-dietary risk factors for nasopharyngeal carcinoma in Guangzhou, China. Int J Cancer 1990; 45:1033-9.

120.   Vaughan TL, Shapiro JA, Burt RD, et al. Nasopharyngeal cancer in a low-risk population: defining risk factors by histological type. Cancer Epidemiol Biomarkers Prev 1996; 5:587-93.

121.   Hildesheim A, Anderson LM, Chen CJ, et al. CYP2E1 genetic polymorphisms and risk of nasopharyngeal carcinoma in Taiwan. J Natl Cancer Inst 1997; 89:1207-12.

122.   Nazar-Stewart V, Vaughan TL, Burt RD, Chen C, Berwick M, Swanson GM. Glutathione S-transferase M1 and susceptibility to nasopharyngeal carcinoma. Cancer Epidemiol Biomarkers Prev 1999; 8:547-51.

123.   Old LH, Boyse EA, Oettgen HF. Precipitation antibody in human serum to an antigen present in cultured Burkitt's lymphoma cells. Proc Natl Acad Sci USA 1966; 56:1699-704.

124.   Wolf H, zur Hausen H, Becker V. EB viral genomes in epithelial nasopharyngeal carcinoma cells. Nat New Biol 1973; 244:245-7.

125.   Andersson-Anvret M, Forsby N, Klein G, Henle W. Relationship between the Epstein-Barr virus and undifferentiated nasopharyngeal carcinoma: correlated nucleic acid hybridization and histopathological examination. Int J Cancer 1977; 20:486-94.

126.   Hording U, Nielsen HW, Albeck H, Daugaard S. Nasopharyngeal carcinoma: histopathological types and association with Epstein-Barr Virus. Eur J Cancer B Oral Oncol 1993; 29B:137-9.

127.   Walter MA, Menarguez-Palanca J, Peiper SC. Epstein-Barr virus detection in neck metastases by polymerase chain reaction. Laryngoscope 1992; 102:481-5.

128.   Tsai ST, Jin YT, Su IJ. Expression of EBER1 in primary and metastatic nasopharyngeal carcinoma tissues using in situ hybridization. A correlation with WHO histologic subtypes. Cancer 1996; 77:231-6.

129.   Wu TC, Mann RB, Epstein JI, et al. Abundant expression of EBER1 small nuclear RNA in nasopharyngeal carcinoma. A morphologically distinctive target for detection of Epstein-Barr virus in formalin-fixed paraffin-embedded carcinoma specimens. Am J Pathol 1991; 138:1461-9.

130.   Lee WY, Hsiao JR, Jin YT, Tsai ST. Epstein-Barr virus detection in neck metastases by in-situ hybridization in fine-needle aspiration cytologic studies: an aid for differentiating the primary site. Head Neck 2000; 22:336-40.

131.   Lo YM, Chan LY, Lo KW, et al. Quantitative analysis of cell-free Epstein-Barr virus DNA in plasma of patients with nasopharyngeal carcinoma. Cancer Res 1999; 59:1188-91.

132.   Lo YM, Chan LY, Chan AT, et al. Quantitative and temporal correlation between circulating cell-free Epstein-Barr virus DNA and tumor recurrence in nasopharyngeal carcinoma. Cancer Res 1999; 59:5452-5.

133.   Shotelersuk K, Khorprasert C, Sakdikul S, Pornthanakasem W, Voravud N, Mutirangura A. Epstein-Barr virus DNA in serum/plasma as a tumor marker for nasopharyngeal cancer. Clin Cancer Res 2000; 6:1046-51.

134.   Lin JC, Chen KY, Wang WY, et al. Detection of Epstein-Barr virus DNA the peripheral-blood cells of patients with nasopharyngeal carcinoma: relationship to distant metastasis and survival. J Clin Oncol 2001; 19:2607-15.

135.   Henle G, Henle W. Epstein-Barr virus-specific IgA serum antibodies as an outstanding feature of nasopharyngeal carcinoma. Int J Cancer 1976; 17:1-7.

136.   Neel HB, 3rd, Pearson GR, Weiland LH, et al. Application of Epstein-Barr virus serology to the diagnosis and staging of North American patients with nasopharyngeal carcinoma. Otolaryngol Head Neck Surg 1983; 91:255-62.

137.   Pearson GR, Weiland LH, Neel HB, 3rd, et al. Application of Epstein-Barr virus (EBV) serology to the diagnosis of North American nasopharyngeal carcinoma. Cancer 1983; 51:260-8.

138.   Chien YC, Chen JY, Liu MY, et al. Serologic markers of Epstein-Barr virus infection and nasopharyngeal carcinoma in Tawanese men. N Engl J Med 2001; 345:1877-82.

139.   Zeng Y, Zhang LG, Li HY, et al. Serological mass survey for early detection of nasopharyngeal carcinoma in Wuzhou City, China. Int J Cancer 1982; 29:139-41.

140.   Zeng Y, Zhong JM, Li LY, et al. Follow-up studies on Epstein-Barr virus IgA/VCA antibody-positive persons in Zangwu County, China. Intervirology 1983; 20:190-4.

141.   Kassim KH, Daley TD. Herpes simplex virus type 1 proteins in human oral squamous cell carcinoma. Oral Surg Oral Med Oral Pathol 1988; 65:445-8.

142.   Shillitoe EJ, Greenspan D, Greenspan JS, Silverman S, Jr. Five-year survival of patients with oral cancer and its association with antibody to herpes simplex virus. Cancer 1986; 58:2256-9.

143.   Califano J, van der Riet P, Westra W, et al. Genetic progression model for head and neck cancer: implications for field cancerization. Cancer Res 1996; 56:2488-92.

144.   Copper MP, Jovanovic A, Nauta JJ, et al. Role of genetic factors in the etiology of squamous cell carcinoma of the head and neck. Arch Otolaryngol Head Neck Surg 1995; 121:157-60.

145.   Foulkes WD, Brunet JS, Sieh W, Black MJ, Shenouda G, Narod SA. Familial risks of squamous cell carcinoma of the head and neck: retrospective case-control study. Bmj 1996; 313:716-21.

146.   Trizna Z, Schantz SP. Hereditary and environmental factors associated with risk and progression of head and neck cancer. Otolaryngol Clin North Am 1992; 25:1089-103.

147.   Lazarus P, Park JY. Metabolizing enzyme genotype and risk for upper aerodigestive tract cancer. Oral Oncol 2000; 36:421-31.

148.   Rebbeck TR. Molecular epidemiology of the human glutathione S-transferase genotypes GSTM1 and GSTT1 in cancer susceptibility. Cancer Epidemiol Biomarkers Prev 1997; 6:733-43.

149.   Goedde HW, Agarwal DP, Fritze G, et al. Distribution of ADH2 and ALDH2 genotypes in different populations. Hum Genet 1992; 88:344-6.

150.   Bartsch H, Nair U, Risch A, Rojas M, Wikman H, Alexandrov K. Genetic polymorphism of CYP genes, alone or in combination, as a risk modifier of tobacco-related cancers. Cancer Epidemiol Biomarkers Prev 2000; 9:3-28.

151.   Oude Ophuis MB, van Lieshout EM, Roelofs HM, Peters WH, Manni JJ. Glutathione S-transferase M1 and T1 and cytochrome P4501A1 polymorphisms in relation to the risk for benign and malignant head and neck lesions. Cancer 1998; 82:936-43.

152.   Lucas D, Menez C, Floch F, et al. Cytochromes P4502E1 and P4501A1 genotypes and susceptibility to cirrhosis or upper aerodigestive tract cancer in alcoholic caucasians. Alcohol Clin Exp Res 1996; 20:1033-7.

153.   Matthias C, Bockmuhl U, Jahnke V, et al. Polymorphism in cytochrome P450 CYP2D6, CYP1A1, CYP2E1 and glutathione S-transferase, GSTM1, GSTM3, GSTT1 and susceptibility to tobacco- related cancers: studies in upper aerodigestive tract cancers. Pharmacogenetics 1998; 8:91-100.

154.   Katoh T, Kaneko S, Kohshi K, et al. Genetic polymorphisms of tobacco- and alcohol-related metabolizing enzymes and oral cavity cancer. Int J Cancer 1999; 83:606-9.

155.   Morita S, Yano M, Tsujinaka T, et al. Genetic polymorphisms of drug-metabolizing enzymes and susceptibility to head-and-neck squamous-cell carcinoma. Int J Cancer 1999; 80:685-8.

156.   Park JY, Muscat JE, Ren Q, et al. CYP1A1 and GSTM1 polymorphisms and oral cancer risk. Cancer Epidemiol Biomarkers Prev 1997; 6:791-7.

157.   Tanimoto K, Hayashi S, Yoshiga K, Ichikawa T. Polymorphisms of the CYP1A1 and GSTM1 gene involved in oral squamous cell carcinoma in association with a cigarette dose. Oral Oncol 1999; 35:191-6.
158.   Sato M, Sato T, Izumo T, Amagasa T. Genetic polymorphism of drug-metabolizing enzymes and susceptibility to oral cancer. Carcinogenesis 1999; 20:1927-31.
159.   Hung HC, Chuang J, Chien YC, et al. Genetic polymorphisms of CYP2E1, GSTM1, and GSTT1; environmental factors and risk of oral cancer. Cancer Epidemiol Biomarkers Prev 1997; 6:901-5.
160.   Gonzalez MV, Alvarez V, Pello MF, Menendez MJ, Suarez C, Coto E. Genetic polymorphism of N-acetyltransferase-2, glutathione S- transferase-M1, and cytochromes P450IIE1 and P450IID6 in the susceptibility to head and neck cancer. J Clin Pathol 1998; 51:294-8.
161.   Ko Y, Abel J, Harth V, et al. Association of CYP1B1 codon 432 mutant allele in head and neck squamous cell cancer is reflected by somatic mutations of p53 in tumor tissue. Cancer Res 2001; 61:4398-404.
162.   Worrall SF, Corrigan M, High A, et al. Susceptibility and outcome in oral cancer: preliminary data showing an association with polymorphism in cytochrome P450 CYP2D6. Pharmacogenetics 1998; 8:433-9.
163.   Lafuente A, Pujol F, Carretero P, Villa JP, Cuchi A. Human glutathione S-transferase mu (GST mu) deficiency as a marker for the susceptibility to bladder and larynx cancer among smokers. Cancer Lett 1993; 68:49-54.
164.   Trizna Z, Clayman GL, Spitz MR, Briggs KL, Goepfert H. Glutathione s-transferase genotypes as risk factors for head and neck cancer. Am J Surg 1995; 170:499-501.
165.   Cheng L, Sturgis EM, Eicher SA, Char D, Spitz MR, Wei Q. Glutathione-S-transferase polymorphisms and risk of squamous-cell carcinoma of the head and neck. Int J Cancer 1999; 84:220-4.
166.   Kihara M, Kubota A, Furukawa M, Kimura H. GSTM1 gene polymorphism as a possible marker for susceptibility to head and neck cancers among Japanese smokers. Cancer Lett 1997; 112:257-62.
167.   Nomura T, Noma H, Shibahara T, Yokoyama A, Muramatusu T, Ohmori T. Aldehyde dehydrogenase 2 and glutathione S-transferase M 1 polymorphisms in relation to the risk for oral cancer in Japanese drinkers. Oral Oncol 2000; 36:42-6.
168.   Deakin M, Elder J, Hendrickse C, et al. Glutathione S-transferase GSTT1 genotypes and susceptibility to cancer: studies of interactions with GSTM1 in lung, oral, gastric and colorectal cancers. Carcinogenesis 1996; 17:881-4.
169.   Jourenkova-Mironova N, Voho A, Bouchardy C, et al. Glutathione S-transferase GSTM1, GSTM3, GSTP1 and GSTT1 genotypes and the risk of smoking-related oral and pharyngeal cancers. Int J Cancer 1999; 81:44-8.
170.   Park LY, Muscat JE, Kaur T, et al. Comparison of GSTM polymorphisms and risk for oral cancer between African-Americans and Caucasians. Pharmacogenetics 2000; 10:123-31.
171.   Matthias C, Bockmuhl U, Jahnke V, et al. The glutathione S-transferase GSTP1 polymorphism: effects on susceptibility to oral/pharyngeal and laryngeal carcinomas. Pharmacogenetics 1998; 8:1-6.
172.   Park JY, Schantz SP, Stern JC, Kaur T, Lazarus P. Association between glutathione S-transferase pi genetic polymorphisms and oral cancer risk. Pharmacogenetics 1999; 9:497-504.
173.   Katoh T, Kaneko S, Takasawa S, et al. Human glutathione S-transferase P1 polymorphism and susceptibility to smoking related epithelial cancer; oral, lung, gastric, colorectal and urothelial cancer. Pharmacogenetics 1999; 9:165-9.
174.   Jourenkova-Mironova N, Voho A, Bouchardy C, et al. Glutathione S-transferase GSTM3 and GSTP1 genotypes and larynx cancer risk. Cancer Epidemiol Biomarkers Prev 1999; 8:185-8.

175. Lazarus P, Sheikh SN, Ren Q, et al. p53, but not p16 mutations in oral squamous cell carcinomas are associated with specific CYP1A1 and GSTM1 polymorphic genotypes and patient tobacco use. Carcinogenesis 1998; 19:509-14.

176. Bosron WF, Lumeng L, Li TK. Genetic polymorphism of enzymes of alcohol metabolism and susceptibility to alcoholic liver disease. Mol Aspects Med 1988; 10:147-58.

177. Coutelle C, Ward PJ, Fleury B, et al. Laryngeal and oropharyngeal cancer, and alcohol dehydrogenase 3 and glutathione S-transferase M1 polymorphisms. Hum Genet 1997; 99:319-25.

178. Harty LC, Caporaso NE, Hayes RB, et al. Alcohol dehydrogenase 3 genotype and risk of oral cavity and pharyngeal cancers. J Natl Cancer Inst 1997; 89:1698-705.

179. Schwartz SM, Doody DR, Fitzgibbons ED, Ricks S, Porter PL, Chen C. Oral squamous cell cancer risk in relation to alcohol consumption and alcohol dehydrogenase-3 genotypes. Cancer Epidemiol Biomarkers Prev 2001; 10:1137-44.

180. Olshan AF, Weissler MC, Watson MA, Bell DA. Risk of head and neck cancer and the alcohol dehydrogenase 3 genotype. Carcinogenesis 2001; 22:57-61.

181. Sturgis EM, Dahlstrom KR, Guan Y, et al. Alcohol dehydrogenase 3 genotype is not associated with risk of squamous cell carcinoma of the oral cavity and pharynx. Cancer Epidemiol Biomarkers Prev 2001; 10:273-5.

182. Bouchardy C, Hirvonen A, Coutelle C, Ward PJ, Dayer P, Benhamou S. Role of alcohol dehydrogenase 3 and cytochrome P-4502E1 genotypes in susceptibility to cancers of the upper aerodigestive tract. Int J Cancer 2000; 87:734-40.

183. Yokoyama A, Muramatsu T, Omori T, et al. Alcohol and aldehyde dehydrogenase gene polymorphisms and oropharyngolaryngeal, esophageal and stomach cancers in Japanese alcoholics. Carcinogenesis 2001; 22:433-9.

184. Schantz SP, Zhang ZF, Spitz MS, Sun M, Hsu TC. Genetic susceptibility to head and neck cancer: interaction between nutrition and mutagen sensitivity. Laryngoscope 1997; 107:765-81.

185. Cloos J, Spitz MR, Schantz SP, et al. Genetic susceptibility to head and neck squamous cell carcinoma. J Natl Cancer Inst 1996; 88:530-5.

186. Zheng Y, Shen H, Sturgis EM, et al. Cyclin D1 polymorphism and risk for squamous cell carcinoma of the head and neck: a case-control study. Carcinogenesis 2001; 22:1195- 9.

187. Sturgis EM, Zheng R, Li L, et al. XPD/ERCC2 polymorphisms and risk of head and neck cancer: a case- control analysis. Carcinogenesis 2000; 21:2219-23.

188. Slaughter DP, Southwick HW, Smejkal W. "Filed cancerization" in oral stratified squamous epithelium: clinical implications of multicentric origin. Cancer 1953; 6:963-8.

189. Licciardello JT, Spitz MR, Hong WK. Multiple primary cancer in patients with cancer of the head and neck: second cancer of the head and neck, esophagus, and lung. Int J Radiat Oncol Biol Phys 1989; 17:467-76.

190. Erkal HS, Mendenhall WM, Amdur RJ, Villaret DB, Stringer SP. Synchronous and metachronous squamous cell carcinomas of the head and neck mucosal sites. J Clin Oncol 2001; 19:1358-62.

191. Jones AS, Morar P, Phillips DE, Field JK, Husband D, Helliwell TR. Second primary tumors in patients with head and neck squamous cell carcinoma. Cancer 1995; 75:1343-53.

192. Fijuth J, Mazeron JJ, Le Pechoux C, et al. Second head and neck cancers following radiation therapy of T1 and T2 cancers of the oral cavity and oropharynx. Int J Radiat Oncol Biol Phys 1992; 24:59-64.

193.   Cooper JS, Pajak TF, Rubin P, et al. Second malignancies in patients who have head and neck cancer: incidence, effect on survival and implications based on the RTOG experience. Int J Radiat Oncol Biol Phys 1989; 17:449-56.
194.   Roberts TJ, Epstein B, Lee DJ. Second neoplasms in patients with carcinomas of the vocal cord: incidence and implications for survival. Int J Radiat Oncol Biol Phys 1991; 21:583-9.
195.   Schwartz LH, Ozsahin M, Zhang GN, et al. Synchronous and metachronous head and neck carcinomas. Cancer 1994; 74:1933-8.
196.   Cooper JS, Scott C, Marcial V, et al. The relationship of nasopharyngeal carcinomas and second independent malignancies based on the Radiation Therapy Oncology Group experience. Cancer 1991; 67:1673-7.
197.   Wang CC, Chen ML, Hsu KH, et al. Second malignant tumors in patients with nasopharyngeal carcinoma and their association with Epstein-Barr virus. Int J Cancer 2000; 87:228-31.
198.   Cianfriglia F, Di Gregorio DA, Manieri A. Multiple primary tumours in patients with oral squamous cell carcinoma. Oral Oncol 1999; 35:157-63.
199.   Day GL, Blot WJ, Shore RE, et al. Second cancers following oral and pharyngeal cancer: patients' characteristics and survival patterns. Eur J Cancer B Oral Oncol 1994; 30B:381-6.
200.   Khuri FR, Kim ES, Lee JJ, et al. The impact of smoking status, disease stage, and index tumor site on second primary tumor incidence and tumor recurrence in the head 10:823-9.
201.   Leong PP, Rezai B, Koch WM, et al. Distinguishing second primary tumors from lung metastases in patients with head and neck squamous cell carcinoma. J Natl Cancer Inst 1998; 90:972-7.
202.   Vikram B. Changing patterns of failure in advanced head and neck cancer. Arch Otolaryngol 1984; 110:564-5.
203.   Guggenheimer J, Verbin RS, Johnson JT, Horkowitz CA, Myers EN. Factors delaying the diagnosis of oral and oropharyngeal carcinomas. Cancer 1989; 64:932-5.
204.   Mackie AM, Epstein JB, Wu JS, Stevenson-Moore P. Nasopharyngeal carcinoma: the role of the dentist in assessment, early diagnosis and care before and after cancer therapy. Oral Oncol 2000; 36:397-403.
205.   Black RJ, Gluckman JL, Shumrick DA. Screening for distant metastases in head and neck cancer patients. Aust N Z J Surg 1984; 54:527-30.
206.   Reiner B, Siegel E, Sawyer R, Brocato RM, Maroney M, Hooper F. The impact of routine CT of the chest on the diagnosis and management of newly diagnosed squamous cell carcinoma of the head and neck. AJR Am J Roentgenol 1997; 169:667-71.
207.   de Bree R, Deurloo EE, Snow GB, Leemans CR. Screening for distant metastases in patients with head and neck cancer. Laryngoscope 2000; 110:397-401.
208.   Halpern J. The value of chest CT scan in the work-up of head and neck cancers. J Med 1997; 28:191-8.
209.   Hong WK, Bromer RH, Amato DA, et al. Patterns of relapse in locally advanced head and neck cancer patients who achieved complete remission after combined modality therapy. Cancer 1985; 56:1242-5.
210.   Induction chemotherapy plus radiation compared with surgery plus radiation in patients with advanced laryngeal cancer. The Department of Veterans Affairs Laryngeal Cancer Study Group. N Engl J Med 1991; 324:1685-90.
211.   Lefebvre JL, Chevalier D, Luboinski B, Kirkpatrick A, Collette L, Sahmoud T. Larynx preservation in pyriform sinus cancer: preliminary results of a European Organization for Research and Treatment of Cancer phase III trial. EORTC Head and Neck Cancer Cooperative Group. J Natl Cancer Inst 1996; 88:890-9.

212. Leibel SA, Scott CB, Mohiuddin M, et al. The effect of local-regional control on distant metastatic dissemination in carcinoma of the head and neck: results of an analysis from the RTOG head and neck database. Int J Radiat Oncol Biol Phys 1991; 21:549-56.

213. Calhoun KH, Fulmer P, Weiss R, Hokanson JA. Distant metastases from head and neck squamous cell carcinomas. Laryngoscope 1994; 104:1199-205.

214. Johnson JT. Proposal of standardization on screening tests for detection of distant metastases from head and neck cancer. ORL J Otorhinolaryngol Relat Spec 2001; 63:256-8.

215. Houghton DJ, Hughes ML, Garvey C, et al. Role of chest CT scanning in the management of patients presenting with head and neck cancer. Head Neck 1998; 20:614-8.

216. Houghton DJ, McGarry G, Stewart I, Wilson JA, MacKenzie K. Chest computerized tomography scanning in patients presenting with head and neck cancer. Clin Otolaryngol 1998; 23:348-50.

217. Mercader VP, Gatenby RA, Mohr RM, Fisher MS, Caroline DF. CT surveillance of the thorax in patients with squamous cell carcinoma of the head and neck: a preliminary experience. J Comput Assist Tomogr 1997; 21:412-7.

218. Martin GF, Gullane PJ, Heeneman H. Radionuclide scans in the assessment of distant metastases from squamous cell carcinoma of the head and neck. J Otolaryngol 1981; 10:383-6.

219. Lindberg R. Distribution of cervical lymph node metastases from squamous cell carcinoma of the upper respiratory and digestive tracts. Cancer 1972; 29:1446-9.

220. Laubenbacher C, Saumweber D, Wagner-Manslau C, et al. Comparison of fluorine-18-fluorodeoxyglucose PET, MRI and endoscopy for staging head and neck squamous-cell carcinomas. J Nucl Med 1995; 36:1747-57.

221. Adams S, Baum RP, Stuckensen T, Bitter K, Hor G. Prospective comparison of 18F-FDG PET with conventional imaging modalities (CT, MRI, US) in lymph node staging of head and neck cancer. Eur J Nucl Med 1998; 25:1255-60.

222. Myers LL, Wax MK, Nabi H, Simpson GT, Lamonica D. Positron emission tomography in the evaluation of the N0 neck. Laryngoscope 1998; 108:232-6.

223. Stuckensen T, Kovacs AF, Adams S, Baum RP. Staging of the neck in patients with oral cavity squamous cell carcinomas: a prospective comparison of PET, ultrasound, CT and MRI. J Craniomaxillofac Surg 2000; 28:319-24.

224. Mendenhall WM, Mancuso AA, Parsons JT, Stringer SP, Cassisi NJ. Diagnostic evaluation of squamous cell carcinoma metastatic to cervical lymph nodes from an unknown head and neck primary site. Head Neck 1998; 20:739-44.

225. Bohuslavizki KH, Klutmann S, Kroger S, et al. FDG PET detection of unknown primary tumors. J Nucl Med 2000; 41:816-22.

226. Safa AA, Tran LM, Rege S, et al. The role of positron emission tomography in occult primary head and neck cancers. Cancer J Sci Am 1999; 5:214-8.

227. Jungehulsing M, Scheidhauer K, Damm M, et al. 2[F]-fluoro-2-deoxy-D-glucose positron emission tomography is a sensitive tool for the detection of occult primary cancer (carcinoma of unknown primary syndrome) with head and neck lymph node manifestation. Otolaryngol Head Neck Surg 2000; 123:294-301.

228. Hanasono MM, Kunda LD, Segall GM, Ku GH, Terris DJ. Uses and limitations of FDG positron emission tomography in patients with head and neck cancer. Laryngoscope 1999; 109:880-5.

229.   Greven KM, Keyes JW, Jr., Williams DW, 3rd, McGuirt WF, Joyce WT, 3rd. Occult primary tumors of the head and neck: lack of benefit from positron emission tomography imaging with 2-[F-18]fluoro-2-deoxy-D- glucose. Cancer 1999; 86:114-8.

230.   Keyes JW, Jr., Chen MY, Watson NE, Jr., Greven KM, McGuirt WF, Williams DW, 3rd. FDG PET evaluation of head and neck cancer: value of imaging the thorax. Head Neck 2000; 22:105-10.

231.   Lonneux M, Lawson G, Ide C, Bausart R, Remacle M, Pauwels S. Positron emission tomography with fluorodeoxyglucose for suspected head and neck tumor recurrence in the symptomatic patient. Laryngoscope 2000; 110:1493-7.

232.   Kitagawa Y, Sadato N, Azuma H, et al. FDG PET to evaluate combined intra-arterial chemotherapy and radiotherapy of head and neck neoplasms. J Nucl Med 1999; 40:1132-7.

233.   Farber LA, Benard F, Machtay M, et al. Detection of recurrent head and neck squamous cell carcinomas after radiation therapy with 2-18F-fluoro-2-deoxy-D-glucose positron emission tomography. Laryngoscope 1999; 109:970-5.

234.   Stokkel MP, Terhaard CH, Hordijk GJ, van Rijk PP. The detection of local recurrent head and neck cancer with fluorine-18 fluorodeoxyglucose dual-head positron emission tomography. Eur J Nucl Med 1999; 26:767-73.

235.   Anzai Y, Carroll WR, Quint DJ, et al. Recurrence of head and neck cancer after surgery or irradiation: prospective comparison of 2-deoxy-2-[F-18]fluoro-D-glucose PET and MR imaging diagnoses. Radiology 1996; 200:135-41.

236.   Charron M, Beyer T, Bohnen NN, et al. Image analysis in patients with cancer studied with a combined PET and CT scanner. Clin Nucl Med 2000; 25:905-10.

237.   Knappe M, Louw M, Gregor RT. Ultrasonography-guided fine-needle aspiration for the assessment of cervical metastases. Arch Otolaryngol Head Neck Surg 2000; 126:1091-6.

238.   Righi PD, Kopecky KK, Caldemeyer KS, Ball VA, Weisberger EC, Radpour S. Comparison of ultrasound-fine needle aspiration and computed tomography in patients undergoing elective neck dissection. Head Neck 1997; 19:604-10.

239.   van den Brekel MW, Castelijns JA, Stel HV, Golding RP, Meyer CJ, Snow GB. Modern imaging techniques and ultrasound-guided aspiration cytology for the assessment of neck node metastases: a prospective comparative study. Eur Arch Otorhinolaryngol 1993; 250:11-7.

240.   Takes RP, Knegt P, Manni JJ, et al. Regional metastasis in head and neck squamous cell carcinoma: revised value of US with US-guided FNAB. Radiology 1996; 198:819-23.

241.   van den Brekel MW. US-guided fine-needle aspiration cytology of neck nodes in patients with N0 disease. Radiology 1996; 201:580-1.

242.   Atula TS, Varpula MJ, Kurki TJ, Klemi PJ, Grenman R. Assessment of cervical lymph node status in head and neck cancer patients: palpation, computed tomography and low field magnetic resonance imaging compared with ultrasound-guided fine-needle aspiration cytology. Eur J Radiol 1997; 25:152-61.

243.   van den Brekel MW. Lymph node metastases: CT and MRI. Eur J Radiol 2000; 33:230-8.

244.   Cortesina G, Gabriele P, Giordano C, et al. Report of an international workshop on perspectives on secondary prevention of laryngeal cancer. Eur J Cancer 1993; 9:1348-52.

245.   Sankaranarayanan R, Mathew B, Jacob BJ, et al. Early findings from a community-based, cluster-randomized, controlled oral cancer screening trial in Kerala, India. The Trivandrum Oral Cancer Screening Study Group. Cancer 2000; 88:664-73.

246. Mehta FS, Gupta PC, Bhonsle RB, Murti PR, Daftary DK, Pindborg JJ. Detection of oral cancer using basic health workers in an area of high oral cancer incidence in India. Cancer Detect Prev 1986; 9:219-25.

247. Warnakulasuriya KA, Nanayakkara BG. Reproducibility of an oral cancer and precancer detection program using a primary health care model in Sri Lanka. Cancer Detect Prev 1991; 15:331-4.

248. Ikeda N, Ishii T, Iida S, Kawai T. Epidemiological study of oral leukoplakia based on mass screening for oral mucosal diseases in a selected Japanese population. Community Dent Oral Epidemiol 1991; 19:160-3.

249. Ikeda N, Downer MC, Ozowa Y, Inoue C, Mizuno T, Kawai T. Characteristics of participants and non-participants in annual mass screening for oral cancer in 60-year-old residents of Tokoname city, Japan. Community Dent Health 1995; 12:83-8.

250. Nagao T, Warnakulasuriya S, Ikeda N, Fukano H, Fujiwara K, Miyazaki H. Oral cancer screening as an integral part of general health screening in Tokoname City, Japan. J Med Screen 2000; 7:203-8.

251. Downer MC, Evans AW, Hughes Hallet CM, Jullien JA, Speight PM, Zakrzewska JM. Evaluation of screening for oral cancer and precancer in a company headquarters. Community Dent Oral Epidemiol 1995; 23:84-8.

252. Jullien JA, Downer MC, Zakrzewska JM, Speight PM. Evaluation of a screening test for the early detection of oral cancer and precancer. Community Dent Health 1995; 12:3-7.

253. Field EA, Morrison T, Darling AE, Parr TA, Zakrzewska JM. Oral mucosal screening as an integral part of routine dental care. Br Dent J 1995; 179:262-6.

254. Talamini R, Barzan L, Franceschi S, Caruso G, Gasparin A, Comoretto R. Determinants of compliance with an early detection programme for cancer of the head and neck in north-eastern Italy. Eur J Cancer B Oral Oncol 1994; 30B:415-8.

255. Banoczy J, Rigo O. Prevalence study of oral precancerous lesions within a complex screening system in Hungary. Community Dent Oral Epidemiol 1991; 19:265-7.

256. Axell T. Occurrence of leukoplakia and some other oral white lesions among 20,333 adult Swedish people. Community Dent Oral Epidemiol 1987; 15:46-51.

257. Bouquot JE, Gorlin RJ. Leukoplakia, lichen planus, and other oral keratoses in 23,616 white Americans over the age of 35 years. Oral Surg Oral Med Oral Pathol 1986; 61:373-81.

258. Frenandez Garrote L, Sankaranarayanan R, Lence Anta JJ, Rodriguez Salva A, Maxwell Parkin D. An evaluation of the oral cancer control program in Cuba. epidemiology 1995; 6:428-31.

259. Hawkins RJ, Wang EE, Leake JL. Preventive health care, 1999 update: prevention of oral cancer mortality. The Canadian Task Force on Preventive Health Care. J Can dent Assoc 1999; 65:617.

260. Santana JC, Delgado L, Miranda J, Sanchez M. Oral Cancer Case Finding Program (OCCFP). Oral Oncol 1997; 33:10-2.

261. Rosenberg D, Cretin S. Use of meta-analysis to evaluate tolonium chloride in oral Cancer screening. Oral Surg Oral Med Oral Pathol 1989; 67:621-7.

262. Leipzig B, Zellmer JE, Klug D. The role of endoscopy in evaluating patients with head and neck cancer. A multi-institutional prospective study. Arch Otolaryngol 1985; 111:589-94.

263. Epstein JB, Oakley C, Millner A, Emerton S, van der Meij E, Le N. The utility of toluidine blue application as a diagnostic aid in patients previously treated for upper oropharyngeal carcinoma. Oral Surg Oral Med Oral Pathol Oral Radiol Endod 1997; 83:537-47.

264.   Franceschi S, Barzan L, Talamini R. Screening for cancer of the head and neck: if not now, when? Oral Oncol 1997; 33:313-6.
265.   Smith RA, Mettlin CJ, Davis KJ, Eyre H. American Cancer Society guidelines for the early detection of cancer. CA Cancer J Clin 2000; 50:34-49.
266.   Screening for oral cancer. U.S. Preventive Task Force. Guide to Clinical Preventive Services 1996.

Chapter 3

ORAL PRENEOPLASIA AND CHEMOPREVENTION OF SQUAMOUS CELL CARCINOMA OF THE HEAD AND NECK

Omer Kucuk, MD, FACN
Barbara Ann Karmanos Cancer Institute
Wayne State University, Detroit, Michigan

INTRODUCTION

In the year 2000, oral, pharyngeal and laryngeal cancers have been estimated to account for 40,300 cases and 11,700 deaths in the United States (1). More than 90% of oral cancers occur in individuals 45 years of age and over (2). The overall five-year survival rate is 53%, which has not changed in the past thirty years (3,4). The low survival rate may be attributed to the fact that these cancers are usually at an advanced stage when they are diagnosed. Furthermore, these cancers and their treatments are extremely disfiguring and often result in morbidity such as inability to swallow and/or impaired speech.

PREVENTION OF SQUAMOUS CELL CANCER OF THE HEAD AND NECK (SCCHN)

Tobacco and alcohol are the major risk factors for SCCHN, accounting for 75% of all cases (5). Other risk factors include malnutrition or poor dietary intake of essential minerals (6,7) and exposure to viruses such as human papillomavirus (8) and Epstein-Barr virus (9). On the other hand, an increased consumption of fruits and vegetables is associated with lower risk of SCCHN (10). Consequently, primary prevention measures for SCCHN include: 1) avoiding tobacco products, 2) limiting alcohol intake, 3) eating a diet rich in fruit and vegetables and 4) avoiding exposure to certain viruses. Secondary prevention measures include visual examination and palpation of the oral cavity for early detection of oral cancer. The American Cancer Society (ACS) recommends an oral cancer examination every 3 years for individuals over age 20 and annually for persons 40 years of age or older (6,11). An oral cancer examination, generally performed by dentists and dental hygienists, is associated with little discomfort. Other health care providers, such as nurse practitioners, physician assistants and physicians, should also make oral cancer examination part of their routine physical examination.

CHEMOPREVENTION

"Cancer chemoprevention" refers to the prevention of invasive cancer with nutritional and pharmacologic agents. The development of invasive cancer from the first initiating event in epithelial cells occurs over many years. Thus progress in chemopreventive agent development is limited by the long natural history of the disease process. Therefore, the identification of surrogate endpoint biomarkers (SEBs) for cancer incidence and treatment effect offers an alternative intermediate endpoint to cancer incidence in clinical cancer chemoprevention trials. There is a great need to identify and validate SEBs, which will help researchers develop new strategies for cancer prevention. Phase II clinical chemoprevention trials offer an opportunity to identify and evaluate novel SEBs. Preneoplastic lesions in the oral cavity, such as leukoplakia, that have a high rate of progression to invasive cancer, have been the "gold standard" intermediate endpoints for phase II cancer chemoprevention trials for head and neck cancer. Increasing knowledge of the molecular events involved in carcinogenesis has provided multiple biomarkers reflecting the pathophysiologic processes occurring early during neoplastic transformation. Potential biomarkers include, but are not limited to, markers of proliferation, apoptosis, differentiation, oncogenes, tumor suppressor genes, cell cycle regulatory proteins, promoter methylation, oxidative stress, inflammation and gap junctional intercellular communication (GJIC).

ORAL PRENEOPLASIA

Due to its unique biology and anatomy, squamous cell carcinoma of the head and neck represents an ideal model system for the study of chemopreventive agent efficacy. Damage to the epithelial cells of upper aerodigestive tract by constituents of tobacco and alcohol results in field cancerization characterized by multiple foci of genetic damage that can progress to cancer (12). Consequently, the rate of second primary cancers after curative treatment of the initial head and neck cancer is 3-7% per year (13). Thus this population is an excellent cohort for prevention studies (13).

Leukoplakia is a well-characterized precursor lesion with a high rate of progression to invasive squamous cell carcinoma of the oral cavity. The incidence of invasive oral cancer in subjects with oral leukoplakia is as high as 31% at ten years, while spontaneous regression occurs in <10% of these lesions (14). The accessibility of the oral cavity for measurement of leukoplakia size and histologic sampling allows for treatment efficacy assessment. As a result, considerable knowledge has been amassed regarding the molecular changes associated with oral leukoplakia. Multiple chemoprevention trials have been performed to determine the efficacy of agents such as beta-carotene or retinoids in reducing the size and degree of dysplasia of oral preneoplastic lesions (15-17). The oral leukoplakia is therefore an excellent model for investigating the efficacy of novel mechanistically targeted chemopreventive agents.

Appearance of carcinogenic injury to oral mucosa includes leukoplakia, erythroplakia and mixed patterns of the two lesions. Leukoplakia, which means "white patch", reflects the presence of keratin overlying epithelial hyperplasia. Although this change has been recognized clinically for many decades, a precise histologic definition of leukoplakia in the oral cavity and its relationship to invasive carcinoma has only recently been well described (18-20). A variety of injuries can result in a whitish mucosal appearance and only rarely these leukoplakic lesions have dysplasia or intraepithelial carcinoma (21). Erythroplakia consists of thin, atrophic epithelium associated with submucosal inflammation and telangiectasia, which accounts for the red appearance. A high frequency of severe dysplasia or carcinoma in situ (CIS) occurs in erythroplakic lesions and a high incidence of invasive carcinoma has been observed in association with these lesions (19,20).

Crissman and Zarbo (21) elected to use the term "squamous intraepithelial neoplasia" (SIN) to reclassify the preneoplastic changes of upper aerodigestive tract in a manner similar to the terminology used in the uterine cervix. They have graded the lesions in groups I-III, where group III represents severe keratinizing or nonkeratinizing dysplasia or classic CIS (Table 1), indicating the severity of the intraepithelial change and its propensity for the development of subsequent carcinoma (21).

Table 1.   **Definitions and grading for squamous intraepithelial neoplasia (21)**

Grade	Synonyms	Interpretation
SIN I	Slight or mild dysplasia	Evidence of injury, either reversible
	Keratosis	or occasionally irreversible
SIN II	Moderate dysplasia	Usually represents intra-epithelial
	Keratosis with atypia	neoplastic transformation; often with recurrence or progression
SIN III	Severe keratinizing or nonkeratinizing dysplasia	Represents mucosal change with high frequency of progression to
	Carcinoma in situ	invasive squamous cell carcinoma

MUTAGEN SENSITIVITY AND SCCHN

While SCCHN is strongly associated with tobacco use, chromosome instability and defective DNA repair may underlie susceptibility to environmental carcinogenesis (22). Hsu suggested that chromosome fragility in the general population exists to varying degrees and indicates genetic instability, and that the individuals who are most genetically sensitive to carcinogens are more likely to develop cancer (23). The number of bleomycin-induced chromosomal breaks in cultured peripheral blood lymphocytes may be a measure of an individual's "mutagen sensitivity", i.e., susceptibility to environmental cancers (22,24). Hsu et al. (24) found wide inter-individual variability in chromatid breakage rates, i.e. genotoxicity induced by bleomycin. Approximately 12% of normal persons were regarded as bleomycin sensitive, while nearly 50% of patients with cancer in the upper aerodigestive tract were found to be sensitive (22). In a prospective study of mutagen sensitivity in patients with upper aerodigestive tract cancer, Schantz et al. (25) found that mutagen sensitivity correlated with the risk of developing second malignant tumors in patients cured of head and neck cancer. A case-control study showed that persons with untreated upper aerodigestive tract cancer express greater sensitivity than do controls, when their cells are exposed to bleomycin in vitro (26). These findings were recently confirmed by Cloos et al. (27) who found increased mutagen sensitivity in head-and-neck squamous-cell carcinoma patients, particularly in those with multiple primary tumors.

Mutagen sensitivity can be modulated in vitro (28) and in vivo (29) by various nutrients. The antioxidant micronutrients, alpha-tocopherol and ascorbic acid have been shown to protect against carcinogen-induced chromosomal breakage (28-31). Since vegetable and fruit consumption has been found to be protective against the development of upper aerodigestive tract cancers (32,33), certain antioxidant micronutrients in the diet may provide protection against DNA damaging carcinogens. Kucuk et al (34) investigated the intra-individual variation in mutagen sensitivity and its possible correlation with plasma nutrient levels in a group of 25 healthy individuals in Hawaii. Mutagen sensitivity, as assessed by bleomycin-induced chromosomal breaks in cultured peripheral blood lymphocytes and plasma nutrient levels were measured monthly for 11 months. Significant inverse correlations were found between mutagen sensitivity scores and the plasma levels of alpha-carotene (r = -0.64), total carotenoids (r = -0.41), and ascorbic acid (r = -0.40). There were also significant inverse associations between monthly mean plasma levels of alpha-carotene (r = -0.58), beta-carotene (r = -0.76) and total carotenoids (r = -0.72) and monthly mean chromosomal breaks. In contrast, there was a significant positive correlation between monthly mean plasma triglyceride level (r = 0.60) and monthly mean mutagen sensitivity. These results suggest that mutagen sensitivity could potentially be reduced by dietary modifications or by supplementing certain micronutrients.

DIET AND SCCHN

Epidemiological data consistently show an inverse relationship between cancer risk and dietary intake of vegetables and fruits or their antioxidant micronutrients (33). Most cancer patients have low micronutrient levels at presentation. Cancer is a disease of aging and micronutrient deficiencies are common among older individuals. Monget et al (35) found that serum concentrations of most micronutrients had an inverse association with age and most nursing home residents had low serum levels of vitamin C, zinc and selenium. Micronutrient deficiency may also be present in pediatric cancer patients. Donma et al (36) found reduced hair zinc levels in children with malignancies compared to healthy children and children with cancers in remission.

Negri et al (37) investigated the relationship between selected micronutrients and oral and pharyngeal cancer risk using data from a case-control study conducted in Italy and Switzerland. Cases were 754 incident, histologically confirmed oral cancers (344 of the oral cavity and 410 of the pharynx) and controls were 1,775 subjects with no history of cancer admitted to hospitals in the same catchment areas. Dietary habits were investigated using a validated food-frequency questionnaire. Odds ratios (ORs) were computed after allowance for age, sex, center, education, occupation, body mass index, smoking and drinking habits and non-alcohol energy intake. ORs were 0.95 for retinol, 0.61 for carotene, 0.91 for lycopene, 0.83 for vitamin D, 0.74 for vitamin E, 0.63 for vitamin C, 0.82 for thiamine, 0.87 for riboflavin, 0.59 for vitamin B6, 0.61 for folic acid, 0.62 for niacin, 0.91 for calcium, 0.88 for phosphorus, 0.65 for potassium, 0.82 for iron, 0.67 for non-alcohol iron and 0.89 for zinc. When the combined intake of vitamins C and E and carotene was considered, the protective effect of each nutrient was more marked or restricted to subjects with low intake of the other two. The association with vitamin C and carotene was independent of smoking and drinking habits, while that with vitamin E was less evident in those heavily exposed to alcohol or tobacco. In general, the more a micronutrient was correlated to total vegetable and fruit intake, the stronger was its protective effect against oral cancer.

Soy isoflavones may also have protective effects against SCCHN. Alhasan et al (38) showed that a soy isoflavone, genistein inhibited cell proliferation, caused cell cycle arrest at the S/G2-M phase and induced apoptosis in a squamous cell carcinoma cell line HN4. These effects appeared to be dose and time dependent, and specific for tumor cells, because genistein did not affect normal keratinocytes. Alhasan et al (39) also observed that these changes were accompanied by down-regulation of Cdk1 and CyclinB1, and up-regulation of p21WAF1, which may be responsible for the induction of cell cycle arrest and apoptosis. The evidence for the induction of apoptosis was supported by the appearance of DNA ladder and the cleavage of poly-ADP-ribose polymerase (PARP), hallmark of apoptosis. This was also accompanied by the up-regulation of Bax, with modest down-regulation of Bcl-2 protein expression, which changes in the balance between pro- and anti-apoptosis molecules in favor of pro-apoptosis. Furthermore, they also observed down-regulation and degradation of Cdc25C, which is a marker of cell proliferation, and plays important role in CyclinB-Cdk1 complex activation. The down-regulation followed by the degradation of Cdc25C is an indicator of G2/M arrest and anti-proliferation effects of genistein. These results suggest that genistein may have a role in the prevention and/or treatment of SCCHN.

TOBACCO AND NUTRIENTS

Tobacco use is a major risk factor for SCCHN. Tobacco use has consistently been associated with increased oxidative stress and decreased serum antioxidant micronutrient levels. Pamuk et al (40) reported on the relationship between current cigarette smoking and serum concentrations of vitamins C, E, and A, and five carotenoids in ninety-one low income, African-American women. Among smokers, serum concentrations of alpha-carotene, beta-carotene, cryptoxanthin, and lycopene averaged 71-79% of the concentrations among non-smokers. Mean serum concentrations of vitamins C and E and lutein/zeaxanthin were only slightly lower among smokers relative to non-smokers. Among current smokers, mean serum concentrations of all five carotenoids had an inverse correlation with the amount smoked. Ross et al (41) determined plasma concentrations of carotenoids, ascorbic acid, alpha-tocopherol and gamma-tocopherol in plasmas from fifty smokers and fifty age-matched never-smoker Scottish men. Significantly less alpha-carotene, beta-carotene, cryptoxanthin and ascorbic acid were found in smokers compared to persons who never smoked. Pakrashi and Chatterjee (42) measured prostatic excretion of zinc in ejaculates of twenty-nine tobacco smokers, twenty-five tobacco chewers and thirty non-users of tobacco. They found reduced levels of zinc in the ejaculates of tobacco smokers compared to tobacco chewers and tobacco non-users. It has been postulated that smoking results in depletion of antioxidant micronutrients by generating oxidative stress. However, low dietary intake of antioxidant micronutrients by smokers may also be a factor in the observed inverse association. For example, Faruque et al (43) observed lower dietary intake of vitamin C, carotenoids and zinc and lower plasma level of vitamin C in 44 male students who smoked compared to 44 male non-smoker students.

Similar to SCCHN, lung cancer is also caused by smoking. Since smoking generates oxidative stress and leads to decreased serum levels of beta-carotene, supplementing the diet with beta-carotene in smokers to prevent lung cancer is reasonable. However, a large clinical study conducted in Finland found just the opposite (44). This unexpected result might have been due to the paradoxical pro-oxidant effect of beta-carotene in lungs where the oxygen tension is high. Studies have shown that beta-carotene, at high concentrations, has a pro-oxidant effect when the oxygen pressure is also high (45). Therefore, in the lungs where the oxygen tension is high, administering large doses of beta-carotene may lead to oxidative DNA damage and higher incidence of cancer. Furthermore, beta-carotene and tobacco smoke interact to increase AP-1 production in ferret lungs (46), which may also explain the increased risk of lung cancer with beta-carotene supplementation in current smokers but not in non-smokers.

ALCOHOL AND NUTRIENTS

Alcohol consumption has also been associated with increased oxidative stress and decreased micronutrient levels. Alcohol and tobacco in combination may result in even more severe micronutrient deficiencies compared to either one used alone. Tsubono et al (47) examined the associations of smoking and alcohol with plasma levels of beta-carotene, alpha-carotene, lutein, lycopene and zeaxanthin in 634 healthy men aged 40-49 years. After controlling for age, serum cholesterol, serum triglycerides, body mass index, and ingestion of green vegetables, yellow vegetables and fruits, there was a significant inverse association between smoking and alcohol consumption and plasma levels of beta-carotene and alpha-carotene; only smoking reduced the level of lutein, and neither smoking nor alcohol significantly reduced the level of lycopene or zeaxanthin. Brady et al (48) in a population based sample of 400 individuals found an association between smoking and alcohol consumption and lower serum levels of alpha-carotene, beta-carotene, beta-cryptoxanthin, and lutein/zeaxanthin. In addition, lower serum lycopene was associated with older age. Lecomte et al (49) measured plasma carotenoid levels in 118 healthy men consuming low or moderate alcohol and 95 alcoholics. Beta-carotene, alpha-carotene, zeaxanthin-lutein, lycopene and beta-cryptoxanthin levels were significantly lower in alcoholics and 21 days after withdrawal plasma levels of all carotenoids increased. However, Leo et al (50) did not find a significant difference in the levels of carotenoids, retinol and alpha-tocopherol from oropharyngeal mucosa samples of eleven chronic alcoholics with oropharyngeal cancer and eleven control subjects.

CANCER TREATMENT AND NUTRIENTS

Nutritional status is known to profoundly impact treatment morbidity, efficacy and overall prognosis in cancer patients (51-58). Various prognostic nutritional indices have been developed to predict treatment complications and overall survival (51,52,55,58). Radiation and chemotherapy are better tolerated and may be more effective in nutritionally sound individuals (51,52). For example, head and neck cancer patients with poor nutritional status are at increased risk for post-operative wound breakdown and infections, fistula formation and flap loss (51,55). These patients frequently present with significant weight loss and chronic protein-calorie malnutrition, which may be exacerbated by an acute weight loss due to decreased intake secondary to tumor-induced dysphagia (51-55). Approximately 30-40% of patients with advanced stage head and neck cancer have severe malnutrition and additional 20-30% have moderate malnutrition at the time of presentation (51-55). Olmedilla et al (59) found that the plasma levels of carotenoids, retinol and vitamin E were significantly lower in patients who had laryngectomy for laryngeal cancer compared to control subjects. After commercial enteral formula feeding carotenoid levels further decreased and retinol and tocopherol levels increased, however the levels remained lower than the controls for all micronutrients (59). Post-operative alterations of the upper aerodigestive tract may further compromise intake, increase metabolic demands and compound the nutritional stress (53,56). Since there are no known zinc stores in the human body, zinc deficiency sets in quickly with malnutrition in these patients (60).

Both radiation therapy and chemotherapy have been associated with increased oxidative stress, which may further deplete tissue levels of antioxidant micronutrients, particularly in smokers and in the presence of inadequate dietary intake. Faber et al (61) measured lipid peroxidation, plasma glutathione and glutathione peroxidase activity, and plasma micronutrient levels in cancer patients before and after doxorubicin-containing chemotherapy. The concentration of lipid peroxidation products, measured as thiobarbituric acid reactant materials, in the plasma of cancer patients was higher than in controls and the level was further increased after chemotherapy. These results indicated that cancer patients had increased oxidative stress at presentation, which was further aggravated by doxorubicin treatment. Cancer patients had lower levels of glutathione, glutathione peroxidase, selenium and zinc levels, but these were not further modified by chemotherapy. Torii et al (62) reported that doxorubicin treatment caused cardiomyopathy and increased lipid peroxidation and lower alpha-tocopherol levels in the myocardium of spontaneously hypertensive rats.

Radiation therapy of malignancies in the head and neck area results in a marked reduction in saliva flow rate and alterations in saliva composition within the first week of therapy and impairs saliva flow throughout the duration of therapy. Decreased secretion of saliva may lead to symptoms such as oral pain and burning sensations, loss of taste and appetite and increased incidence of oral disease. These symptoms may affect eating and increase the risk of inadequate nutritional intake. Backstrom et al (63) investigated the average nutritional intake of 24 patients treated for malignancies in the head and neck region who had dry mouth symptoms that had persisted for at least four months after the completion of radiation therapy. The average caloric intake was 1925 calories in the irradiated patients with dry mouth symptoms compared to 2219 calories in the age- and sex-matched controls. The average intakes of vitamin A, beta-carotene, vitamin E, vitamin B6, folic acid, iron and zinc were significantly lower in the irradiated patients than in controls.

Abnormal dark adaptation also has been related to a deficiency of zinc in humans (64). Zinc supplementation to zinc deficient sickle cell anemia patients is known to correct this abnormality (64). Decreased dark adaptation has recently been identified as the dose-limiting toxicity for fenretinide (4-hydroxyphenylretinamide), a cancer chemopreventive retinoid currently under clinical investigation. Clinical trials should be conducted with combination of zinc and fenretinide to determine if the combination has reduced toxicity and enhanced chemopreventive activity.

CHEMOPREVENTIVE AGENTS

In epidemiologic studies, consumption of certain dietary micronutrients and phytochemicals has been associated with decreased risk of head and neck cancer. In vitro and animal studies have shown potent anti-tumor activity of numerous dietary chemicals. Therefore, human studies have been conducted with nutritional and botanical compounds with potential cancer preventive effects. There are numerous compounds with chemopreventive effects against head and neck cancer in animal models and in vitro studies. Carotenoids and retinoids have received the most attention with promising early results but disappointments in recent clinical trials.
  Current clinical studies are investigating other nutritional and pharmaceutical compounds in the chemoprevention of head and neck cancer. Table 2 shows a list some of the chemopreventive agents under investigation.

Table 2. **Chemopreventive compounds**

Group	Compounds
Retinoids	13-cRA, 4-HPR, ATRA, 9-cRA
Carotenoids	beta-carotene, lycopene, lutein, astaxanthin
Tocopherols	alpha-tocopherol, gamma-tocopherol
Flavonoids, polyphenols	genistein, EGCG
Minerals	selenium, zinc
DME modulators	oltipraz
Cycloxygenase inhibitors	celecoxib, rofecoxib
Anti-proliferative agents	ODC inhibitors (DFMO)
PPAR-gamma inhibitors	thiazolidinones
Pro-apoptotic agents	exisulind
Others	curcumin, ellagic acid, Bowman-Birk inhibitor

13-cRA, 13-cis-retinoic acid; 4-HPR, 4-hydroxyphenylretinamide; ATRA, all-trans-retinoic acid; 9-cRA, 9-cis-retinoic acid; EGCG, epigallactocathecingallate; DME, drug metabolizing enzyme; ODC, ornithine decarboxylase; DFMO, difluoromethylornithin

RETINOIDS

Retinoids have previously been used to treat oral premalignant conditions in multiple investigations. Koch used three retinoic acid analogs to treat three divided groups of 75 patients with multifocal leukoplakia (65). Response rates (complete responders + partial responders) were 50%, 87% and 91% for the three respective groups. Later Hong et al. (66) performed a randomized trial using 13-cis-retinoic acid on 44 patients with either histologically-proven premalignant oral lesions (mild dysplasia, moderate dysplasia or severe dysplasia/carcinoma-in-situ) or lesions without cytologic abnormalities (acanthoses, keratoses and parakeratoses which accounted for 21/44 or, more than 47% of subjects entered). Of subjects randomized to the treatment arm, 67% experienced significant regression of the clinical lesions and 54% had reversal of "dysplasia" (dysplasia + atypical hyperplasia). Of greatest interest, however, was the histologic reversal of the three cases of severe dysplasia in the retinoic treatment group. These data have been generally supported by other studies (67,68).

ALPHA-TOCOPHEROL

While epidemiological evidence relating alpha-tocopherol intake to cancer risk in humans is scarce, there is some evidence suggesting that low serum levels of alpha-tocopherol might be associated with an increased risk (69-71). Benner et al. (72) conducted a clinical trial of alpha-tocopherol in patients with oral intraepithelial neoplasia and found a complete response rate of 23% and partial response rate of 23%. Further clinical trials are needed to study the efficacy of alpha-tocopherol either alone or in combination with other potential chemopreventive agents, particularly other antioxidant micronutrients, in the prevention of oral and other neoplasia.

BETA-CAROTENE

Carotenoids have been shown to prevent cancer formation and induce regression of cancers in the oral mucosa of animals (73,74). Many epidemiologic studies have reported an inverse correlation between beta-carotene and cancer (75-79). Beta-carotene is safe at moderate levels and does not have the side effects and toxicity associated with retinoids (76,80,81).

The results of clinical trials suggest that beta-carotene is effective in the treatment of oral intraepithelial neoplasia (82-88) resulting in complete remissions ranging from 8% to 33%, partial remissions ranging from 11% to 63%, and overall response rates ranging from 44% to 71%. Garewal et al. (87) reported a 71% response rate in 24 patients with oral leukoplakia who were given 30 mg of beta-carotene daily for 6 months. There was no significant toxicity requiring drug discontinuation or dose reduction. Stich et al. (88)

reported a 15% complete remission rate in oral leukoplakia after administration of beta-carotene 180 mg/week for 6 months to betel nut /tobacco chewers in India. They have also shown significant suppression of micronucleated cells in buccal mucosa. However, a clinical trial using beta-carotene in the maintenance phase of a prevention study in patients with head and neck cancer found it to be ineffective (89). The results of a large chemoprevention study suggested that beta-carotene administration may even lead to an increase in the incidence of lung cancer (90). Thus, the role of beta-carotene in cancer chemoprevention is still uncertain and needs to be further studied with clinical trials in different populations of patients.

COMBINATION OF BETA-CAROTENE AND ALPHA-TOCOPHEROL

Epidemiologic data show that individuals who have low serum levels of either beta-carotene (91) or vitamin E (92) are at a high risk of developing cancer. It is particularly noteworthy that serum vitamin E and vitamin A levels were significantly lower in patients with second primary tumors than in patients with a single head and neck cancer (93). Experimental cancers in animals can be prevented by administration of either beta-carotene (86,94) or vitamin E (95) or the combination of the two agents (73). Combined oral administration of alpha-tocopherol and beta-carotene caused regression of experimental squamous cell carcinomas in hamster buccal mucosa (73).

NON-STEROIDAL ANTI-INFLAMMATORY DRUGS (NSAIDS)

Intake of NSAIDs has been associate with reduced incidence of cancer at a variety of organ sites in epidemiologic studies in humans and carcinogenesis studies in rodents (96,97). While this link is the strongest for colorectal carcinoma, the potential for NSAIDs to prevent cancer has also been shown in multiple other cancers, including breast, bladder, and lung in animal carcinogenesis models (98-100).

NSAIDs inhibit the cyclooxygenase family of enzymes, which metabolise arachidonic acid to prostaglandins, prostacyclin, and thromboxanes. Prostaglandins, particularly PGE2, have been implicated in carcinogenesis due to their capacity to increase cell growth, inhibit cell apoptosis, promote angiogenesis, and cause local immunosuppresion. The COX-1 isoform is constitutively expressed in many normal tissues and mediates a variety of functions such as gastric mucosal cytoprotection and platelet aggregation. The COX-2 isoform is induced by cytokines and growth factors and is expressed in inflammatory, preneoplastic, and cancer tissues. Recent data showed that selective COX-2 inhibition by celecoxib in patients with familial adenomatous polyposis results in reduction in the number of colorectal polyps (101). This led to the FDA approval of celecoxib for chemoprevention of colon cancer in this patient population. Current clinical trials are investigating the chemopreventive effects of NSAIDs in other tissues, such as superficial bladder cancer, sporadic colorectal adenomas, and actinic keratosis.

Mechanisms of action of NSAIDs may also include signaling pathways other than cyclooxygenases. He et al. (102) have shown that sulindac down-regulates the transcriptional activity of the nuclear peroxisome proliferator-activated receptor gamma (PPAR-gamma) and that the apoptotic effect of sulindac on colon cancer cells is at least in part mediated by PPAR-gamma (102). NSAID-induced apoptosis is also mediated by 15-lipoxygenase-1 (103) independently of COX-2 in colon cancer cells (103). Recent studies have shown that sulindac sulfone, a sulindac derivative devoid of COX inhibitory activity, induces apoptosis in colon cancer cells via activation of protein kinase G (104). Several NSAIDs, such as indomethacin and flufenamic acid, directly bind to and stimulate the transcriptional activity of another member of the PPAR family, PPAR-gamma (105). Activation of PPAR-gamma mediates differentiation, growth arrest, and apoptosis in vitro in a variety of cancer cell types, including lung, colon, breast and oral cavity (106-109). A negative feedback loop mediated by activation of PPAR-gamma controls COX-2 expression in endothelial cells and macrophages (110). NSAIDs are very promising agents that may prevent cancer in a variety of epithelial sites.

The presence of chronic inflammation and prostaglandins in tumors of upper aerodigestive tract is well documented (111). The local and systemic levels of prostaglandin E2 (PGE2), a metabolite of the COX pathway, are higher in head and neck cancer patients than in control subjects. COX-2 has been shown to be upregulated up to 150-fold in SCCHN and up to 50-fold in the normal appearing tissues of patients with SCCHN compared with normal control subjects (112). High levels of expression of COX-2 have also been reported in oral leukoplakia and dysplasia (112). Furthermore, NSAIDs prevent SCCHN in animal models (113). Recent data also show that PPAR-gamma may have a role in head and neck carcinogenesis, providing an additional mechanism for NSAIDs in SCCHN (109).

ZINC

Zinc deficiency causes a profound reduction in the activity of a thymic hormone, thymulin. Prasad et al found decreased production of interleukin-2 and interferon-gamma by TH1 cells, reduced NK cell activity and decreased recruitment of T cell precursors in zinc deficient subjects (114). Mocchegiani observed a significant increase or stabilization in body weight of AIDS patients who received zinc supplement in addition to AZT, associated with an increase in CD4 cells and plasma thymulin and decrease in the frequency of opportunistic infections (115). Abdulla et al observed that plasma zinc was decreased and the copper:zinc ratio in the plasma was significantly higher in 13 patients with SCCHN in comparison to the healthy controls (116). The patients who showed a marked decrease in plasma zinc levels died within twelve months. The authors suggested that plasma zinc and copper/zinc ratio may be of value as a potential screening and predicting test in patients with head and neck cancer. However, Garofalo et al observed no significant difference in serum zinc and observed no diagnostic or prognostic value in these parameters in patients with head and neck cancer (117).

Zinc deficiency is known to cause weight loss, abnormal cellular immune functions, hypogeusia, and difficulty in wound healing, all of which commonly occur in malnourished head and neck cancer patients. Wound healing is in many respects analogous to growth and in as much as zinc deficiency affects growth adversely, it is not surprising that zinc deficiency also causes impaired wound healing (118-120), and that zinc supplementation promotes wound healing in zinc deficient subjects (118-120). Zinc deficient rats show a significant reduction in total collagen, a reduction in the total dry weight of the sponge connective tissue and the non-collagenous protein content, a decrease in RNA/DNA, and a depletion of polyribosomes in sponge connective tissue, suggesting that the proliferation of fibroblasts is impaired as a result of zinc deficiency (121).

Prasad et al (122) described the zinc levels in plasma, lymphocytes, and granulocytes in zinc deficient and zinc sufficient subjects with head and neck cancer and healthy volunteers. By the cellular zinc criteria, a mild deficiency of zinc was observed in 25% of the normal healthy volunteers and 48% of the head and neck cancer subjects. Productions of IL-2 and TNF-α were significantly decreased in zinc deficient subjects in both groups (cancer and healthy volunteers), whereas the productions of IL-4, IL-5 and IL-6 were not affected by zinc status. The mean IL-4 production in cancer patients was higher than in non-cancer subjects, but statistically the difference was not significant. In zinc deficient subjects of both groups, the production of IL-1β was significantly increased in comparison to the zinc sufficient subjects. NK cell activity was decreased in zinc deficient subjects in comparison to zinc sufficient subjects in both groups. The ratios of CD4+/CD8+ and CD4+CD45RA+/CD4+CD45R0+ cells were decreased in zinc deficient subjects. 57% (27/47) patients were classified as nutritionally deficient (NUTR-) whereas 43% (20/47) were nutritionally sufficient (NUTR+) based on their PNI indices. Zinc status was inversely associated with both tumor size (p=0.002), disease stage (p=.04) and unplanned hospital days (p=.04). Zinc deficiency and cell mediated immune dysfunction are present in a large percentage of head and neck cancer patients at initial presentation (122). Zinc and nutrition interaction was significant for post-operative febrilc days (p = 0.03) and for disease free interval (p=0.01). Fifty percent of the morbidities (pulmonary and non-pulmonary) were due to infectious episodes. Thus, they observed that zinc status of head and neck cancer patients affects significantly cell-mediated immune functions and clinical morbidities. The results showed that the functions of TH1 cells were compromised as evidenced by decreased production of IL-2 and IFN-γ in zinc deficient head and neck cancer patients, whereas the TH2 cytokines were unaffected. NK cell lytic activity was also decreased in zinc deficient patients. Thus, there is an imbalance between the functions of TH1 and TH2 cells, which may have been responsible for cell mediated immune function disorders in zinc deficient cancer patients. Further research must be carried out in order to document the effect of zinc supplementation in zinc deficient patients with squamous cell carcinoma of head and neck.

The disease free interval is longest for the group with zinc-sufficient and nutrition-sufficient status. If these results are confirmed in larger studies, zinc supplementation may be recommended for head and neck cancer patients at presentation to reduce treatment- and disease-related morbidity, to improve immune function, to delay disease recurrence and to prevent second primary tumors.

PHYTOCHEMICALS

Since major factors associated with cancer are pro-oxidant in nature, it is hypothesized that administration of anti-oxidant supplements would prevent cancer. Increased consumption of fruits and vegetables, which contain numerous anti-oxidant micronutrients, has consistently been associated with a lower risk of cancer in epidemiological studies. However, vegetables and fruits contain numerous cancer preventive compounds with different mechanisms of action, and they are all taken together in small quantities as a part of a complex diet. It is therefore inappropriate to extrapolate from epidemiological studies and conclude that just because a micronutrient has an inverse association in epidemiological studies it would result in cancer risk reduction when taken as a dietary supplement. Clinical studies are needed to investigate the mechanisms of action as well as efficacy and toxicity of each micronutrient, alone and in combination with other micronutrients. Multiple chemopreventive agents, when taken together, may have synergistic or antagonistic interactions or no interactions with each other. Examples of promising nutritional chemopreventive compounds in clinical trials include vitamin E, selenium, lycopene, folic acid, and soy isoflavones. The importance of conducting clinical chemoprevention trials has become very clear recently, when several clinical trials showed that the agents hypothesized to prevent cancer did exactly the opposite (44,123). A large chemoprevention study conducted to determine whether beta-carotene and/or alpha-tocopherol would prevent lung cancer showed that beta-carotene supplementation increased the risk of lung cancer (44). These unexpected results highlight the importance of conducting well-designed, prospective, randomized clinical trials before making recommendations to the public regarding the use of supplements.

CONCLUSIONS

Micronutrients and phytochemicals modulate genetic pathways of carcinogenesis and inhibit the initiation and progression of SCCHN. These compounds may have a role in the prevention of cancer in high-risk populations, such as tobacco smokers, as well as in the prevention of disease progression or relapse. Clinical studies investigating the use of these agents in the prevention of SCCHN should be a high priority.

REFERENCES

1.   Greenlee, RT, Hill-Harmon, MB, Murray, T, and Thun, M. Cancer statistics, 2001. CA Cancer J Clin, 51:15-36, 2001.
2.   Ries, L. A. G., C. L. Kosary, et al. SEER Cancer Statistics Review, 1973-1996, National Cancer Institute, 1999.
3.   Swango, P. A. Cancer of the oral cavity and pharynx in the United States: an epidemilogic overview. J Public Health Dent 56(6): 309-318, 1996.
4.   Schantz, SP, Harrison, LB, and Forastiere, AA. Tumors of the nasal cavity and paranasal sinuses, nasopharynx, oral cavity, and oropharynx. VT DeVita, S Hellman, SA Rosenberg, eds., Cancer: Principles and Practice of Oncology. Lippincott Williams & Wilkins, NY, 797-860, 2001.
5.   Wynder, E. L., M. H. Mushinski, et al. Tobacco and alcohol consumption in relation to the development of multiple primary cancers. Cancer 40(4 Suppl): 1872-8, 1977.

6.   Horowitz, A. M., H. S. Goodman, et al. The need for health promotion in oral cancer prevention and early detection. J Public Health Dent 56(6): 319-30, 1996.

7.   Devesa, S. S., W. J. Blot, et al. Cohort trends in mortality from oral, esophageal, and laryngeal cancers in the United States [see comments]. Epidemiology 1(2): 116-21, 1990.

8.   Gillison, M. L., W. M. Koch, et al. Human papillomavirus in head and neck squamous cell carcinoma: are some head and neck cancers a sexually transmitted disease? Curr Opin Oncol 11: 191-199, 1999.

9.   Yu MC, H. B. Nasopharyngeal Cancer. Cancer Epidemiology and Prevention. F. J. Schottenfeld D. New York, Oxford University Press: 603-618, 1996.

10. Potter, J. D., A. Chavez, et al. (1997). Food, nutrition and the prevention of cancer: a global perspective. Washington DC, World Cancer Research Fund/American Institute of Cancer Research.

11. Update January 1992: the American Cancer Society guidelines for cancer-related check-up.(1992). CA-Cancer J Clin 42: 44-45.

12. Slaughter, DP, Southwick, HW, Smejkal, W. Field cancerization in oral stratified squamous epithelium: Clinical implications of multicentric origin. Cancer, 6:963-968, 1953.

13. Lippman, SM and Hong, WK. Not yet standard: Retinoids versus second primary tumors. J Clin Oncol, 11:1204-1207, 1993.

14. Lee, JJ, Hong, WK, Hittelman, WN, et al. Predicting cancer development in oral leukoplakia: Ten years of translational research. Clin Cancer Res, 6:1702-1710, 2000.

15. Hong, WK, Endicott, J, Itri, LM, et al. 13-cis-retinoic acid in the treatment of oral leukoplakia. N Eng J Med, 315:1501-1505, 1986.

16. Lippman, SM, Batsakis, JG, Toth, BB, et al. Comparison of low-dose isotretinoin with beta carotene to prevent oral carcinogenesis. N Eng J Med, 328:15-20, 1993.

17. Garewal, HS, Katz, RV, Meyskens, F, et al. Beta-carotene produces sustained remissions in patients with oral leukoplakia. Arch Otolaryngol Head Neck Surg, 125:1305-1310, 1999.

18. Waldron CA, Shafer WG: Leukoplakia revisited. A clinico-pathologic study of 3,256 leukoplakias.Cancer 36:1386-1392, 1968.

19. Mashberg A. Erythroplakia: the earliest sign of asymptomatic oral cancer. J Am Dent Assoc 96:615-620,1978.

20. Shafer WG, Waldron CA. Erythroplakia of the oral cavity. Cancer 36:1021-1028, 1975.

21. Crissman JD, Zarbo RJ: Dysplasia, in situ carcinoma and progress to invasive squamous cell carcinoma of the upper aerodigestive tract. Am J Surg Pathol 13 (Suppl):5-16, 1989.

22. Hsu, T.C., Spitz, M.R., and Schantz, S.P. (1991). Mutagen sensitivity: A biological marker of cancer susceptibility. Cancer Epidemiol. Biomarkers Prev. 1, 83-89.

23. Hsu, T.C. (1983). Genetic instability in the human population: a working hypothesis. Hereditas 98, 1-9.

24. Hsu, T.C., Johnston, D.A., Cherry, L.M., Ramkisson, D., Schantz, S.P., Jessup, J.M., Winn, R.J., Shirley, L., and Furlong, C. (1989). Sensitivity to genotoxic effects of bleomycin in humans: Possible relationship to environmental carcinogenesis. Int. J. Cancer 43, 403-409.

25.   Schantz, S.P., Spitz, M.R., and Hsu, T.C. (1990). Mutagen sensitivity in head and neck cancer patients: a biologic marker for risk of multiple primary malignancies. J. Natl. Cancer Inst. 82, 1773-1775.

26.   Spitz, M.R., Fueger, J.J., Halabi, S., Schantz, S.P., Sample, D., and Hsu, T.C. (1993). Mutagen sensitivity in upper aerodigestive tract cancer: A case-control analysis. Cancer Epidemiol. Biomarkers Prev. 2, 329-333.

27.   Cloos, J., Braakhuis, B.J.M., Steen, I., Copper, M.P., DeVries, N., Nauta, J.J.P. and Snow, G.P. (1994). Increased mutagen sensitivity in head-and-neck squamous-cell carcinoma patients, particularly those with multiple primary tumors. Int. J. Cancer. 56, 816-819.

28.   Trizna, Z., Schantz, S.P., and Hsu, T.C. (1991). Effects of N-acetyl-L-cysteine and ascorbic acid on mutagen-induced chromosomal sensitivity in patients with head and neck cancers. Am. J. Surg. 162, 294-298.

29.   Pohl, H.,and Reidy, J. (1989). Vitamin C intake influences the bleomycin-induced chromosome damage assay: Implications for detection of cancer susceptibility and chromosome breakage syndromes. Mutat. Res. 224, 247-252.

30.   Trizna, Z., Hsu, T.C., and Schantz, S.P. (1992). Protective effects of vitamin E against bleomycin-induced genotoxicity in head and neck cancer patients in vitro. Anticancer Res. 2, 325-328.

31.   Shamberger, R.L., Baughman, F.F., Kalchert, S.L., et al. (1973). Carcinogen-induced chromosomal breakage decreased by antioxidants. Proc. Natl. Acad. Sci. USA 70, 1461-1463.

32.   LaVecchia, C., Negri, E., D'Avanzo, B., Franchesci, S., Decarli, A., and Boyle, P. Dietary indicators of laryngeal cancer risk. Cancer Res., 50:4497-4500, 1990.

33.   Block, G., Patterson, B., and Subar, A. (1992). Fruits, vegetables, and cancer prevention: A review of epidemiological evidence. Nutr. Cancer 18, 1-29.

34.   Kucuk, O., Pung, A., Franke, A., Custer, L., Wilkens, L., LeMarchand, L., Higuchi, C., Cooney, R., and Hsu, T.C. (1995). Variability of mutagen sensitivity in healthy adults: Correlations with plasma nutrient levels. Cancer Epidemiol. Biomarkers Prev. 4, 217-221.

35.   Monget, A. L., Galan, P., Preziosi, P., Keller, H., Bourgeois, C., Arnaud, J., Favier, A., and Hercberg, S. (1996). Micronutrient status in elderly people. Int. J. Vit. Nutr. Res. 66, 71-76.

36.   Donma, M. M., Donma, O., and Tas, M. A. (1993). Hair zinc and copper concentrations and zinc:copper ratios in pediatric malignancies and healthy children from southeastern Turkey. Biol. Trace Element Res. 36, 51-63.

37.   Negri, E., Franceschi, S., Bosetti, C., Levi, F., Conti, E., Parpinel, M., and La Vecchia, C. (2000). Selected micronutrients and oral and pharyngeal cancer. Int. J. Cancer 86, 122-127.

38.   Alhasan, S. A., Pietrasczkiwicz, H., Alonso, M. D., Ensley, J., and Sarkar, F. H. (1999). Genistein-induced cell cycle arrest and apoptosis in a head and neck squamous cell carcinoma cell line. Nutr. Cancer 34, 12-19.

39.   Alhasan, S. A., Ensley, J. F., and Sarkar, F. H. (2000). Genistein induced molecular changes in a squamous cell carcinoma of the head and neck cell line. Int. J. Oncol. 16, 333-338.

40.   Pamuk, E. R., Byers, T., Coates, R. J., Vann, J. W., Sowell, A. L., Gunter, E. W., and Glass, D. (1994). Effects of smoking on serum nutrient concentrations in African-American women. Am. J. Clin. Nutr. 59, 891-895.

41.   Ross, M. A., Crosley, L. K., Brown, K. M., Duthie, S. J., Collins, A. C., Arthur, J. R., and Duthie, G.G. (1995). Plasma concentrations of carotenoids and antioxidant vitamins in Scottish males: influences of smoking. Eur. J. Clin. Nutr. 49, 861-865.

42.   Pakrashi, A., and Chatterjee, S. (1995). Effect of tobacco consumption on the function of male accessory sex glands. Int. J. Androl. 18, 232-236.

43. Faruque, M. O., Khan, M. R., Rahman, M. M., and Ahmed, F. (1995). Relationship between smoking and antioxidant micronutrient status. Br. J. Nutr. 73, 625-632.

44. Albanes, D., Heinonen, O. P., Taylor, P. R., Virtamo, J., Edwards, B. K., Rautalahti, M., Hartman, A. M., Palmgren, J., Freedman, L. S., Haapakoski, J., Barrett, M. J., Pietinen, P., Malila, N., Tala, E., Liippo, K., Salomaa, E. R., Tangrea, J. A., Teppo, L., Askin, F. B., Taskinen, E., Erozan, Y., Greenwald, P., Huttunen, J. K. (1996). Alpha-Tocopherol and beta-carotene supplements and lung cancer incidence in the alpha-tocopherol, beta-carotene cancer prevention study: effects of base-line characteristics and study compliance. J. Natl. Cancer Inst. 88, 1560-1570.

45. Palozza, P., Luberto, C., Calviello, G., Ricci, P., and Bartoli, G.M. (1997). Antioxidant and prooxidant role of beta-carotene in murine normal and tumor thymocytes: effects of oxygen partial pressure. Free Rad. Biol. Med. 22, 1065-1073.

46. Wang, X.D., Liu, C., Bronson, R.T., Smith, D.E., Krinsky, N.I., and Russell, M. (1999). Retinoid signaling and activator protein-1 expression in ferrets given beta-carotene supplements and exposed to tobacco smoke. J. Natl. Cancer Inst. 91, 60-66.

47. Tsubono, Y., Tsugane, S., and Gey, K. F. (1996). Differential effects of cigarette smoking and alcohol consumption on the plasma levels of carotenoids in middle aged Japanese men. Jap. J. Res. 87, 563-569.

48. Brady, W. E., Mares-Perlman, J. A., Bowen, P., and Stacewicz-Sapuntzakis, M. (1996). Human serum carotenoid concentrations are related to physiologic and lifestyle factors. J. Nutrition 126, 129-137.

49. Lecomte, E., Grolier, P., Herbeth, B., Pirollet, P., Musse, N., Paille, F., Braesco, V., Siest, G., and Artur, Y. (1994). The relationship of alcohol consumption to serum carotenoid and retinol levels. Effects of withdrawal. Int. J. Vit. Nutr. Res. 64, 170-175.

50. Leo, M. A., Seitz, H. K., Maier, H., and Lieber, C. S. (1995). Carotenoid, retinoid and vitamin E status of the oropharyngeal mucosa in the alcoholics. Alcohol & Alcoholism 30, 163-170.

51. Goodwin, W. J., and Torres, J. (1984). The value of prognostic nutritional index in the management of patients with carcinoma of the head and neck. Otolaryngol. Head Neck Surg. 6, 932-937.

52. Brooks, G. B. (1985). Nutritional status- a prognostic indicator in head and neck cancer. Otolaryngol. Head Neck Surg. 93, 69-74.

53. Williams, E. F., and Meguid, M. M. (1989). Nutritional concepts and considerations in head and neck surgery. Head Neck Surg. 11, 393-399.

54. Bassett, M. R., and Dobie, R. A. (1983). Patterns of nutritional deficiency in head and neck cancer. Otolaryngol. Head Neck Surg. 91, 119-125.

55. Hooley, R., Levine, H., Flores, T.C., Wheeler, T., and Steiger, E. (1983). Predicting postoperative complications using nutritional assessment. Arch. Otolaryngol. 109, 83-85.

56. Sobol, S. M., Conoyer, J. M., and Sessions, D. G. (1979). Enteral and parenteral nutrition in patients with head and neck cancer. Ann. Otolaryngol. 88, 495-501.

57. Mullen, J. L., Gertner, M. H., Buzby, G.P., Goodhart, G.L., and Rosato, E. F. (1979). Implications of malnutrition in the surgical patient. Arch. Surg. 114, 121-125.

58. Buzby, G. P., Mullen, J. L., Matthews, D. C.; Hobbes, C. I., and Rosato, E. F. (1980). Prognostic nutritional index in gastrointestinal surgery. Am. J. Surg. 139, 160-167.

59. Olmedilla, B., Granado, F., Blanco, I., and Rojas-Hidalgo, E. (1996). Evaluation of retinol, alpha- tocopherol, and carotenoids in serum of men with cancer of the larynx before and after commercial enteral formula feeding. J. Parenteral Enteral Nutr. 20, 145-149.

60.   Prasad, A. S. (1993). Biochemistry of zinc. Plenum Press, New York.

61.   Faber, M., Coudray, C., Hida, H., Mousseau, M., and Favier, A. (1995). Lipid peroxidation products, and vitamin and trace element status in patients with cancer before and after chemotherapy, including Adriamycin. A preliminary study. Biol. Trace Element Res. 47, 117-123.

62.   Torii, M., Ito, H., and Suzuki, T. (1992). Lipid peroxidation and myocardial vulnerability in hypertrophied SHR myocardium. Exp. Mol. Pathol. 57, 29-38.

63.   Backstrom, I., Funegard, U., Andersson, I., Franzen, L., and Johansson, I. (1995). Dietary intake in head and neck irradiated patients with permanent dry mouth symptoms. Oral Oncol. Eur. J. Cancer 31B, 253-257.

64   Warth, J. A., Prasad, A. S., Zwas, F., and Frank, R. N. (1981). Abnormal dark adaptation in sickle cell anemia. J. Lab. Clin. Med. 98, 189-194.

65.   Koch H: Biochemical treatment of precancerous oral lesions; the effectiveness of various analogues of retinoic acid. J Maxillofac Surg 6:59-63, 1978

66.   Hong WK, Endicott J, Itri LM, et al: 13-cis-retinoic acid in the treatment of oral leukoplakia. N Engl J Med 315:1501-1505, 1986

67.   Condero AA, Allevato MAJ, Barclay CA, et al: Treatment of lichen planus and leukoplakia with the oralretinoid Ro10-0359. In: Orfanos CE, et al, eds. Retinoids. Basel:Springer-Verlag, 1981:273-278

68.   Shah JP, Strong EW, DeCrosse JJ, et al: Effect of retinoids on leukoplakia. Am J Surg 146:466-470, 1983

69   Wald NJ, Boreham J, Hayward JL, Bulbrook RD. Plasma retinol, beta-carotene and vitamin E levels in relation to the future risk of breast cancer. Br J Cancer 49:321-324, 1984.

70.   Stahelin HB, Rosel F, Buess E, Brubacher G. Cancer, vitamins and plasma lipids: prospective Basel study. J Natl Cancer Inst 73:1463-1468, 1984.

71.   Salonen JT, Salonen R, Lapapetelaianean R, Alfthan G, Puska P. Risk of cancer in relation to serum concentrations of selenium and vitamins A and E: matched case-control analysis of prospective data. Br Med J 290:417-420, 1985.

72.   Benner SE, Winn RW, Lippman SM, et al. Regression of oral leukoplakia with alpha-tocopherol: a community clinical oncology program chemoprevention study. J Natl Cancer Inst 85:44-47, 1993.

73.   Shklar G, Schwartz J, Trickler D and Reid S. Regression of experimental cancer by oral administration of combined alpha-tocoperol and beta-carotene. Nutr Cancer 12:321-325, 1989.

74.   Suda D, Schwartz J and Shklar G. GGT reduction in beta-carotene inhibition of hamster buccal pouch carcinogenesis. Eur J Cancer Clin Oncol 23:43-46,1987.

75.   Nomura AM, Stemmermann GM, Heilbrun LK et al. Serum vitamin levels and risk of cancer of specific sites in men of Japanese ancestry in Hawaii. Cancer Res 45:2369-2372, 1983.

76.   Peto R, Doll R, Buckley JD, Sporn MB. Can dietary beta-carotene materially reduce human cancer rates? Nature 290:201-208, 1981.

77.   Omenn GS, Goodman G, Rosenstock L, Barnhart S, Lund B, Thornquist M, Feigl P. Cancer chemoprevention with vitamin A and beta-carotene in populations at high risk for lung cancer. In Cerutti PA, Nygaard OF, Simic M (eds), 1987, pp. 279 -283.

78.   Hennekens CH. Beta-carotene and chemoprevention of cancer. In Cerutti PA, Nygaard OF, Simic MG (eds), 1987, pp. 269-277,1987.

79.   Ziegler RG. A review of the epidemiologic evidence that carotenoids reduce the risk of cancer. J Nutr 119:116-122, 1988.

80.   Neiman C, Obbink HJR. The biochemistry and pathology of hypervitaminosis A. Vitam Horm 12:69-99, 1954.

81.   Hennekens CH, Mayrent SL, Willett W. Vitamin A, Carotenoids, and Retinoids. Cancer 58:1837-1841,1986.

82. Kaugars GE, Silverman S Jr, Lovas JGL, Brandt RB, Riley WT, Dao Q, Singh VN, Gallo J. A clinical trial of antioxidant supplements in the treatment of oral leukoplakia. Oral Surg Oral Med Oral Pathol 78:462- 468,1994.

83. Malaker K, Anderson BJ, Beecroft WA, Hodson DI. Management of oral mucosal dysplasia with beta-carotene and cis-retinoic acid: a pilot crossover study. Cancer Detect Prev 15:335-340, 1991.

84. Toma S, Benso S, Albanese E, Palumbo R, Nicolo G, Mangiante P. Response of oral leukoplakia to beta-carotene treatment. In: Vitamins and Cancer Prevention. Baton Rouge: Louisiana StateUniversity Press; 1991.

85. Garewal HS, Katz RV, Meyskens F, Pitcock J, Morse D, Friedman S, Peng Y, Pendrys DG, Mayne S, Alberts D, Kiersch T, Graver E. Beta-carotene produces sustained remissions in patients with oral leukoplakia: results of a multicenter prospective trial. Arch Otolaryngol Head Neck Surg. 125(12):1305-10, 1999.

86. Garewal HS. Potential role of beta-carotene in prevention of oral cancer. Am J Clin Nutr 53:294S-297S, 1991.

87. Garewal HS, Meyskens FL, Jr., Killen D, Reeves D, Kiersch TA, Elletson H, Strosberg A, King D, Steinbronn K. Response of oral leukoplakia to beta-carotene. J Clin Oncol 8:1715-1720, 1990.

88. Stich HF, Rosin MP, Hornby AP, Matthew B, Sankaranarayana R, Nair MK. Remission of oral leukoplakias and micronuclei in tobacco/betel quid chewers treated with beta-carotene and with beta-carotene plus vitamin A. Int J Cancer 42:195-199, 1988.

89. Lippman SM, Batsakis JG, Toth BB, et al. Comparison of low-dose isotretinoin with beta-carotene to prevent oral carcinogenesis. N Engl J Med 328:15-20,1993.

90. The Alpha-tocopherol and Beta-carotene Cancer Prevention Study Group. The effect of vitamin E and beta-carotene on the incidence of lung cancer and other cancers in male smokers. N Engl J Med 330:1029-1035, 1994.

91. Stahelin HB, Gey KF, Eichholzer M, Ludin E. Beta-carotene and cancer prevention: The Basel study. Am J Clin Nutr 53:265S-269S, 1991.

92. Knekt P, Aromaa A, Maatela J, Aaran R-K, Nikkari T, Hakama M, Hakulinen T, Peto R, Teppo L. Vitamin E and cancer prevention. Am J Clin Nutr 53:283S -286S, 1991.

93. de Vries N, Snow GB. Relationship of Vitamins A and E and beta-carotene serum levels to head and neck cancer patients with and without second primary tumors. Eur Arch Otorhinolaryngol 247:368-370, 1990.

94. Krinsky NI. Effects of carotenoids in cellular and animal systems. Am J Clin Nutr 53:238S-246S, 1991.

95. Shklar G. Oral mucosal carcinogenesis inhibition by Vitamin E. J Natl Cancer Inst. 68:791-797, 1982.

96. Schreinemachers, DM and Everson, RB. Aspirin use and lung, colon, and breast cancer incidence in a prospective study. Epidemiol, 5:138-146, 1994.

97. Beazer-Barclay, Y, Levy, DB, Moser, AR, et al. Sulindac suppresses tumorigenesis in the Min mouse. Carcinogenesis, 17:1757-1760, 1996.

98. Harris, RE, Alshafie, GA, Abou-Issa, H, et al. Chemoprevention of breast cancer in rats by celecoxib, a cyclooxygenase 2 inhibitor. Cancer Res, 60:2101-2103, 2000.

99. Rao, KV, Detrisac, CJ, Steele, VE, et al. Differential activity of aspirin, ketoprofen and sulindac as cancer chemopreventive agents in the mouse urinary bladder. Carcinogenesis, 17:1435-1438, 1996.

100. Jalbert, G and Castonguay, A. Effects of NSAIDs on NNK-induced pulmonary and gastric tumorigenesis in A/J mice. Cancer Lett, 66:21-28, 1992.

101.   Steinbach, G, Lynch, PM, Phillips, RKS, et al.   The effect of celecoxib, a cyclooxygenase-2 inhibitor, in familial adenomatous polyposis.   N Eng J Med, 342:1946-52, 2000.

102.   He, T-C, Chan, TA, Vogelstein, B, et al.   PPAR-gamma is an APC-regulated target of nonsteroidal anti inflammatory drugs.   Cell, 99:335-345, 1999.

103.   Shureiqi, I, Chen, D, Lotan, R, et al.   15-Lipoxygenase-1 mediates nonsteroidal anti-inflammatory drug-induced apoptosis independently of cyclooxygenase-2 in colon cancer cells.   Cancer Res, 60:6846-6850, 2000.

104.   Sohm J-W, Mao, Y, Kim, M-G, et al.   Cyclic GMP mediates apoptosis induced by sulindac derivatives via activation of c-Jun NH2-terminal kinase 1.   Clin Cancer Res, 6:4136-4141, 2000.

105.   Lehmann, JM, Lenhard, JM, Oliver, BB, et al.   Peroxisome proliferator-activated receptors alpha and gamma are activated by indomethacin and other non-steroidal anti-inflammatory drugs.   J Biol Chem, 272:3406-3410, 1997.

106.   Chang, T-S and Szabo, E.   Induction of differentiation and apoptosis by ligands of peroxisome proliferator-activated receptor-gamma in non-small cell lung cancer.   Cancer Res, 60:1129-1138, 2000.

107.   Sarraf, P., Mueller, E., Jones, D., et al.   Differentiation and reversal of malignant changes in colon cancer through PPAR-gamma.   Nat. Med., 4: 1046-1052, 1998.

108.   Mueller, E., Sarraf, P., Tontonoz, P., et al.   Terminal differentiation of human breast cancer through PPAR-gamma.   Mol. Cell, 1: 465-470, 1998.

109.   Silver, R and Ondrey, F.   Functional RXR alpha mediated PPAR activation decreases upper aerodigestive squamous cell cancer (SCCA) proliferation.   Proc AACR, 2001.

110.   Inoue, H, Tanabe, T, and Umesono, K.   Feedback control of cyclooxygenase-2 expression through PPAR-gamma.   J Biol Chem, 275:28028-28032, 2000.

111.   Ondrey, FG.   Arachidonic acid metabolism: A primer for head and neck surgeons.   Head & Neck, 20:334-349, 1998.

112.   Chan, G, Boyle, JO, Yang, EK, et al.   Cyclooxygenase-2 expression is up-regulated in squamous cell carcinoma of the head and neck.   Cancer Res, 59:991-994, 1999.

113.   Tanaka, T, Nishikawa, A, Mori, Y, et al.   Inhibitory effects of non-steroidal anti-inflammatory drugs, piroxicam and indomethacin on 4-nitroquinoline 1-oxide-induced tongue carcinogenesis in male ACI/N rats.   Cancer Lett, 48:177-182, 1989.

114.   Prasad, A. S., Beck, F. W. J., Grabowski, S. M., Kaplan. J. and Mathog, R. H. (1997). Zinc deficiency: Changes in cytokine production and T-cell subpopulations in patients with head and neck cancer and in non-cancer subjects. Proc. Asso. Am.. Physicians 109, 68-77.

115.   Mocchegiani, E., Veccia, S., Ancarani, F., Scalise, G., and Fabris, N. (1995). Benefit of oral zinc supplementation as an adjunct to zidovudine (AZT) therapy against opportunistic infections in AIDS. Int. J. Immunopharmacol. 17, 719-727.

116.   Abdulla, M., Biorklund, A., Mathur, A., and Wallenius, K. (1979). Zinc and copper levels in whole blood and plasma from patients with squamous cell carcinomas of head and neck. J. Surg. Oncol. 12, 107-113.

117.   Garofalo, J. A., Erlandson, E., Strong, E. W., Lesser, M., Gerold, F., Spiro, R., Schwartz, M., and Good, R. A. (1980). Serum zinc, serum copper, and the Cu/Zn ratio in patients with epidermoid cancers of the head and neck. J. Surg. Oncol. 15, 381-386.

118.   Wacker, WEC. 1976. Role of zinc in wound healing: A critical review. 1976. In: Prasad AS (Ed).   Trace Elements in Human Health and Disease, Vol. I. New York, Academic Press, pp 107-113.

119.   Strain, W. H., Pories, W. J., and Hinshaw, J. R. (1960). Zinc studies in skin repair. Surg. Forum 11, 291-292.

120.   Pories, W. J., and Strain, W. H. (1966). Zinc and wound healing. In: "Zinc Metabolism" (A. S. Prasad, Ed.), pp. 378-394. Charles C Thomas, Springfield, IL.

121.   Fernandez-Madrid, F., Prasad, A. S., and Oberleas, D. (1973). Effect of zinc deficiency on nucleic acid, collagen and non-collagenous protein of the connective tissue. J. Lab. Clin. Med. 82, 951-961.

122.   Prasad, A. S., Beck, F. W. J., Doerr, T. D., Shamsa, F. H., Penny, H. S., Marks, S. C., Kaplan, J., Kucuk, O., and Mathog, R. H. (1998). Nutritional status of head and neck cancer patients; zinc deficiency and cell mediated immune functions. J. Am. Coll. Nutr. 5, 409-418.

123.   Omenn, G. S., Goodman, G. E., Thornquist, M. D., Balmes, J., Cullen, M. R., Glass, A., Keogh, J. P., Meyskens, F. L. Jr, Valanis, B., Williams, J. H. Jr, Barnhart, S., Cherniack, M. G., Brodkin, C. A., and Hammar, S. (1996). Risk factors for lung cancer and for intervention effects in CARET, the Beta-Carotene and Retinol Efficacy Trial. J. Natl. Cancer Inst. 88, 1550-1559.

Chapter 4

EARLY STAGE HEAD AND NECK CANCER – SURGERY

Steven J. Charous, M.D.
Rush-Presbyterian-St. Luke's Medical Center & Evanston Northwestern Healthcare Hospitals

Early stage head and neck cancer is a highly curable disease. As are the goals of treating any disease process, the goal of treating head and neck cancer is to eradicate the cancer while minimizing the associated morbidity of the treatment. Since eating, breathing, and speaking are all crucial functions regulated by the head and neck regions involved with cancer, finding the appropriate treatment often becomes a significant challenge.

The goal of this chapter is to acquaint the reader with appropriate diagnostic and treatment plans for early stage head and neck cancer from the perspective of the surgeon. Given the limitations imposed because of the breadth of the topic involved, the following assumptions and limitations will be held. It will be assumed that the type of cancer to be treated will be squamous cell carcinoma. Since this particular type of cancer represents over 90% of all head and neck cancers, this assumption should not limit the information the reader obtains. In addition, only cancers arising from the oral cavity, oropharynx, hypopharynx and larynx will be addressed. Thus tumors arising from the nasal cavity or paranasal sinuses, ear or temporal bone, skin or any salivary gland, will not be discussed. Again, cancers arising from the areas to be discussed account for the vast majority of cancers of the head and neck and the limitations imposed will hopefully only help to better focus on the main issues.

In order to proceed in a logical and comprehensive fashion, this chapter will be divided into sections based on the anatomic site of origin of the cancer. Therefore, there will be four sections consisting of the oral cavity, oropharynx, hypopharynx and larynx. Each of these sections will review the anatomy involved, possible surgical resections and reconstruction options, and rehabilitation. A final section will discuss the indications, types, implications and controversies of neck dissections in the treatment of early stage head and neck cancers. However, before proceeding any further, a definition of what comprises "early" head and neck cancer is necessary.

The tumor, node, metastasis (TNM) staging system proposed by the American Joint Committee on Cancer (AJCC) divides cancers of the head and neck into four stages. Stages I and II are considered "early" stages, while stages III and IV are considered "late" stages. To broadly simplify cancer staging into "early" vs. "late" in the head and neck, consider the following statements. 1) A distant metastasis (M_1) creates a late stage carcinoma. 2) Clinical or radiographic evidence of nodal metastasis in the neck (N_{1-3}) creates a late-staged carcinoma. 3) T_3 and T_4 tumors are considered late-staged tumors. Thus, only T_1 and T_2 carcinomas with no clinical or radiological evidence of regional or distant metastases are considered early stage carcinomas of the head and neck

To simplify our thinking regarding classifying the tumor (T) stage, consider the following. With the exception of laryngeal cancers, tumors less than 2 cm. in its greatest dimension and limited to only one anatomic subsite are considered T_1 cancers. Tumors greater than 2 cm. but less than 4 cm. in their greatest dimension are considered T_2 cancers. T_2 cancers can invade a second subsite, but neither T_1 nor T_2 lesions invade underlying bone or cartilage. (Of note: one underlying difficulty of defining the T stage is that the surface dimension is often the dimension measured because of its accessibility, whereas the deep aspect of the tumor may be its greatest dimension.) CT and/or MRI can often aid in staging although they often fall short because of subtle infiltration that is difficult to detect with imaging. Combining both physical examination and radiographic analysis is the best method in accurately predicting the size and extent of the tumor.

ORAL CAVITY CANCERS

Anatomy

The anterior border of the oral cavity begins at the vermilion borders of the upper and lower lips. The posterior border extends to the junction of the hard and soft palate above, and the circumvallate papillae of the tongue below. The subsites of the oral cavity consist of the lips, buccal mucosa, floor of mouth, upper and lower alveolar ridges, retromolar trigone, hard palate and the anterior two-thirds of the tongue. Sensory innervation is provided by all three branches of the fifth (trigeminal) cranial nerve and motor innervation to the tongue is provided by the twelth (hypoglossal) cranial nerve. Blood supply arises from branches of the external carotid artery including branches from the lingual artery, the facial artery, and the maxillary artery.

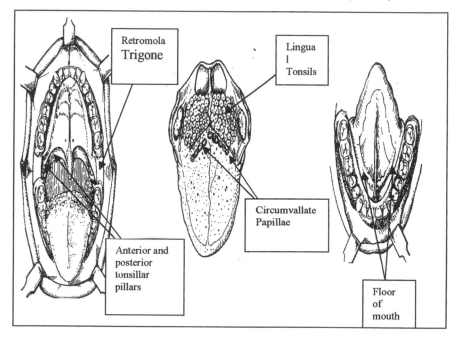

Figure 1. **Anatomy of the Oral Cavity and Oropharynx**

Lymphatic drainage is crucial to understanding oral cavity cancer spread because of the way these tumors tend to spread. Regional metastatic squamous cell carcinoma tends to spread first to lymph nodes that drain the upper regions of the neck such as the ones located in the submental, submandibular and upper-deep jugular regions. As multiple lymph nodes become involved, spread to the middle and lower jugular regions occurs. It is unusual for a oral cavity cancer to spread first to a lower or posterior neck lymph node without first invading more superior ones.

Evaluation of cancers of the oral cavity begins with a careful history. A significant history of tobacco and alcohol use increases suspicion for a malignancy. Floor of mouth and buccal mucosal cancers are more common in patients who chew tobacco. Weight loss and odynophagia are common presenting complaints. Other symptoms of oral cavity cancer include oral pain, otalgia, hemoptysis and articulation problems.

In general, surgical treatment and radiation treatment for T1 and T2 squamous cell carcinomas of the oral cavity have similar cure rates that range from 80-95%. There are several benefits of surgical treatment. One, treatment is accomplished in a single stage. This is in contrast to the usual five days a week for six weeks protocols of the standard radiation treatments. In addition, a three to six month healing time is necessary to resolve the mucositis after radiation therapy. Thus compliance with the surgical treatment is not an issue whereas it is with radiation therapy. Secondly, although there may be some impairment from the surgical resection, the long-term oral dryness that accompanies radiation therapy is often severely bothersome to the patients. Lastly, surgical resection allows for the use of radiation therapy in the future should a second primary in the oral cavity occur. In general, the larger the tumor, the more radical the surgery, the more complex the reconstruction, the more advantage there is in radiation therapy. What constitutes the right treatment? The right treatment depends upon the patient, the tumor location and the tumor extent; a common theme in head and neck cancer treatment. The following is a site-by-site overview of oral cavity cancers.

Lips

Given the fact that the lips are always uncovered and highly visible, diagnosis of lip cancer is usually made in the early stages. Direct measurement and palpation allows easy assessment of the extent of the tumor. Examination of the inner sulcus of the lip may be needed to evaluate for mandibular involvement. Hypesthesia or anesthesia of the chin may signify mental nerve involvement and a more aggressive cancer. Incisional biopsies can be performed in the office to confirm the diagnosis.

Once a diagnosis has been confirmed, a treatment plan can be formulated depending upon the extent and exact location of the tumor, as well as the patient's health status and wishes. In general, surgery and radiation therapy for these smaller tumors have similar cure rates and range from 80-95%. Surgery may be preferred because of the often low morbidity, few side effects and possible need for radiation therapy in the future for second primary cancers of the oral cavity (which may occur in up to 40% of patients with lip cancer).

The specific procedure needed to excise a lip cancer depends upon the clinical nature of the tumor. Of utmost and primary importance independent of which surgical procedure is performed, is the ability to achieve negative margins. Failure to do so will likely lead to treatment failure. However, what constitutes adequate margins is somewhat controversial. Whereas some may accept a few millimeters margin as adequate especially for small lesions[i], others suggest at least a 1 – 2 cm. margin especially for larger lesions[ii, iii] Consideration is then secondarily given to lip cosmesis and function. Function requires the complete sphincter mechanism of the orbicularis oris muscle to achieve oral continence. This can only be achieved if less than two-thirds of the lip is resected. Reconstruction also must not decrease the oral opening so much as to create microstomia.

Most lip cancers require full-thickness excision as anything less then full thickness risks a positive deep margin in invasive squamous carcinoma. The most common configuration of the excision for a lesion less than half of the length of the lip is either a V or W-shaped with the apex of the resection coming to the mental crease for lower lip lesions or the nasolabial crease for upper lip lesions.

Reconstruction of the lip defect depends upon the extent and location of the defect. If possible, direct reapproximation is performed as it is both a simple and effective means of reconstruction. This can be achieved when up to one-third of the lip is removed. Attempts should be made to preserve the mental nerves and thus lip sensation. Careful closure of all layers and accurate approximation of the vermilion border leaves an excellent cosmetic and functional result.

Larger lesions require more sophisticated reconstructions. There are a multitude of advancement flaps and rotation flaps that are useful in lip reconstruction. For example, a cross-lip flap takes a portion of the normal lip directly opposite the defect and rotates it into the defect. Or an advancement flap can be created by extending the inferior border of the defect bilaterally into the nasolabial creases and thus allow more movement medially of the edges so as to close the defect. Commissure defects are in general more difficult to reconstruct in a manner as to allow both adequate function and acceptable cosmesis.

Cure rates for lip cancers less than 2 cm. in diameter exceed 90%[iv]. Cure rates for lesions 2-4 cm. in diameter range from 50-80% [2]. Lesions that carry a worse prognosis include those lesions that involve the oral commissure and the upper lip[2]. This may be due to the fact that lesions involving the commissure or upper lip are more likely to metastasize than those of the lower lip.

Buccal Mucosa

Resection of buccal mucosal lesions is usually straight forward and with minimal morbidity. Small cancers less than 2 cm. can usually be excised and closed primarily. For slightly larger lesions where closure is difficult, split thickness skin grafts can be used effectively. For lesions between 3 - 4 cm. or involving the full thickness including skin, radial forearm free flap are excellent means of reconstruction. Lesions that extend anteriorly to the oral commissure are more difficult to reconstruct functionally. Lesions that extend onto Stenson's duct may require its reimplantation. Early cancers involving the buccal mucosa have low likelihood of cervical metastases.

Hard Palate and Alveolous

Hard palate tumors differ from that those found elsewhere in the oral cavity in that 50% of the malignant tumors are squamous cell carcinomas and 50% are of minor salivary gland origin. Preoperative evaluation should include CT scanning to evaluate for bony invasion. Dental evaluation preoperatively may be of benefit in planning for post-operative prosthetics and/or dentures. Bony invasion may be difficult to detect clinically and significant understaging of the tumor results if it is not identified. Early staged tumors require only local resection. Reconstruction is not necessary as the mucosal defects of the hard palate will heal-in by secondary intention. The incidence of neck metastases from early hard palate tumors is low and neck dissections are not necessary.

Floor of Mouth

The floor of mouth is a semilunar area extending from the inner margin of the lower alveolus to the ventral aspect of the tongue. Its posterior border is the anterior tonsillar pillars. A muscular diaphragm forms the support of the floor of mouth and contains the sublingual gland, Wharton's duct (the submandibular gland's duct), and the lingual nerve (which brings taste and sensation to the anterior two-thirds of the tongue). Thus tumors involving this area can easily spread deeply to involve a number of important structures and have direct extension into the neck.

Likewise, resection of tumors of the floor of the mouth can cause significant morbidity by compromising important nearby structures. Injury to the above named structures (Wharton's duct, sublingual gland, and the lingual nerve) may bring about minor complaints. Of more importance is the hypoglossal nerve whose injury results in significant speech and swallowing problems. Also of significant importance is the amount of scarring that can occur between the tongue and the floor of mouth with even small resections. Scarring of the lateral and anterior tongue can lead to speech impediments and difficulty swallowing. Proper surgical planning can minimize these problems. In surgical planning for floor of mouth tumors, careful bimanual palpation of the tumor should be performed. Deep infiltration through the loose submucosal planes can be deceptive in the small mucosal lesion. Tongue movement should be evaluated as impaired tongue movement can signify either hypoglossal nerve involvement and/or invasion of the tongue musculature. Mobility of the tumor should be assessed to help determine mandibular invasion. Again, CT scanning can be very helpful in determining the extent of the tumor as well as mandibular invasion.

Resection of early floor of mouth tumors is relatively straightforward. Mucosal margins are usually easy to obtain. The deep margins are often more ill-defined and intra-operative frozen sections can be of help in determining an adequate resection. Removal of the alveolus and/or mandibular periosteum is often required to ensure complete tumor removal. Invasion of the periosteum signifies a more aggressive tumor and if mandibular involvement has occurred, it is a late-staged tumor and a type of mandibulectomy is necessary depending upon the extent of involvement. Care should be taken to preserve the hypoglossal nerve.

Closure of the resulting defect may be critical to the functional outcome for the patient. A number of different reconstructive techniques are available to decrease the morbidity of floor of mouth and tongue scarring. For very small lesions, healing by secondary intention or primary closure may be all that is necessary. Split thickness skin grafts are next-in-line for the simple reconstructive option. However, these grafts often fail in the floor of mouth and thus are often not the best alternative.

Three reconstructive alternatives are probably best-suited for floor of mouth defects. Each of these are vascularized flaps and therefore they will contract minimally and not scar significantly. The nasolabial flap, based on the facial artery, is taken from the skin around the nasolabial fold of the face and rotated into the floor of the mouth. It is easily accessible and reliable. The platysma musculocutaneous flap is taken from the skin and platysma muscle of the lower, lateral aspect of the neck and rotated upward into the defect. It is more suited for patients who are simultaneously undergoing neck dissection. The last option is the radial forearm free flap. Based on the radial artery of the forearm, is it anastamosed to a neck artery and vein. It is reliable, thin, and pliable (all qualities beneficial for reconstruction of floor of mouth defects) but it is technically more difficult and usually requires a second surgeon to perform the harvesting and anastamotic aspects of the flap.

Postoperative evaluation and therapy with speech and swallowing therapists is often very beneficial to the patients. Parenteral nutrition may be necessary until healing has resolved. Aspiration is not an issue.

Tongue

The most common site for squamous cell carcinoma of the oral cavity is the tongue. Presenting symptoms are as described above. CT scanning of small anterior tongue lesions is of limited value in evaluating the primary tumor but is of help in determining the possibility of neck metastases.

Most T1 and T2 cancers of the tongue can be excised perorally with a wedge excision and can either closed primarily or can be allowed to heal by secondary intention. If the excision involves portions of the floor of the mouth, then the same considerations of scarring, impaired mobility and resulting morbidities must be addressed. Please refer to the above section on floor of mouth tumors for a more complete discussion.

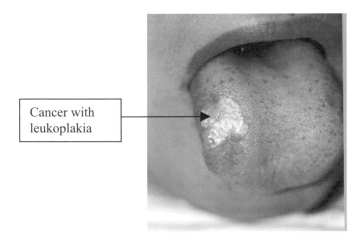

Cancer with leukoplakia

Figure 2. **T1 Cancer of Tongue**

Overall, surgical excision of T1 and T2 lesions of the tongue have a cure rate of 80-95%. This is comparable to radiation therapy treatments.

OROPHARYNGEAL CANCERS

Anatomy

The oropharynx is the extension of the oral cavity. The plane of the junction of the hard and soft palate above and the circumvallate papillae below forms its anterior border and the plane of the hyoid bone forms its inferior border. The superior border is at the level of the soft palate where the oropharynx joins the nasopharynx. The base of tongue extends to the vallecula where it meets the base of the epiglottis and includes the pharyngoepiglottic and glossoepiglottic folds. The four subsites of the oropharynx are: 1) the base of tongue, 2) the soft palate, 3) the tonsillar fossae and pillars, and 4) the posterior pharyngeal wall.

Tumors of the oropharynx generally metastasize initially to lymph nodes high in the jugular chain and then proceed to involve lymph nodes lower in the neck. Clinical evidence of adenopathy by imaging or palpation in the lower neck only usually is accompanied by subclinical or microscopic involvement of upper level lymph nodes. Bilateral adenopathy is not uncommon in midline tumors or in tumors with extension deep into the tissues. Previous neck surgery or previous radiation therapy to the neck may alter the normal lymphatic drainage pathway and thus alter the order of spread of any metastases.

Soft Palate Tumors

The soft palate is a dynamic structure which functions to allow airflow from the nose into the upper airway. It elevates to close off the oropharynx from the nasopharynx. It closes to prevent regurgitation of food and liquid into the nasopharynx and nasal cavity, and it closes during speech to help create a variety of sounds. Excessive resection of the soft palate therefore results in hypernasal speech and nasal regurgitation of food and/or liquids.

Palate tumors arise on the anterior surface of the soft palate. As they spread, they extend laterally onto the tonsillar pillars and tonsils, inferiorly onto the base of tongue and posteriorly and superiorly into the nasopharynx.

Imaging with CT or MRI is useful in determining the extent of soft palate tumors which may extend beyond what is seen clinically. Imaging is also helpful in determining any neck disease.

Small lesions of the palate are amenable to transoral resection. T1 lesions can be excised with an adequate margin and the soft palate can be reapproximated with primary closure with minimal morbidity. However, as the tumor enlarges, the complexity of the surgery increases as does the morbidity associated with it. Resection of large portions of the soft palate are difficult to reconstruct and thus large resections often result in significant speech and swallowing disorders. Reconstruction can be attempted with local flaps from the oral cavity, distant flaps such as the pectoralis myocutaneous flap or free flaps such as the radial forearm free flap. However, because no reconstruction can return the dynamic function of the soft palate, the reconstruction will usually attempt to close off the nasopharynx from the oropharynx completely leaving one or two small ports laterally to allow secretions to drain and to allow a degree of nasal breathing to take place.

An alternative to reconstruction is oral appliances or prostheses. Although a prosthetic can be easily made for the hard palate, a soft palate prosthesis is difficult to make well. Too long of a prosthestic results is significant gagging and discomfort by the patient, and too short of a prosthetic results is excessive regurgitation and hypernasality. In summary, small tumors of the soft palate can be excised adequately and simply, but larger tumor resections result in significant morbidity and are therefore, these tumors are more amenable to radiation therapy if possible.

Base of Tongue

Base of tongue tumors are less common than tumors of the anterior two-thirds of the tongue and unfortunately, base of tongue tumors usually present at later stages. Patients often present with vague symptoms of sore throat, "lump in the throat" feeling, referred otalgia, or a neck mass. Pain usually presents only with deeper muscle infiltration by the tumor. The base of tongue is difficult to examine in the office and sometimes only careful and persistent examination of the area with a dental mirror or fiberoptic scopes leads to identification of the tumor. Palpation of the area can identify an indurated portion of the tongue and is often crucial in identifying the tumor. Late symptoms and difficult examination often leads to delayed referrals, delayed treatment and a poorer prognosis. Thus high levels of suspicion for throat pain that persists in patients with a smoking history is imperative.

Surgical excision of T1 and T2 tumors of the base of tongue are seldom performed because of the fact that these tumors usually present in the later stages for reasons just described. For those tumors that are resectable in the early stages excision is possible, as follows:

A mandibulotomy is sometimes necessary for exposure. This can be performed either anteriorly through a lip-split incision or through a lateral mandibulotomy[vi]. The mandibulotomy allows adequate access for tumor excision and most often has little post-operative morbidity associated with it. Once the tumor has been exposed, it is resected with adequate margins. The most difficult margin to assess is the deep margin as its borders are often unclear. Intra-operative frozen sections of the margins are of great help in assuring negative margins. Identification and preservation of the hypoglossal nerve, if possible, is helpful in preserving post-operative function of the tongue. Periosteum of the mandible is often resected with the tumor as it often acts as the barrier to bony invasion. Invasion of the mandible represents a later stage tumor and resection will not be discussed here.

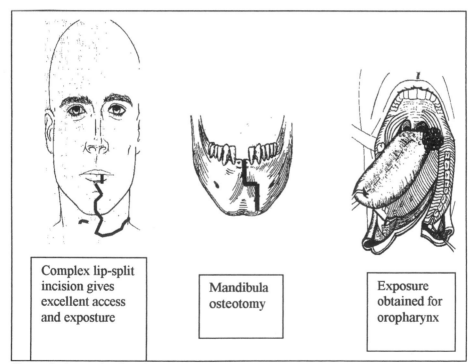

Complex lip-split incision gives excellent access and exposture

Mandibula osteotomy

Exposure obtained for oropharynx

Figure 3. **Access for Oropharyngeal Tumors**

Another option for surgical resection is utilizing the endoscopic laser approach. The technique is described in more detail in the section on laryngeal tumors below. In brief, a laryngoscope and binocular microscopy are used for visualization of the tumor and a CO_2 laser is used to excise it. Bleeding can be troublesome and because the deep margin can often be nebulous, this method of resection is reserved for only T1 tumors.

Reconstruction of the early base of tongue lesions is usually kept simple. Primary closure and healing by secondary intention are common for these lesions. If more than one-third of the base of tongue is resected, reconstruction is necessary to avoid tongue tethering that leads to impaired speech and swallowing. Skin grafts are quick, easy and are the first line of reconstruction for the tongue base. Though portions of the graft often fail, they usually suffice in preventing fistulas and excessive tethering caused by scarring. Local flaps using the remaining tongue are an option, but often are associated with impaired speech and deglutition. Other local flaps using the buccal mucosa or the lateral pharyngeal walls can be used with minimal morbidity. For larger defects, myocutaneous flaps such as the pectoralis myocutaneous flap have been used. However, these are usually too bulky are not a great option. The radial forearm free flap is a pliable thin flap with excellent success in reconstruction and minimal morbidity. The high degree of technical expertise as well as the need for a second surgical team make this reconstruction more complicated and costly, but it is the state-of-art for today's reconstruction options.

Tonsil and Tonsillar Pillar Tumors

This region is the most common site for tumors of the oropharynx. As these tumors grow, they can invade multiple anatomic structures. Which structures structures are involved and to what extent they are involved determines the appropriate intervention. Medial growth results in soft palate involvement. Superior growth involves the lateral pharyngeal wall and the nasopharynx. Inferior and medial growth of the tumor can result in base of tongue and hypopharyngeal involvement. Deep infiltration by the tumor can result in carotid sheath invasion and/or invasion of the pterygoid musculature. Neck metastases from the tonsillar area most often involves the upper jugular chain lymph nodes first and then descend along the lower jugular chains later. As a result of the multiple areas of possible invasion, these patients can present with a myriad of symptoms including but not limited to throat pain, referred otalgia or swallowing problems. Invasion of the pterygoid muscles or mandible results in trismus. Patients may first present with a metastatic lymph node as their only sign or symptom.

As has been described above, imaging with CT and/or MRI scanning is greatly beneficial in evaluating the extent of the tumor as well as helping in determine the presence of neck metastases. Mandibular invasion and the depth of invasion by the tumor are especially important in planning the surgical resection and reconstruction and can only be determined preoperatively with CT or MRI. Lesions thought to be small based upon inspection, can often have deeper penetration than is thought clinically. This can often be demonstrated using CT or MRI modalities.

Small T1 lesions of the tonsil or tonsillar pillar can be resected transorally with minimal morbidity. However, a word to the wise! These tumors are infrequently found in the early stages and improper surgical planning results in inadequate resections. Tonsillar carcinomas often infiltrate deeper than expected and attempts to extirpate the tumor without adequate exposure can easily lead to significant complications such as carotid artery injury and grossly positive margins. The carotid artery lies in close proximity to the tonsils and its location must be known for safe resection. It is for these reasons that all but the smallest, most superficial cancers, must be excised with adequate exposure obtained through a mandibulotomy. The exposure, concepts, and reconstructive options are similar as that described for base of tongue resections. However several other salient points need to be considered. Excision with adequate margins often requires removal of a significant portion of the soft palate. The notable sequalae of this is described above in the section on soft palate tumors. Often significant portions of the base of tongue require resection. The potential serious morbidity associated with this can be reviewed in the above section on base of tongue tumors. In addition, resection of the pterygoid musculature can result in significant, permanent trismus postoperatively.

It is for these reasons that only T1 and small T2 lesions that do not significantly affect the soft palate are considered good surgical candidates. Involvement of the neck by the tumor signifies a later stage tumor and will not be discussed here.

Posterior Pharyngeal Wall

Tumors arising primarily from the posterior pharyngeal wall are very uncommon whereas tumors arising from other sites of the oropharynx that invade the posterior pharyngeal wall are not uncommon. Primary tumors of the posterior pharyngeal wall usually present in the late stages and can present with dysphagia, throat pain and/or a neck mass. Surgical resection is most often not the primary treatment because of the late stages these tumors are diagnosed and the significant morbidity associated with any resection. Only the smallest most superficial of tumors are excised. Excision is usually made with the deep margin the prevertebral fascia. If possible, transoral excision is performed. Skin grafts and healing by secondary intention are the most common means of reconstruction.

Lateral to the oropharynx lies the parapharyngeal space which contains the internal carotid artery, internal jugular vein and cranial nerves IX, X, XI and XII. Invasion of this space can lead to multiple cranial neuropathies and vascular compromise. Also lateral to this region lie the pharyngeal constrictor muscles and the mandible. Trismus is associated with invasion of these structures. Posterior to the oropharynx lies the prevertebral space. The deep aspect of the posterior pharyngeal wall consists of the buccopharyngeal fascia. This fascia usually acts as a barrier to invasion of the prevertebral space and allows for a margin of resection around the tumor. However, once the buccopharyngeal fascia is invaded, tumors will often invade the vertebra and make the tumor unresectable.

Lymphatic drainage from the oropharynx region involves jugulodigastric, retropharyngeal and parapharyngeal lymph nodes. The base of tongue and midline palate tend to drain bilaterally and thus bilateral metastatic spread is not uncommon with tumors arising from this region. Blood supply to the oropharynx is mainly from branches of the lingual, facial, and internal maxillary arteries.

HYPOPHARYNX

Anatomy

The hypopharynx is the tube that connects the oropharynx superiorly with the esophagus inferiorly excluding the larynx. There are three subsites of the hypopharynx: 1) the pyriform fossae, 2) the postcricoid area, and 3) the posterior pharyngeal wall.

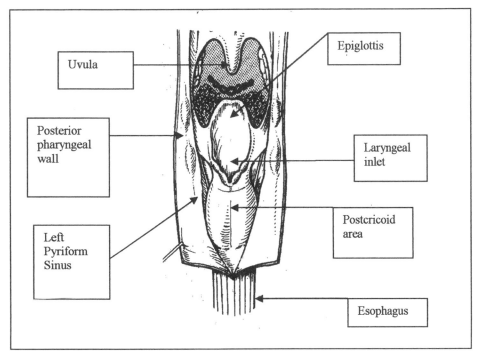

Figure 4. **Anatomy of the Hypopharynx** (posterior view)

The vast majority of tumors of the hypopharynx present in the late stages. These are usually aggressive, fast growing tumors that often present with neck metastases. Other symptoms at presentation include throat pain, dysphagia, otalgia and weight loss. Hoarseness, shortness of breath and symptoms of aspiration indicate laryngeal involvement and advanced disease.

Evaluation of the tumor involves several modalities. Physical examination in the office, even with fiberoptic laryngoscopy, does not adequately assess the extent and location of these tumors. Therefore direct laryngoscopy, esophagoscopy and bronchoscopy is necessary to determine the exact location and extent of these tumors. CT or MRI imaging is also helpful in determining spread within the pharynx, larynx and neck metastases. However, CT or MRI may complement but cannot at this time replace the value of direct visualization from intraoperative endoscopy. Often times, submucosal spread can be extensive and unappreciated in all modalities. (See Table 1 for staging)

Table 1. **Classification of Hypopharyngeal Cancer**

T1	Tumor limited to one subsite of hypopharynx and 2 cm or less in greatest dimension
T2	Tumor involves more than one subsite of hypopharynx or an adjacent site, or measures more than 2 cm. but not more than 4 cm. in greatest diameter without fixation of hemilarynx
T3	Tumor measures more than 4 cm. in greatest dimension or with fixation of hemilarynx
T4	Tumor invades adjacent structures (e.g., thyroid/cricoid cartilage, carotid artery, soft tissues of neck, prevertebral fascia/muscles, thyroid and/or esophagus)

From American Joint Committee on Cancer: AJCC Cancer Staging Manual, 5th ed. Philadelphia: Lippincott-Raven, 1997

Surgical excision of early cancers of the hypopharynx is uncommon for two main reasons. First, early detection of these tumors is uncommon. Most hypopharyngeal tumors are diagnosed when the disease has already spread beyond the confines of the hypopharynx and thus precludes conservative surgical management. The second reason surgical intervention is uncommon is that even if a lesion is detected early, the strategic anatomic location of the hypopharynx will only allow resections of significant morbidity. In these situations, radiation with or without chemotherapy is the treatment of choice. Site-by-site examples of hypopharyngeal tumors and the resections they require follow.

Post-cricoid Tumors

The postcricoid area forms the anterior wall of the hypopharynx and the posterior wall of the larynx. It joins with the cervical esophagus inferiorly, and is in close proximity to the recurrent laryngeal nerves laterally. Tumors of this area account for approximately 20% of hypopharyngeal tumors. At the time of presentation they will often be large and have invaded the cricoid cartilage, the intrinsic laryngeal muscles and a recurrent laryngeal nerve. Because of their location, tumors of the post-cricoid area, no matter how big or small, require total laryngectomies and either partial or total pharyngectomies. Reconstruction is performed with either myocutaneous pedicled flaps or free flap reconstruction. Given today's organ preservation therapy alternatives, surgical therapy is most often not recommended for these patients.

Pyriform Sinus Tumors

The pyriform sinus extends from the level of the hyoid bone superiorly to the cervical esophagus inferiorly. The right and left pyriform sinuses have lateral, medial and anterior walls that funnel inferiorly towards an apex which then terminates into the cervical esophagus.

The pyriform sinus is the most common site for hypopharyngeal tumors. Like postcricoid lesions, they are aggressive tumors which grow quickly and metastasize early. With medial growth they invade the larynx, and with anterior and/or lateral growth they tend to invade the thyroid cartilage. Inferiorly the esophagus may be invaded and skip areas of involvement in the esophagus can occur. CT or MRI imaging aid in the identification of paraglottic space spread as well as thyroid cartilage involvement.

Because late-staged disease is most commonly discovered, surgical resection for the early-staged tumor is uncommon. Like postcricoid tumors, even smaller tumors of the pyriform sinuses are difficult to excise without significant morbidity. At least a partial laryngectomy, partial pharyngectomy for even the earliest of tumors is necessary. These resections result in a compromised voice and increased risk of aspiration. Only those patients with adequate pulmonary function and in otherwise relatively good health are candidates. However, radiation therapy with or without chemotherapy is the better alternative treatment for these tumors.

Posterior Pharyngeal Wall

The posterior pharygeal wall extends from the level of the hyoid bone superiorly to the cervical esophagus inferiorly where it joins the pyriform sinuses. Like the other hypopharyngeal tumors, these tend to present late in their course. Most often they spread superiorly, inferiorly and deeply and metastasize early to the jugular chain lymph nodes. Early tumors are detected more frequently at this site of the hypopharynx. Surgical resection for smaller tumors can be curative. Either a transoral approach or approaching the tumor through a lateral pharyngotomy can be used for access. Once excised, small defects can heal by secondary intention. Skin grafts can be used for slightly larger defects and local muscle rotation flaps can be used for some defects. Invasion of a pyriform sinus, lateral extension of the tumor or cervical esophagus involvement makes the "simple" resection impossible. The morbidity of the "simple" resection can include aspiration but most often this resolves with time. In summary, only T1 lesions of the posterior hypopharyngeal wall warrant consideration for tumor resection as the primary treatment modality. Other lesions, if given the choice, are better served with radiation with or without chemotherapy.

LARYNX

Anatomy

The larynx occupies the central component of the neck and is located anterior to, or strictly speaking, within the hypopharynx. Lateral to the larynx are the pyriform sinuses, the pharyngeal recesses that are the primary route for food to pass into the esophagus. The basic framework of the larynx consists of the thyroid, cricoid, epiglottic and arytenoid cartilages, and the hyoid bone. The shield-like thyroid cartilage supports the soft tissues of the larynx. The epiglottic cartilage is leaf-shaped and forms the anterior wall of the laryngeal entranceway. Its main portion projects posterior to the tongue base and as it folds downward over the larynx during swallowing, it aids in the protection of the laryngeal opening from aspiration.

Innervation to the intrinsic laryngeal muscles is via the recurrent laryngeal nerve, a branch of the vagus nerve (cranial nerve X). Only the cricothyroid muscle is innervated by the external branch of the superior laryngeal nerve, also a branch of the vagus nerve.

The larynx can be divided into three subsites. The supraglottic larynx is defined as that portion of the larynx extending from the tip of the epiglottis to the laryngeal ventricle. It consists of the epiglottis, arytenoid cartilages, false vocal folds and the ventricles. The glottic larynx contains the true vocal cords and extends approximately 5-7mm inferiorly. The subglottis extends from the inferior glottis to the inferior edge of the cricoid cartilage.

As noted in the introduction, the primary function of the larynx is to protect the airway from the aspiration of food particles. With each swallow, the larynx elevates, the aryepiglottic folds squeeze medially, the epiglottis folds posteriorly over the larynx and the true and false vocal folds close tightly. This allows the food bolus to pass around the larynx, into the pyriform sinuses and subsequently into the esophagus. Any alteration or disturbance in the reflex arc may predispose to aspiration.

Phonation occurs with adduction of the vocal cords as air passes from the trachea through the vocal cords. The mucosa overlying the muscles of the vocal cords undulates and the two vibrating vocal cords produce sound. Anything that alters the mucosal wave of the vocal cords, impairs adduction, or changes the configuration of vocal cord alignment will cause decreased phonatory performance. (Note: mucosal wave abnormalities can only be observed with videostroboscopy of the larynx.) Conditions such as inflammation, thickened mucous, vocal cord paralyis, and tumors, can change a voice. One must to careful and define hoarseness as a <u>change</u> in vocal quality, as what may be normal for one person, may not be for another.

The larynx also is crucial in respiratory activity. Inspiration signals the recurrent laryngeal nerve to stimulate vocal cord abduction. Impairment in abduction unilaterally or bilaterally can lead to respiratory compromise.

Subglottis

Primary subglottic carcinomas comprise only 4% to 6% of laryngeal cancers. This is fortunate given the fact that these tumors usually present in the late stages of disease and are associated with a high mortality rate. Cancers of this area may present with hoarseness if they invade the vocal folds above or may present with dyspnea and stridor as they often obstruct the airway. (see Table 2 for staging)

Table 2. **Classification of Subglottic Cancer**

T1	Tumor limited to the subglottis
T2	Tumor extends to vocal cord(s) with normal or impaired mobility
T3	Tumor limited to larynx with vocal cord fixation
T4	Tumor invades through cricoid or thyroid cartilage and/or extends to other tissues beyond the larynx (e.g., trachea, soft tissues of neck, including thyroid, esophagus)

From American Joint Committee on Cancer: AJCC Cancer Staging Manual, 5th ed. Philadelphia: Lippincott-Raven, 1997.

The only surgical option for the treatment of subglottic carcinomas regardless of the stage is total laryngectomy with neck dissections. A total laryngectomy is necessary because the cricoid cartilage is the foundation of the larynx and any significant resection of it results in a non-functional larynx. Paratracheal lymph node dissection accompanies the laryngectomy as that is the area most susceptible to metastases.

Given the above facts, radiation with or without chemotherapy is the treatment of choice for early and late subglottic carcinomas.

Glottic Carcinomas

Cancers of the vocal cords often present early because of the significant hoarseness that accompanies these tumors. In addition, minimal lymphatic drainage to this area decreases the incidence of neck metastases. Because of this, there are often several good treatment options.

The tumor (T) staging for glottic carcinomas is different from other head and neck carcinomas and reviewing it is helpful prior to evaluating treatment strategies (see Table 1). Probably the greatest weakness of the tumor staging is the lack of inclusion of depth of invasion. T1 lesions may involve only the most superficial mucosa or they may invade the underlying musculature of the vocal cord. The surgical option chosen will differ depending upon the depth of invasion and the exact location of the tumor. This will in turn affect the post-operative functional result.

Table 3. **Classification of Glottic Carcinomas**

T1	Tumor limited to vocal cord(s) (may involve anterior or posterior commissures) with normal mobility T1a: Tumor limited to one vocal cord T1b: Tumor involves both vocal cords
T2	Tumor extends to supraglottis and/or subglottis, and/or with impaired vocal cord mobility
T3	Tumor limited to the larynx with vocal cord fixation
T4	Tumor invades through thyroid cartilage and/or to other tissues beyond the larynx, e.g., trachea, soft tissues of neck, including thyroid, pharynx

From American Joint Committee on Cancer: AJCC Cancer Staging Manual, 5th ed. Philadelphia: Lippincott-Raven, 1997.

Because of the great significance attributed to location and depth of invasion, accurate preoperative assessment of the cancer is imperative. Videostroboscopy of the larynx, an in-office procedure using fiberoptic scopes and stroboscopic evaluation of the vocal cords, is very helpful in evaluating and documenting the stage of the disease. By allowing an evaluation of the mucosal wave of the vocal cords, it can determine whether the tumor has extended deep into the vocal fold musculature. It also allows detailed analysis of vocal cord movement and thus detects impaired movement better than conventional office laryngoscopy. Direct laryngoscopy performed in the operating as a diagnostic procedure is invaluable in determining the extent of the tumor. Direct laryngoscopy provides access to biopsy the tumor for a definitive diagnosis, and it permits visualization and manipulation of the tumor to better determine its borders and extent. Appreciation of invasion into the laryngeal ventricle and subglottis is often only done with direct laryngoscopy. CT scanning is also helpful in all but the smallest of laryngeal tumors. Its great contributions to defining laryngeal tumor extent are its ability to determine spread within preepiglottic and paraglottic spaces of the larynx, to help determine thyroid cartilage invasion and to evaluate the neck for regional metastases.

For superficial T1 squamous cell carcinomas limited to the membranous portion of the true vocal cords, surgical excision via direct microlaryngoscopy with or without the use of the laser is an excellent means for curing the disease.[vii] The procedure can be performed as an outpatient. Unlike other tumor extirpations, these lesions require only a 2mm to 3mm margin. Little post-operative recuperation is necessary and voice outcome following resection is usually excellent.

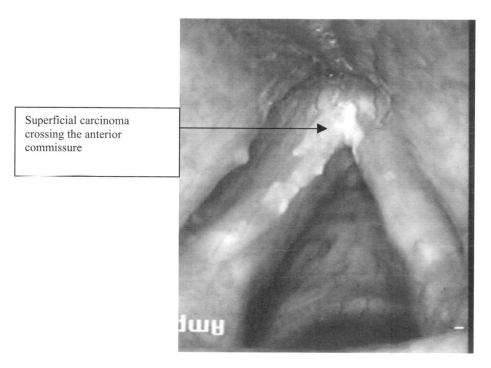

Superficial carcinoma crossing the anterior commissure

Figure 5. **T1b Squamous Cell Carcinoma of the Vocal Cords**

For deeper tumors, the same procedure just described can be performed. However, once invasion and thus resection of the vocalis ligament and thyroarytenoid musculature has occurred, the voice quality post-operatively is not as good. The degree to which voice quality suffers and comparison of voice quality post-operatively to post-radiation therapy is highly controversial and articles supporting each therapeutic modality as having the better vocal quality post-treatment abound.

Tumors that involve the anterior commissure require a different approach. This is because the anterior commissure ligament directly abuts the thyroid cartilage without interposed perichondrium. This makes direct extension and invasion of the thyroid cartilage by the tumor more likely. In addition, a margin from the contralateral vocal cord is now necessary to obtain an adequate margin. Thus for these tumors, as well as for tumors involving the arytenoid cartilages, a vertical hemilaryngectomy is performed. A vertical hemilaryngectomy is performed under general anesthesia. A temporary tracheotomy is performed first and the patient can usually be decannulated before discharge home 5 to 7 days post-operatively. A transverse neck incision is performed and half of the thyroid cartilage along with the affected vocal cord and part or all of an arytenoid cartilage excised. A margin of the contralateral vocal cord may also be taken. The resected vocal cord is usually reconstructed with either strap muscles or an epiglottic flap.

Postoperatively, temporary nasogastric feedings are necessary until edema decreases and compensatory swallowing mechanisms are learned. Voice quality is significantly worse compared with the endoscopic technique only because the extent of resection is much greater.

Surgical removal of T2 glottic tumors is more controversial. T2 tumors that invade the supraglottis by crossing the ventricle are referred to as transglottic tumors. Purists will state that adequate removal of transglottic cancers is only possible with a total laryngectomy because once the tumor has crossed the ventricle, it has access to and can spread to the paraglottic and preepiglottic spaces. The classic vertical hemilaryngectomy does not include complete removal of these spaces. Other surgeons will perform extended hemilaryngectomies for limited T2 lesions and attempt to remove a large portion of the paraglottic and preepiglottic tissue.

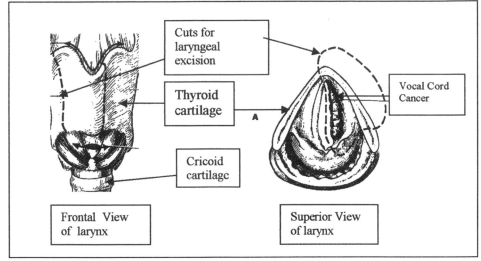

Figure 6. **Vertical Hemilaryngectomy**

T2 lesions that extend inferiorly and invade the subglottis may be amenable to surgical excision. The standard vertical hemilaryngectomy in these cases is altered to incorporate the cricothyroid membrane and even portions of the cricoid cartilage. However extension beyond 1 cm anteriorly or 0.5cm posteriorly into the subglottis disallows the ability to perform a hemilaryngectomy.

There are several benefits of surgical therapy over radiation therapy in treatment of early glottic carcinoma. The one stage procedure does not require patient compliance and is more cost-effective. Saving radiotherapy for second primaries or recurrences is another benefit of performing surgical excision on an easily removable lesion. The patient's age, health status, exact tumor extent, as well as the patient's wishes and biases are all important in forming the appropriate treatment plan.

Supraglottic Carcinomas

The supraglottis extends from the tip of the epiglottis superiorly to the laryngeal ventricles inferiorly and includes the epiglottis, false vocal folds, aryepiglottic folds, laryngeal surface of the arytenoids and the laryngeal ventricles. These tumors spread locally from one subsite to another and also invade the paraglottic and preepiglottic spaces. Lymphatic drainage occurs through the thyrohyoid membrane and neck metastases occur in the deep jugular chain of lymph nodes.   Contralateral spread is not uncommon especially in patients with ipsilateral metastases.

Like the staging system used for glottic cancers, the tumor (T) staging system for supraglottic cancers is unlike the tumor classifications for other regions in the head and neck as the stage depends upon invasion of other surrounding structures and not the size of the tumor (see Table 2). Workup for supraglottic cancers is the same as that described above for glottic cancers and thus will not be reiterated.

Table 4. **Classification of Supraglottic Cancer**

T1	Tumor limited to one subsite of supraglottis with normal vocal cord mobility
T2	Tumor invades mucosa of more than one adjacent subsite of supraglottis or glottis or region outside the supraglottis (e.g., mucosa of base of tongue, vallecula, medial wall of pyriform sinus) without fixation of the larynx
T3	Tumor limited to larynx with vocal cord fixation and/or invades any of the following: postcricoid area, preepiglottic tissues
T4	Tumor extends through the thyroid cartilage, and/or extends into soft tissues of the neck, thyroid and/or esophagus

From American Joint Committee on Cancer: AJCC Cancer Staging Manual, 5th ed. Philadelphia: Lippincott-Raven, 1997.

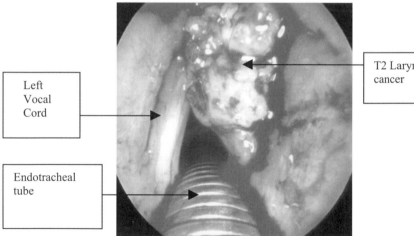

Figure 7. **T2 Supraglottic Carcinoma**

Surgical treatment for early supraglottic cancers can be divided into either endoscopic methods or the open traditional supraglottic laryngectomy. Since the popularization of endoscopic laser techniques, the possible indications for endoscopic excision of supraglottic tumors has greatly increased.[viii] Because no skin incision or extensive dissection is necessary with the endoscopic technique, some surgeons have found that the recovery time is faster. In addition, because microscopic excision is performed, the possibility of increased precision and the preservation of more non-involved tissue are achieved.[ix] The con of this method is that accessibility endoscopically may make some patients ineligible. In addition, this method though straightforward for smaller lesions, can be technically challenging for larger tumors. In brief, most surgeons will thus use the endoscopic technique for smaller lesions and reserve the standard supraglottic laryngectomy for larger tumors.

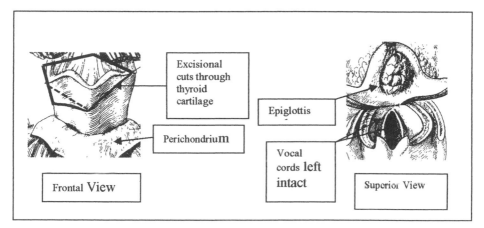

Figure 8. **Supraglottic Laryngectomy**

The endoscopic technique will not be described here as the basics are similar to any microlaryngoscopic procedure including that described above for glottic tumors. The following is a brief description of the supraglottic laryngectomy. A temporary tracheotomy is performed. A transverse skin incision is made in the lower central aspect of the neck and skin flaps are elevated. The strap muscles are divided and the thyroid cartilage is cut transversely at a level just superior to the true vocal cords. The thyroid cartilage, epiglottis, and false vocal folds are excised along with the hyoid bone. The remaining larynx including the true vocal cords is reapproximated to the tongue base to close the defect. Modifications and extensions are possible depending upon the site and extent of the tumor.

Because the true vocal folds are left completely intact, voice in patients after a supraglottic laryngectomy is usually excellent. Swallowing difficulties including aspiration can occur and patients often need swallowing rehabilitation before starting oral intake again. However, most patients do well once proper techniques of swallowing have been learned. Other postoperative complications such as wound breakdown, fistulas and infections are most common in patients status-post radiation therapy or in patients with diabetes or significant malnutrition.

Cure rates for patients undergoing treatment for T1 and T2 supraglottic cancers are the same whether they undergo surgery or radiation. The benefits of surgery over radiation for these types of tumors are described in the section on glottic cancers and will not be discussed here.

Neck Dissection

By definition, early stage head and neck carcinomas do not have clinical or radiological evidence of neck metastases and are staged as N0. Then why have a discussion on neck dissection for these cancers? Because even without clinical and radiological evidence of metastasis, there is still a significant percentage of occult or micro-metastases in some of these tumors. CT scans can miss from 46% to 67% of malignant lymph nodes[x,xi]. Thus, the neck dissection for the N0 neck has dual purposes. It functions to remove any micro-cancer that has not been detected, and it identifies occult disease so that decisions about post-operative radiation therapy can be made based on pathologic staging. (For an excellent discussion and review of neck dissections for early squamous cell carcinomas, refer to Pillsbury and Clark's article[xii].) Neck dissections with pathologically proven multiple metastases or extranodal spread are usually indicated for post-operative radiation therapy.

There are several types of neck dissections and the decision of which one is performed depends upon the location and size of the primary tumor as well as the presence of neck metastases. The radical neck dissection involves excision of lymph nodes from levels I – V and includes removal of the internal jugular vein, the sternocleidomastoid muscle, the submandibular gland and the spinal accessory nerve (cranial nerve XI). The greatest morbidity from this procedure or any neck dissection for that matter results from injury to the spinal accessory nerve. This causes significant shoulder weakness and discomfort and often requires physical therapy for rehabilitation. The modified radical neck dissection removes lymph nodes from the same levels as the radical neck dissection but preserves at least one of the structures described above. A supraomohyoid neck dissection removes lymph nodes from levels I – III of the neck and is typically used in early tumors of the oral cavity. A selective neck dissection is a neck dissection that is curtailed to the location of the primary tumor and removes lymph nodes from the areas the tumor is most likely to metastasize to. In general, the literature supports that the efficacy of a selective neck dissection is comparable to more comprehensive lymphadenectomy surgeries [xiii, xiv, xv]With the exception of a neck scar and a cosmetically thinned neck, the resulting morbidity of any neck dissection is minimal unless the spinal accessory nerve is removed or injured.

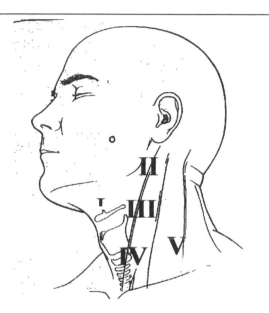

Figure 9. **Levels of Neck Lymph Nodes**

When is a neck dissection indicated for N0 necks in early head and neck cancer? The answer is neck dissection is performed when the risk of occult metastases is significant. What is a significant risk of metastases? Most clinicians agree that a risk of metastasis greater than 25-30% is significant and warrants a neck dissection. Some define this risk as low as 10-15%. Clinically, T1 cancers do not have that high of a risk of metastasis and thus do not warrant neck dissections. However, many T2 lesions do carry that risk and thus a neck dissection is warranted in these cases. In addition, those cancers that have a propensity for bilateral or contralateral spread (such as the base of tongue or supraglottis) may be indicated for bilateral neck dissections.

What does the future hold for diagnosing and treating neck disease? In diagnosis, positron emission tomography, by detecting the high metabolic rate of proliferating tumor cells, has been shown in one study to be more accurate in identifying lymph node metastases than MRI[xvi]. Surgically the role of sentinel node localization in head and neck metastases is being actively investigated in a number of centers. The somewhat unpredictability and complexity of lymphatic drainage is the great barrier to success for this technique. Various success has been shown in studies for this techniques's predictive value in identifying lymph node metastases.[xvii, xviii, xix]

CONCLUSION

Early stage head and neck cancer is a highly curable disease when the appropriate treatment is administered. The decision as to which treatment, radiation or surgery, is utilized is dependent upon multiple factors including the location and size of the tumor, the health and bias of the patient, as well as the experience and biases of the head and neck multidisciplinary cancer team.

REFERENCES

1. [1] Brodland DG, Zitelli JA. Surgical margins for excision of primary cutaneous squamous cell carcinoma. J Am Acad Dermatol 1992;27:241-248.
2. 1987;80:787-791.
3. [1] Luce EA: Carcinoma of the lower lip. Surg Clin North Am; 1986;66:3-11.
4. [1] Baker SR, Krause CJ. Carcinoma of the lip. Laryngoscope 1980;90:19-27.
5. [1] Lydiatt DD, Robbins DT, Byers RM, Wolf PF. Treatment of stage I and II oral tongue cancer. Head Neck 1993;15:308-315.
6. [1] Thawley SE, Panje WR, Batsakis JG, Lindberg RD. Comprehensive Management of Head and Neck Tumors. WB Saunders 1999, Chapter 42:861-876.
7. [1] Shapshay SM, Hybels RL, Bohigian RK. Laser Excision of Early Vocal Cord Carcinoma: Indications, Limitations, and Precautions. Ann Otol Rhinol Laryngol 1990;99:46-50.
8. [1] Pellitteri PK, Kennedy TL, Vrabec DP, et al. Radiotherapy: The mainstay in the treatment of early glottic carcinoma. Arch Otolaryngol Head Neck Surg 1991; 117:297-301.
9. [1] Mcguirt WF, Blalock MA, Koufman JA, et al. Voice analysis of patients with endoscopically treated early laryngeal carcinoma. Ann Otol Rhinol Laryngol 1992;101:142-146.
10. [1] Voice quality after narrow-margin laser cordectomy compared with laryngeal irradiation. Otolaryngol- Head Neck Surg 1999;121(5):528-533.
11. [1] Davis RK, Kelly SM, Hayes J. Endoscopic CO_2 Laser Excisional Biopsy of Early Supraglottic Cancer. Laryngoscope 1991; 101:680-683.
12. [1] Zeitels SM, Vaughan CW, Domanowski GF. Endoscopic Management of Early Supraglottic Cancer. Ann Otol Rhinol Laryngol 1990;99:951-956.
13. [1] Friedman M, Roberts N, Kirshenbaum G, et al. Nodal size of metastatic squamous cell carcinoma of the neck. Laryngoscope 1993;103:854-6.
14. [1] Don D, Yoshimi A, Lufkin R, Fu Y, Calcaterra T. Evaluation of cervical lymph node metastasis in squamous cell carcinoma of the head and neck. Laryngoscope 1995:105:669-74.
15. [1] Pillsbury HC, Clark M. A rationale for therapy of the N0 neck. Laryngoscope 1997;107:1294-1315.

16. [1] Clayman GL, Frank DK. Selective neck dissection of anatomically appropriate levels is as efficacious as modified radical neck dissection for elective treatment of the clinically negative neck in patients with squamous cell carcinoma of the upper respiratory and digestive tracts. Arch Otolaryngol Head Neck Surg 1998;124:348-352.

17. [1] Ferlito A, Rinaldo A. Selective lateral neck dissection for laryngeal cancer with limited metastatic disease: is it indicated? J Laryngol Otol 1998;112:1031-1033.

18. [1] Hosal AS, Carrau RL, Johnson JT, Myers EN. Selective Neck Dissection in the Management of the Clinically Node-Negative Neck. Laryngoscope 2000;110:2037-2040.

19. [1] Laubenbacher C, Saumweber D, Wagner-Manslau C, Kau RJ, Herz M, Avril N, Ziegler S, Kruschke C, Arnold W, Schwaiger M. Comparison of fluorine-18-flourdeoxyglucose PET, MRI and endoscopy for staging head nad neck squamous cell carcinomas. J Nucl Med 1995;36:1747-57.

20. [1] Sentinel Node Localization in Oral Cavity and Oropharynx Squamous Cell Cancer. Taylor RJ, Wahl RL, Sharma PK, Bradford CR, Terrell JE, Teknos TN, Heard EM, Wolf GT, Chepeha DB. Arch Otolaryngol Head Neck Surg 2001.

21. [1] Koch WM, Choti MA, Civelek AC, Eisele DW, Saunders JR. Gamma probe-directed biopsy of the sentinel node in oral squamous cell carcinoma. Arch Otolaryngol Head Neck Surg 1998; 124:455-459.

22. [1] Pitman KT, Johnson JT, Edington H, et al. Lymphatic mapping with isosulfan blue dye in squamous cell carcinoma of the head and neck. Arch Otolarygol Head Neck Surg 1998;124:790-793.

Chapter 5

RADIATION THERAPY IN THE MANAGEMENT OF EARLY-STAGE HEAD AND NECK CANCER

Russell W. Hinerman, MD, William M. Mendenhall, MD,
Robert J. Amdur, MD
University of Florida College of Medicine, Gainesville, Florida

INTRODUCTION

This chapter presents a concise overview of the role of radiation therapy in the management of early (stage I and II) squamous cell carcinoma of the head and neck. Treatment guidelines and results for the relatively common head and neck cancer sites with clinical N0 neck disease are included.

TREATMENT SELECTION

Radiation therapy is a local-regional treatment modality that may be used in the management of head and neck cancer to preserve function and avoid the morbidity associated with a major operation. A course of radiation therapy is often less expensive than an operation, or it may be combined with surgery to destroy known or suspected residual cancer after resection. Radiation therapy may also be used before surgery to render an advanced, unresectable cancer amenable to complete surgical removal. This chapter will be limited to a discussion of definitive radiotherapy as a primary treatment modality for early-stage head and neck cancer. Results of treatment with radiotherapy for various subsites of head and neck cancer at the University of Florida are listed in each section. Generally, local control is quite good, since all data pertains to T1 and T2 primary cancers. The broad experience of the physicians at this institution in treating these malignancies has likely also contributed to these results. The reader desiring further detail about radiation treatment techniques or the management of relatively uncommon head and neck tumors is referred to a more comprehensive text.

GENERAL PRINCIPLES

Radiation Therapy Modalities

Most patients receiving radiation therapy for head and neck cancer are treated with external beam radiation for all or part of their treatment. Megavoltage photon beams are used for management of most cancers arising in the oral cavity, pharynx, or larynx; ^{60}Co or a 4- to 6-MV linear accelerator is ideal. A megavoltage X-ray beam delivers a relatively low dose to the skin surface and is associated with a high exit dose; as the beam energy increases, the surface dose decreases and the exit dose increases. In contrast, an electron beam delivers a relatively high dose to the skin and subcutaneous tissues; after one to several centimeters, the dose falls off very rapidly, and the exit dose is quite low. As the energy of the electron beam increases, the surface dose increases and the exit dose increases. Orthovoltage X-ray beams, with energies varying from 100 to 250 kV, deliver a maximal dose at the skin surface, and the depth dose falls off less steeply than that of an electron beam. Orthovoltage radiation is used for the treatment of most skin cancers of the head and neck, although an electron beam is preferable for skin cancers on the forehead and the scalp because the dose to the underlying calvarium and the brain may be limited more effectively. Intraoral cone radiation therapy is a form of external-beam irradiation that is given with an orthovoltage or electron beam through a cone placed into the oral cavity or the oropharynx to deliver a boost dose to relatively early cancers arising in these sites.

Interstitial implants may be used to deliver all or part of the treatment for cancers of the oral cavity and the oropharynx. It is necessary to define the tumor precisely and encompass it with the radioactive sources in order to perform a satisfactory implant. The advantages of interstitial treatment are that the high dose may be limited to a small volume of tissue and the treatment is delivered over a short overall time, producing a high probability of tumor control and a relatively low risk of complications. Cesium needles and iridium wires are frequently used for implantation in treating head and neck cancers (Figs. 1, 2, and 3) (1-3).

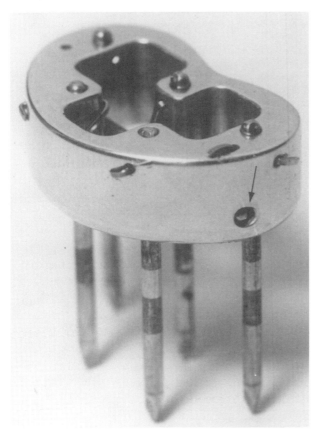

Figure 1. **Custom-made implant device for stage T1-T2 cancers of the floor of the mouth. Note the single crossing needle through center of device. The devices are currently machined from nylon. Usually, cesium needles with a 2.25-cm active length (a 3.2-cm actual length) are used: the intensity of the needles is adjusted so that a dose rate of approximately 0.4 to 0.5 Gy/hour is delivered to the tumor. To ensure a adequate surface dose, the height of the implant device (9 mm) is such that 3 mm of the active ends of the cesium needles extends above the mucosal surface. The crossing needle is also 3 mm above the mucosal surface (i.e., at the active ends of the needles). Reprintedwith permission from ref. (1).**

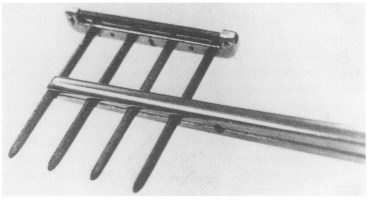

Figure 2. **Radium needles mounted in a rigid device for implantation of oral tongue cancer. The holders were originally fashioned from stainless steel or aluminum, but more recently nylon has proved more satisfactory. The needles are secured to the bar with half-hard stainless steel wire passed through the eyelets. An Allen forceps has been drilled to grasp the needles. Crossing needles may be attached to the bar or inserted separately. Cesium needles have replaced the radium sources. Reprinted with permission from ref. (2).**

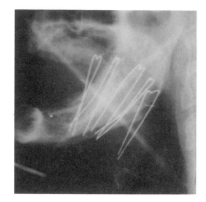

Figure 3. Lateral view of ^{192}Ir implant for carcinoma (stage T2N0) of the left side of the oral tongue. The lesion measured 3.5 × 2.0 × 2.0 cm, with submucosal extension to within 0.5 cm of the midline of the tongue. Treatment consisted of a dose of 30 Gy given in 10 fractions followed 1 week later by the implant. With the patient in a sitting position, the gutter-guide technique along with a combination of local anesthesia and regional nerve block was used. Fluoroscopy was used in the operating room to verify accurate source spacing and alignment. The implant sources were 4 cm long. A gauze pack was secured in the lateral floor of the mouth to displace the tongue medially away from the mandible. The implant remained in place for 73 hours and delivered 40 Gy tumor dose to the area of gross disease (0.55 Gy per hour). The patient died of a second primary cancer 6½ years after radiotherapy. Reprinted with permission from ref. (3).

Dose-Fractionation Considerations

In general, the probability of tumor control and complications increases with increasing dose, dose per fraction, volume irradiated and decreasing overall treatment time (4,5). Split-course radiation therapy should be avoided because it is associated with a decreased probability of tumor control and does not appreciably lower the risk of late complications (6,7). A conventionally fractionated course of radiation therapy is composed of one treatment per day, 5 days per week, with a fraction size of 1.8 to 2.0 Gy. The final dose depends on the volume of tumor irradiated, the radiosensitivity of adjacent normal tissues, and the probability of complications. Acutely responding tissues, such as the normal mucosa and carcinoma, respond similarly to radiation. Therefore, treatment schedules that are associated with a minimum of mucositis and its attendant symptoms have a relatively small chance of eradicating a head and neck cancer.

The probability of late complications is not related to the acute effects of radiation except at the very extremes of acute reactions; it does tend to increase with increasing tumor volume because of destruction of normal tissue by the tumor. It is necessary to accept a low risk (≤ 5%) of severe late complications in order to have a reasonable probability of disease control with treatment (4,8). A very low risk (1%) of severe complications is desirable in the treatment of early cancers for which the chance of cure is high and an acceptable treatment alternative exists (e.g., T1 or T2 vocal cord cancer suitable for a hemilaryngectomy). However, a higher risk of severe complications (5% to 10%) is acceptable for more advanced lesions in which the chance of cure is lower or the surgical alternative is associated with a significant functional or cosmetic deficit (e.g., a bulky, endophytic laryngeal cancer for which the surgical alternative would be total laryngectomy).

Twice-a-day radiation therapy involving a lower dose per fraction (such as 1.2 Gy) may be used to increase the probability of tumor control with a similar or lower risk of late complications in selected patients (9,10). Dose-fraction schedules for treatment of various T-stage lesions with external-beam irradiation alone are outlined in Table 1 (11); these are approximations and vary according to the primary site and cell type (e.g., lymphoepithelioma requires a lower dose than does squamous cell carcinoma). Twice-a-day treatment schedules usually entail a higher total dose than do conventional treatment schedules. At our institution, most primary head and neck cancers treated primarily with radiotherapy receive hyperfractionated treatment (1.2 Gy twice a day) with a minimum 6-hour interfraction interval. Exceptions to this are low-volume T1 or T2 tumors for which the local control rate is acceptable with once-daily fractionation, (e.g., T1 vocal cord carcinomas which generally received 63 Gy at 2.25 Gy per day), or in patients for whom two treatments per day is logistically unfeasible.

Table 1. **Radiation Therapy Alone: Doses and Fractionation Schedules***

	Once-a-Day Fractionation		Twice-a-Day Fractionation
T Stage	1.8 Gy/Fraction	2.0 Gy/Fraction	1.2 Gy/Fraction
T1	65	60	No data
T2	70	64	74.4
T3	70	70	76.8
T4	75	70	79.2

*These are general treatment schedules and will vary with primary site and tumor cell type. Reprinted with permission from ref. (11).

Data Analysis

It is imperative that an accepted staging system (such as that of the American Joint Committee on Cancer) (12,13) is used when clinical data are collected and reported so that the end results for various treatment modalities can be compared stage for stage. The minimal follow-up necessary depends on how quickly a particular tumor is likely to recur after treatment. Approximately 90% of head and neck squamous cell carcinomas that recur do so within 2 years of treatment, and essentially all recurrences are noted within

5 years of treatment. Therefore, the minimal follow-up for all patients included in reported series analyzing end results should be 2 years. Although survival after treatment is the "bottom line," it is also necessary to analyze control of disease at the primary site (local control) and in the neck lymph nodes (neck control) to assess the effectiveness of a local-regional treatment modality such as radiation therapy or surgery. Local-regional control rates should be calculated by excluding from the analysis those patients who die within 2 years of treatment with the site or sites in question continuously disease-free, because these patients have not survived long enough for the efficacy of treatment to be determined (14). Alternatively, the data may be analyzed by use of an actuarial method. All patients should be included in analyses of complications and survival.

TREATMENT GUIDELINES AND RESULTS

Neck

Clinically Negative Neck. Decisions about management of the neck depend on the plan of management for the primary lesion. The clinically negative neck is treated electively if the anticipated risk of occult neck disease is 20% or greater (Table 2) (15). If the primary lesion is to be irradiated, the neck is electively irradiated. If the primary lesion is to be treated surgically, the neck is electively dissected. Resection of the primary lesion should not be combined with radiation therapy for the sole purpose of electively irradiating the neck because radiation therapy may be required at some time in the future for treatment of a second primary head and neck cancer.

Table 2. **Clinically Negative Neck: Definition of Risk Groups**

Group	Estimated Risk of Subclinical Neck Disease	T Stage	Site
I Low risk	< 20%	T1	Floor of mouth, retromolar trigone, gingiva, hard palate, buccal mucosa, glottic larynx
		T2	Glottic larynx
II Intermediate risk	20%–30%	T1	Oral tongue, soft palate, pharyngeal wall, supraglottic larynx, tonsil
		T2	Floor of mouth, oral tongue, retromolar trigone, gingiva, hard palate, buccal mucosa
III High risk	> 30%	T1–T4	Nasopharynx, pyriform sinus, base of tongue
		T2–T4	Soft palate, pharyngeal wall, supraglottic larynx, tonsil
		T3–T4	Floor of mouth, oral tongue, retromolar trigone, gingiva, hard palate, buccal mucosa

Reprinted with permission from ref. (15).

Elective neck irradiation and elective neck dissection are equally and highly effective in managing subclinical neck disease (Tables 3 and 4) (15,16). The morbidity associated with elective neck irradiation is negligible. The likelihood of salvage after isolated neck failure in an unirradiated neck is approximately 50% if the primary site remains continuously disease free. This percentage drops significantly if the neck has received prior radiation (17) or if there is recurrent disease at the primary site.

Table 3. **Clinically Negative Neck Nodes: Prevention of Treatment Failure in the Neck by Initial Therapy**

Risk Group	No ENI	Partial ENI	Total ENI
I (< 20%)	13/15 (87%)	16/17 (94%)	1/1 (100%)
II (20%–30%)	6/9 (67%)	34/38 (89%)	10/11 (91%)
III (> 30%)	3/4 (75%)	32/33 (97%)	61/62 (98%)

ENI, elective neck irradiation (no. controlled/no. treated).
Reprinted with permission from ref. (15).

Table 4. **Failure of Initial Neck Treatment: 596 Patients with Carcinoma of the Tonsillar Fossa, Base of Tongue, Supraglottic Larynx, or Hypopharynx (M.D. Anderson Hospital 1948-1967)**

Treatment	No Treatment	Partial Treatment	Complete Treatment	N1	N2a	N2b	N3a	N3b
Irradiation	—	15%	2%	15%	27%	27%	38%	34%
Surgery	55% (16/29)	35%	7%	11%	8%	23%	42%	41%
Combined	—	1/5	0/6	0	0	0	23%	25%

Reprinted with permission from ref. (16).

Oral Cavity

Oral Tongue. Early (T1, T2) oral tongue cancer may be treated with either radiation therapy or surgery with an equal likelihood of cure (18). Although the risk of a significant radiation therapy complication is low, surgery is the preferred treatment in the authors' institution because of a smaller risk of severe bone exposure or soft tissue necrosis that may persist for months or years after radiation therapy (19). Patients are treated primarily with radiation therapy if they decline surgery or are at high risk for operative complications.

Early (stage I and II) oral tongue cancer is irradiated with use of a short, intensive course of external-beam treatment combined with either an interstitial implant or an intraoral cone boost. The latter significantly lessens the risk of mandibular complications (18). Brachytherapy, however, is the mainstay of treatment for most oral tongue cancers with radiotherapy. Overall treatment time is usually 3 to 4 weeks, and should be completed in as short a time as possible (<40 days) (19,20). At least half the total dose is administered by interstitial implant. Local control rates after 50 Gy of external beam radiation combined with interstitial implant (20 to 25 Gy) are significantly worse than those achieved with either implant alone or moderate dose external beam treatment plus high-dose implant (20-24). We currently recommend using 1.6 Gy per fraction with twice-daily external-beam irradiation to a total of 32 Gy followed within 1 to 2 weeks by an implant of approximately 35 to 40 Gy or preceded by intraoral cone irradiation (Fig. 4) (18). Control rates after external beam radiotherapy alone are poor even for T1 and T2 tumors (Figs. 2, 3, and 5) (25-28).

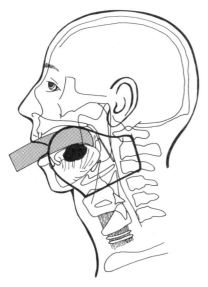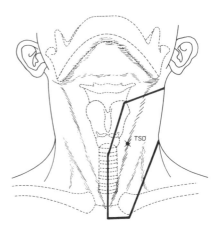

Figure 4. **Well lateralized squamous cell carcinoma of the oral tongue (neck stage N0). (A) A single ipsilateral field is used. The field encompasses the submaxillary and subdigastric lymph nodes; the entire width of the vertebral body is included to ensure adequate posterior coverage of the subdigastric lymph nodes. Stainless steel pins are usually inserted into the anteriormost and posteriormost aspects of the lesion to aid in localizing the cancer on the treatment planning (simulation) roentgenogram and to confirm coverage by the interstitial implant. For lesions smaller than 2.0 cm in diameter, the low neck is not irradiated (unless the histology is poorly differentiated squamous cell carcinoma). The larynx is excluded from the radiation field. The anterior submental skin and subcutaneous tissues are shielded, when possible, to reduce submental edema and late development of fibrosis. The upper border is shaped to exclude most of the parotid gland. An intraoral lead block (stippled area) shields the contralateral mucosa. The block is coated with beeswax to prevent a high-dose effect on the adjacent mucosa resulting from scattered low-energy electrons from the metal surface. The usual preinterstitial tumor dose is 32 Gy using 1.6 Gy per fraction, twice-a-day fractionation. For larger lesions, which extend near the midline, treatment is applied by means of parallel opposed portals with no intraoral lead block. (B) For well lateralized lesions greater than 2.0 cm in patients with a stage N0 neck, only the ipsilateral low neck is irradiated. Reprinted with permission from ref. (18).**

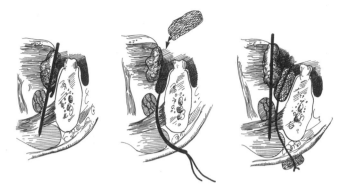

Figure 5. **The use of packing to reduce dose to mandible. (Left) Implant without packing. (Center) Large curved needle inserted through skin to floor of the mouth, (Right) Gauze pack tied to suture and secured between mandible and tongue after implant is completed. Reprinted with permission from ref.** (29).

The actuarial probabilities of local control at 2 years for 18 patients treated with radiotherapy alone at our institution before and after surgical salvage for T1 lesions are 79% and 93%, respectively. The corresponding probabilities for 48 patients with T2 tumors are 72% and 83%, respectively. Actuarial cause-specific survival rates for AJCC stages I and II at 5 years are 88% and 82%, respectively. The risk of severe bone or soft tissue complications necessitating surgical intervention was 6% and 13%, respectively, for T1 and T2 tumors (19).

Floor of Mouth. Until the late 1970's, most early floor of mouth cancers seen at our institution were treated with radiotherapy, reserving surgery for radiation failures. With the advent of rim resection, however, it became possible to resect these lesions with relatively little morbidity. Local control and survival rates after rim resection of early-stage cancers are similar to those achieved with radiotherapy (18,30). The late morbidity of radiotherapy is greater than with surgery because mandibular and soft-tissue necrosis, although usually temporary, is not uncommon after treatment with primary radiation. Accordingly, T1 and T2 tumors are now generally treated surgically, particularly if the tumor abuts the gingiva. Radiotherapy is added only if adverse pathologic factors are present. Patients who decline surgery or are at high risk for operative complications are still treated with primary radiotherapy.

The ideal candidate for treatment with radiation alone has a lesion that can be managed by use of an intraoral cone for all or part of the treatment; this produces a low risk of mandibular necrosis. The patient should be edentulous, ideally for a number of years, resulting in a decreased mandibular height which facilitates cone placement.

Interstitial implant is essential if intraoral cone therapy is not possible. The time-dose factors are less critical than with oral tongue lesions, and the required doses are slightly lower. Lesions smaller than 1 cm in diameter and < 4 mm thick may be treated with intraoral cone or implant alone. Larger tumors have a 20-30% risk of subclinical disease in the neck and require external beam irradiation in addition to treatment with oral cone or implantation. The neck and primary site are generally treated to a dose of 45-50 Gy, followed by a 25-Gy implant. If an oral cone is used, it should precede the megavoltage portion of treatment to allow for optimal tumor visualization and patient comfort (Fig. 6)

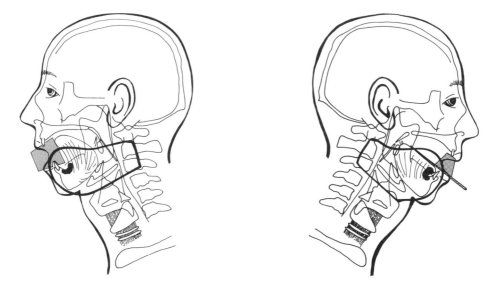

Figure 6. **Portals for radiotherapy of floor-of-mouth cancer. (A) Limited anterior floor-of-mouth carcinoma (no tongue invasion and N0 or N1 neck disease). Two notches are cut on a cork so that it can be held in the same position between the patient's upper and lower incisors during every treatment session: the tip of the tongue is displaced from the treatment field. The anterior border of the field covers the full thickness of the mandibular arch. The lower field edge is at the thyroid cartilage, ensuring adequate coverage of the submandibular lymph nodes. The subdigastric lymph nodes will be adequately covered by treating the entire width of the vertebral bodies posteriorly. The superior border is shaped so that much of the oral cavity, oropharynx, and parotid glands are out of the portal. The minimum tumor dose is specified at the primary site (i.e., not along the central axis of the portal) with the aid of computer dosimetry. (B) Carcinoma of the floor of mouth with tongue invasion. The tongue is depressed into the floor of the mouth with a tongue blade and cork as shown. Reprinted with permission of ref. (18).**

The local control rates (direct method) for 73 patients treated with radiotherapy alone at our institution for T1 and T2 lesions are 86% and 69%, respectively. The corresponding ultimate rates of local control after surgical salvage of radiation failures are 94% and 86%, respectively. Actuarial cause-specific survival probabilities for AJCC stages I and II at 5 years are 96% and 70%, respectively. The incidence of severe bone or soft tissue complications necessitating surgical intervention was 5% for 117 patients with T1-T4 primary tumors treated with irradiation alone. Forty-two percent experienced mild to moderate complications (30).

Oropharynx

The philosophy at the University of Florida is to treat all oropharyngeal cancer with radiation therapy alone. There is no compelling evidence to suggest that the likelihood of local control or survival is improved by combining surgery with radiation therapy (31-33).

Tonsillar Area. T1 and T2 cancers of the anterior tonsillar pillar have, until recently, been treated at our institution with external-beam irradiation combined with an intraoral cone or interstitial boost. The trend recently, however, has been to use external hyperfractionated radiation alone on all early (T1 and T2) cancers of the tonsillar fossa and anterior tonsillar pillar. Intraoral cone irradiation is still used as a boost if the tumor can be adequately encompassed within the cone because tumors involving the anterior pillar have a worse prognosis than more posterior lesions.

Treatment portals used for tonsillar cancer automatically cover the first-echelon lymph nodes down to the level of the thyroid notch. The risk of spread to the submandibular nodes increases if there is significant extension to the anterior tonsillar pillar or retromolar trigone. The lower two-thirds of the larynx is not included in the primary fields. Most early tumors are well-lateralized and can be treated with an ipsilateral wedge-pair setup or an ipsilateral mixed-beam consisting of a combination of high energy electrons and photons (Fig. 7). We have been inclined to use the wedge-pair technique if there is no tongue invasion and no significant involvement of the medial soft palate. The advantage of the wedge pair compared with the mixed-beam technique is the ability to treat lesions whose medial extent is more than 4.5 cm from the skin surface. A separate low neck field is generally added, as well.

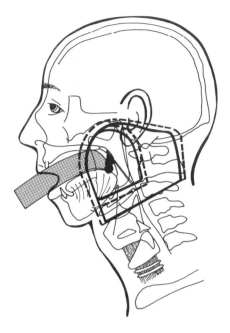

Figure 7. **Mixed beam radiotherapy portals for tonsillar cancer. Early, well lateralized lesions of the tonsillar region may be treated by an ipsilateral mixed-beam technique consisting of a combination of high energy electrons and high energy X rays. If tumor extends deeper than approximately 4.5 cm, the technique is generally not used because of rapid falloff in dose from the electron beam. The technique has the advantage of delivering a low dose to the contralateral parotid gland and contralateral mucosal surfaces. An intraoral lead block is commonly used to further reduce the dose of radiation to the contralateral mucosa and to shield some of the minor salivary glands from the beam. Because the effective treatment area is constricted with electrons compared with X rays, the perimeter of the electron beam portals (dashed lines)is larger by 1 cm except at the inferior border, which adjoins the lower neck field. Because these lesions lie behind the dense mandible, an extra 1.0 to 1.5 cm is added for the purpose of making depth-dose calculations for the electron portion of the treatment to compensate for shadowing of the tumor by the mandible. If the neck is clinically negative, only the ipsilateral nodes require radiotherapy (50 Gy given dose in 25 fractions).(See Fig. 4(B)). In patients with N0 disease, the nodes in the lateral supraclavicular fossa are at very low risk and are not irradiated electively. Reprinted with permission of ref. (33).**

The actuarial probabilities of local control at 5 years for 56 patients treated for T1 lesions with radiotherapy alone at our institution before and after surgical salvage were 83% and 92%, respectively. The corresponding probabilities for 150 patients with T2 tumors were 81% and 89%, respectively. Five year local control rates for anterior tonsillar pillar versus tonsillar fossa/posterior tonsillar pillar were as follows: T1, 70% and 90%, and T2, 73% and 88%, respectively. Actuarial cause-specific survival rates for AJCC stages I and II at 5 years were 100% and 86%, respectively. The risk of severe bone or soft tissue complications necessitating surgical intervention was 5% in 400 patients treated with T1-T4 primary tumors (32).

Soft Palate. T1 and T2 soft palate cancers are treated with external-beam irradiation combined with an intraoral cone boost or with external-beam irradiation alone. Interstitial implantation is also used occasionally for amenable lesions. Treatment portals are similar to those incorporated for other oropharyngeal sites, except that ipsilateral set-ups are seldom used unless the tumor is well lateralized (Figures 8 and 9) (33).

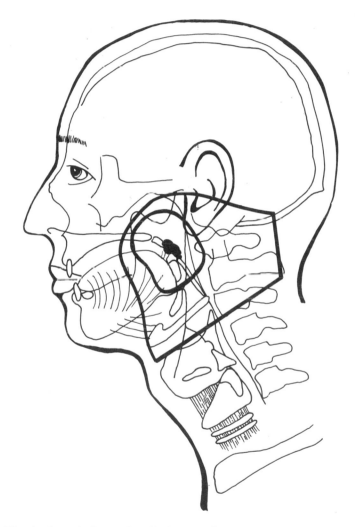

Figure 8. **The basic technique of radiotherapy for soft palate cancer using parallel opposed portals. The minimum treatment volume for early cancers includes the entire soft palate and the adjacent pillars. The timing and extent of field reductions after 45 Gy depend on the status of the neck as well as the configuration of the primary lesion. If the primary lesion extends to the midline or if clinically positive lymph nodes are present, both sides of the lower neck are irradiated. Reprinted with permission from ref. (33)**

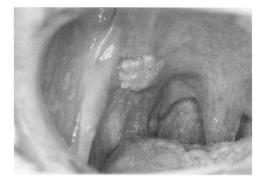

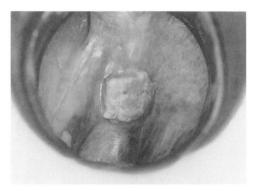

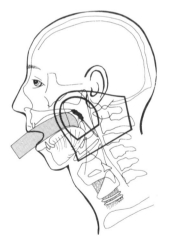

Figure 9. **Exophytic invasive squamous cell carcinoma, 1.5 cm, of the soft palate. (A) Very discrete soft palate lesions in cooperative patients can be given 15 to 20 Gy (2.5 to 3 Gy per fraction) with an intraoral cone before external beam radiotherapy. (B) Photograph through intraoral cone shows adequate coverage of the lesion. (C) If the lesion is well lateralized and the neck is negative, treatment is completed by an ipsilateral ^{60}Co portal that encompasses the primary lesion and upper neck nodes plus a low neck portal as shown in Figure 4B. After a given dose of approximately 54 Gy with ^{60}Co (50 Gy tumor dose at 2.0 cm), the primary portal is reduced off the neck nodes to encompass only the primary lesion. An intraoral lead block is used to reduce irradiation to the contralateral mucosa. If the lesion is close to the midline, parallel opposed portals are used (see Fig. 8). Reprinted with permission from ref. (33)**

The actuarial 5-year local control probabilities for 65 patients with T1 or T2 lesions treated with radiotherapy alone at our institution are 86% and 91%, respectively. Actuarial cause-specific survival probabilities for AJCC stages I and II at 5 years are 84% and 91%, respectively. The incidence of severe bone or soft tissue complications necessitating surgical intervention was 3% for 107 patients with T1-T4 primary tumors treated with radiotherapy alone or followed by planned neck dissection (34).

Base of Tongue. Patients with T1 and T2 base-of-tongue cancers are treated with high-dose external-beam irradiation alone. The addition of an interstitial implant offers no improvement in local control rates in comparison with external-beam therapy alone (35). The primary treatment portals for base-of-tongue cancer are shown in Figure 10 (33). Parallel-opposed lateral fields are virtually always used, since the tongue base is a midline structure with a significant risk of spread to bilateral nodal areas in the neck. A submental boost has been used occasionally at our institution in amenable tumors, allowing for sparing of the mandible and adjacent soft tissues.

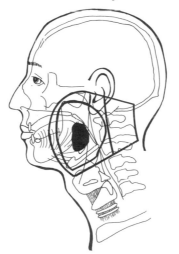

Figure 10. **The usual initial treatment volume for base of tongue cancer treated by parallel opposed portals. Included are the base of tongue, valleculae, suprahyoid epiglottis, upper preepiglottic space, pharyngeal walls, and a portion of the oral tongue, depending on the anterior extent of disease. One of the common errors in planning external beam radiotherapy is a failure to recognize the anterior extension of tumor; palpation through the lateral floor of mouth is the best method to determine anterior extension. A small stainless steel pin is commonly inserted into the anteriormost extent of the cancer or into the base of the anterior tonsillar pillar before simulation; the pin serves as a useful landmark on the treatment-planning (simulation) radiograph. The superior border is approximately 3 cm above the tip of the mastoid in order to encompass the junctional lymph nodes near the base of the skull. Spread to the spinal accessory lymph nodes is frequent enough to justify their inclusion in the initial treatment volume, even in patients with N0 cancer. The posterior submaxillary nodes are included. Most of the larynx is excluded unless tumor invades the supraglottic larynx, hypopharynx, or preepiglottic space. The skin and subcutaneous tissues in the submental midline are shielded unless the patient is very thin or has tumor that palpably extends into the submental area. A reduction is made off the spinal cord at 45 Gy, and further reductions are made as possible. It is usually possible to shield most of the aryepiglottic fold from the reduced fields. Reprinted with permission from ref. (33).**

Stage for stage, the probability of local control is better for base of tongue cancer than for oral tongue cancer. The actuarial 5-year local control probabilities for 105 patients with T1 or T2 lesions treated with radiotherapy alone at our institution are 96% and 91%, respectively. The actuarial cause-specific survival probability for AJCC stages I and II is 100% at 5 years. The incidence of severe bone or soft tissue complications necessitating surgical intervention was 3.7% for 217 patients with T1-T4 primary tumors treated with radiotherapy alone or followed by planned neck dissection (35).

Supraglottic Larynx

Stage I and II supraglottic cancers may be treated with either radiation therapy alone or a supraglottic laryngectomy with bilateral selective neck dissections. Transoral laser excision is also an acceptable alternative in experienced hands for selected lesions (36-38). A substantial proportion of patients whose lesions are anatomically suitable for a supraglottic laryngectomy are not candidates for the procedure because of cardiac or pulmonary disease or both; they are best managed with radiation therapy alone.

Initial treatment portals for patients with Stage I and II disease are parallel-opposed, extending from the bottom of the cricoid cartilage inferiorly to roughly 2 cm above the angle of the mandible superiorly.

This arrangement includes the primary nodal areas at highest risk, i.e., the inferior level II and level III groups (Figure 11) (39). A strip of skin can sometimes be spared anteriorly to reduce the risk of edema, although care must be taken to select patients carefully for this technique to avoid shielding tumor in the preepiglottic space or at the petiolus/anterior commissure.

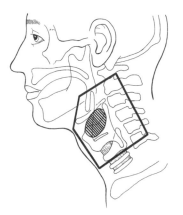

Figure 11. **Example of portal for lesions of the lower epiglottis or false vocal cord and a clinically negative neck. The subdigastric nodes are included but not the junctional nodes. Depending on the anatomy and tumor extent, the anterior border off the beam may fall off (i.e., "flash") or a small strip of skin may be shielded. Reprinted with permission from ref.** (39).

The actuarial 5-year local control probabilities for 147 patients with T1 or T2 lesions treated with radiotherapy at our institution are 100% and 86%, respectively. Actuarial cause-specific survival probabilities for 91 patients with AJCC stage I and II disease at 5 years are 100% and 93%, respectively. There is a trend towards improved local control for those patients with normal vocal cord mobility, those whose tumor volume is calculated to be < 6 cm^3 and/or in those treated with twice-daily rather than once-daily fractionation. Salvage laryngectomy was successful in over half of those patients that it was attempted. The incidence of severe complications necessitating surgical intervention was 4% for 274 patients with T1-T4 primary tumors treated with radiotherapy alone or followed by planned neck dissection (40).

GLOTTIC LARYNX

Carcinoma in Situ

Lesions diagnosed as carcinoma in situ may sometimes be controlled by stripping of the cord. However, it is difficult to exclude the possibility of microinvasion on these specimens, recurrence is frequent, and the cord may become thickened and the voice harsh with repeated stripping.

We usually recommend early radiation therapy for carcinoma in situ, realizing that most patients with this diagnosis eventually receive this treatment and that earlier use of irradiation means a better chance of preserving a good voice.

Many of the patients with a diagnosis of carcinoma in situ have obvious lesions that probably contain invasive carcinoma. We have often proceeded with radiation therapy rather than put the patient through a repeated biopsy procedure.

Early Vocal Cord Carcinoma

The goals of treatment for early vocal cord cancer include cure, laryngeal voice preservation, and optimal voice quality with minimal morbidity, expense, and inconvenience. The treatment of choice is controversial. Options include radiation therapy (41), open partial laryngectomy (42), and transoral laser excision (36-38). The probability of obtaining local control is similar for the three modalities. Selection of treatment depends on the location and extent of the tumor, the medical condition of the patient, the philosophy of the physicians involved, and patient preference. A proportion of T1 and T2 vocal cord cancers are unsuitable for a conservative operation because of the anatomic extent of the lesion or the medical condition of the patient. In the authors' experience, 10% of T1 lesions and 56% of T2 cancers were anatomically unsuitable for a conservative laryngectomy (11).

Radiation therapy is the treatment of choice for all previously untreated T1 and T2 vocal cord cancers at our institution because it results in better voice quality and is less expensive than open conservative surgery. Local control rates after RT for early lesions vary considerably in the literature. The likelihood of local control decreases with impaired vocal cord mobility and increasing T stage (41). Overall treatment time has also been shown to be significantly related to the likelihood of local control after RT for a variety of head and neck cancers. Indeed, reduction of overall treatment time to diminish tumor repopulation during the RT course is one of the major features of altered fractionation schedules that have been shown to be superior to conventional once-daily irradiation (9). Although the reduction in the probability of local control with a protracted treatment course is probably greatest for locally advanced tumors, an adverse effect has even been seen in patients with T1 glottic malignancies (7). Sufficient evidence exists to indicate that once-daily schedules of 1.8 Gy per treatment, 5 days per week, are suboptimal. It has been our practice to treat T1 and T2 vocal cord cancers at 2.25 Gy per fraction once-daily or, in recent years, some patients with T2 lesions with hyperfractionated RT (41). Patients are treated in the lateral the table by the attending physician. Alternatively, setting the patient up supine and treating through opposed lateral portals is acceptable, and the standard of care at most other centers. The typical borders for a T1 lesion involving the anterior two-thirds of one or both cords would be the middle of the thyroid notch, the bottom of the cricoid cartilage, 1 cm behind the posterior border of the thyroid ala, and "falling off" 1.5 cm anteriorly. Fields are enlarged depending on extension off of the true vocal cord for patients with T2 tumors (Fig. 12) (43,44).

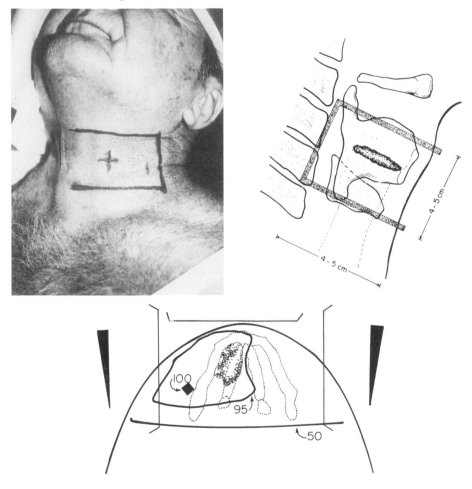

Figure 12. Patients with a T1N0 squamous cell carcinoma confined to the anterior two thirds of the vocal cord. (A) Patient in the lateral "chicken wing" position for treatment. (B) Schematic diagram of the field, which extends from the middle of the thyroid notch to the bottom of the cricoid cartilage, 1 cm posterior to the cartilage and with 1½ cm falloff anteriorly. (C) Computer-generated dosimetry; the dose is specified at the 95% isodose line. Reprinted with permission from ref. (44) (Part A) and ref. (43) (Parts B and C).

A 3-field technique has been used consistently at our institution the past 20 years, consisting of parallel-opposed portals to deliver approximately 90% of the dose and an anterior field to give the remainder. Fields are weighted 3:2 for lateralized cancers, with the anterior field being centered on the tumor. The dose is specified at an isodose line that just encompasses the cancer and usually is 95% of the maximum dose. Patients have predominantly been treated with ^{60}Co or 2 MV X-rays, although a 6 MV beam has been incorporated more frequently in recent years.

Local control after RT and ultimate local control after salvage surgery in 519 patients treated at the University of Florida is depicted in Figures 13 and 14 (41).

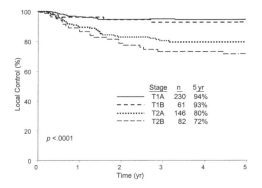

Figure 13. **Local control after radiation treatment for vocal cord carcinoma. Local control rates at 5 years were as follows: T1A, 94%; T1B, 93%; T2A, 80%; and T2B, 72%. . Reprinted with permission from ref. (41).**

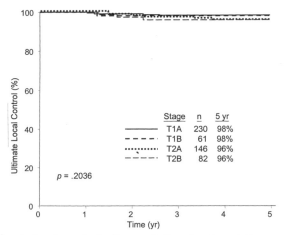

Figure 14. **Ultimate local control after radiation treatment for vocal cord carcinoma. Ultimate local control rates at 5 years were as follows: T1A, 98%; T1B, 98%; T2A, 96%; and T2B, 96%. Reprinted with permission from ref. (41).**

The 5-year local control rates for 182 patients with T2 cancers treated after December 1977 with once-daily versus twice-daily fractionation is as follows: T2A, 82% and 83% (p =. 88); and T2B, 71% and 69% (p = .80), respectively (41). Control of nodal disease in the neck after RT to limited fields is shown in Figure 15 (41)

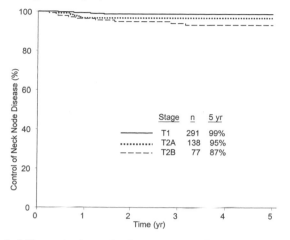

Figure 15. **Control of disease in the neck after treatment for vocal cord carcinoma. The 5-year rates of neck disease control for patients who did not receive elective neck irradiation were as follows: T1A and T1B, 99%; T2A, 95%; and T2B, 87%. Reprinted with permission from ref. (41).**

Actuarial cause-specific survival probabilities at 5 years are shown in Figure 16 (41).

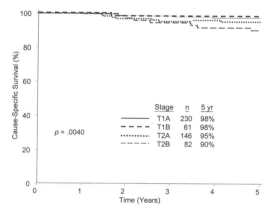

Figure 16. **Cause-specific survival after treatment for vocal cord cancer. The 5-year cause-specific survival rates were as follows: T1AN0, 98%; T1BN0, 98%; T2AN0, 95%; and T2BN0, 90%. Reprinted with permission from ref. (41).**

The incidence of severe complications necessitating surgical intervention was 0.8% (4 of 519) for patients with T1 or T2 tumors treated with radiotherapy at our institution.

Hypopharynx

Pyriform Sinus. A variety of treatment options are currently available for patients with T1 and T2 carcinomas of the pyriform sinus (45). At one end of the spectrum is radical surgery with removal of the larynx and the involved portion of the hypopharynx. Such an approach results in a high probability of tumor control, but also in a high risk of morbidity from disruption of speech and swallowing. The results of conservation surgery are encouraging and suggest that selected patients are likely to be cured with partial laryngopharyngectomy. T1 and favorable T2 cancers may also be managed with radiation therapy. Patients with favorable T2 lesions exhibit the following characteristics: exophytic tumor, good airway, normal cord mobility, and uninvolved apex. At the University of Florida, almost all of these cancers are treated with radiation therapy alone because there are fewer problems with aspiration after irradiation than after partial laryngopharyngectomy.

Parallel-opposed lateral portals are used to encompass the primary lesion and regional nodes on both sides. The superior border is placed 2 to 3 cm above the tip of the mastoid to cover junctional lymph nodes. The retropharyngeal lymph nodes located at the anterior edge of C1 and C2 and must be included as well. The posterior border encompasses the spinal accessory lymph nodes. The anterior border is usually placed about 1 cm behind the anterior skin edge, although care must be taken so as not to shield tumor with this technique. The inferior border is placed at least 1 to 2 cm below the inferior border of the cricoid, and sometimes lower depending on tumor location (Fig. 17) (3,46).

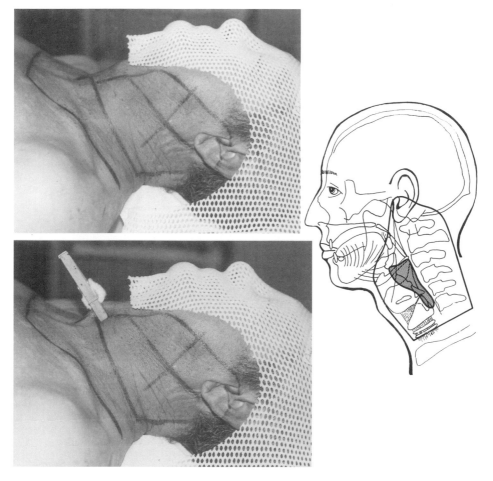

Figure 17. (A) **Portals used for the initial treatment volume in a patient with carcinoma (stippled area) of the pyriform sinus. Superiorly, the portal covers lymph nodes at the base of the skull and then sweeps anteroinferiorly to cover posterior tongue base and jugulodigastric lymph nodes. Anteriorly, at least 1 cm of skin and subcutaneous tissues (as viewed from lateral projection) is usually spared. Inferior border is 2 to 3 cm below bottom of cricoid cartilage and is slanted to facilitate matching with low neck portal and to avoid irradiating shoulders. Posterior field edge usually encompasses spinous process of C2 vertebral body. As treatment progresses, several field reductions are made (to shield spinal cord and to limit volume of mucosa that receives high dose irradiation).(B)Primary treatment fields for carcinoma of the pyriform sinus. (C) A clothespin is used to increase the amount of subcutaneous tissue spared anteriorly. Reprinted with permission from ref. (3) (Part A) and ref. (48) (Parts B and C).**

Severe complications may include laryngeal edema necessitating a permanent tracheostomy or laryngectomy for chondronecrosis. Severe late sequelae related to the initial course of radiotherapy developed in 9% (9/101) of patients treated at our institution for T1 or T2 pyriform sinus cancers (47).

Actuarial rates of initial and ultimate local control after radiotherapy for 22 T1 and 79 T2 patients with tumors treated at our institution are shown in Figure 18 (47). Actuarial cause-specific survival rates are depicted in Figure 19 (47).

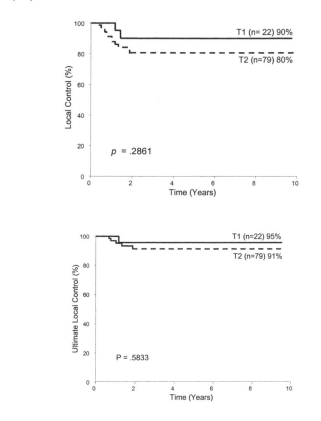

A

B

Figure 18. Actuarial rates of initial (A) (p > .1) and ultimate (B) (p > .1) local control after treatment for pyriform sinus carcinoma. Five-year values were as follows: initial control— stage T1, 90%; stage T2, 80%; ultimate control—stage T1, 95%; stage T2, 91%. Reprinted with permission from ref (47)

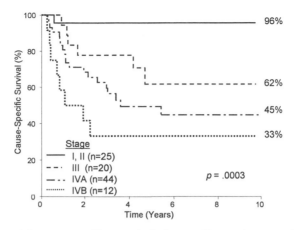

Figure 19. **Actuarial cause-specific survival for pyriform sinus carcinoma. Five-year survival rate for stage I-II was 96%. All patients had T1 and T2 primary cancers. Reprinted with permission from ref. (47).**

Pharyngeal Wall. Lesions arising from the pharyngeal wall are usually advanced at presentation, and the patients have a relatively poor prognosis regardless of treatment. The tumors do not extend off the pharyngeal wall until they are quite extensive and are therefore staged by tumor size according to the AJCC staging system for oropharyngeal cancer. The policy at the University of Florida is to treat essentially all pharyngeal wall cancers with external-beam irradiation alone. There is no definite benefit to combining external-beam irradiation with an interstitial implant.

The irradiation technique for posterior pharyngeal wall lesions is opposed lateral fields to include the primary lesion and the regional nodes. Since these tumors tend to have mucosal skip areas, the entire posterior pharyngeal wall is included initially. The jugular chain, spinal accessory, and retropharyngeal lymph nodes are treated even if the neck is clinically uninvolved. The anterior border does not flash and spares the anterior one-third of the larynx. The isocenter is placed over the posterior edge of the cervical vertebral bodies so that the off-cord reductions have an essentially coplanar posterior border just anterior to the spinal cord to ensure adequate treatment of the mucosal surfaces and retropharyngeal nodes (Fig. 20) (49).

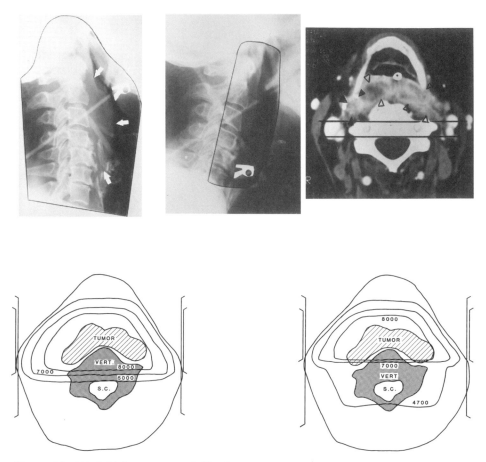

Figure 20. (A) **Initial treatment fields for squamous cell carcinoma of the posterior pharyngeal wall. Arrowheads indicate the superior and inferior margins of the tumor. The anterior border of the field does not flash the skin of the anterior aspect of the neck, thus sparing the anterior portion of the larynx. (B) Treatment field after reducing off the spinal cord. Note that the posterior edge of the field is at the posterior aspect of the vertebral bodies (C) Computerized tomogram before treatment. The open arrowheads denote the primary tumor and the closed arrowheads indicate a retropharyngeal node. Note that there is tumor extending posterior to the anterior surface of the vertebral body. The anterior line indicates the posterior edge of the reduced field if it is designed to split the vertebral bodies. Note that tumor is on the edge of the field. The posterior line indicates the field margin if it is placed at the posterior edge of the vertebral bodies. These lines do not account for beam divergence and are drawn as if the central axis of the beam is placed at the posterior edge of the field. (D) Computerized dosimetry for 45.5 Gy, 8 MV X ray, weighted 1:1, followed by reduction off of the spinal cord and 33.6 Gy, 17 MV X ray, weighted 1:1 (specified total dose = 79.2 Gy). The posterior edge of the reduced field is placed at the anterior aspect of the spinal cord. (E) As in (D) except that the posterior edge of the reduced field splits the vertebral bodies. Reprinted with permission from ref. (49)**

The actuarial probabilities of local control and ultimate local control after salvage for 41 patients with T1 and T2 pharyngeal wall primaries treated with radiation at our institution are shown in Table 5 (50). Cause-specific survival rates at 5 years for AJCC (12,13) stage I and II were 100% and 72%, respectively. Severe complications developed in 11% (11 of 99) of patients with T1-T4 primary tumors treated with radiotherapy.

Table 5. **Pharyngeal Wall Carcinoma: Two-Year and Five-Year Probability of Local Control with Continuous-Course External Beam**

		Local Control After Radiotherapy		Ultimate Local Control After Salvage	
Stage	No. Pts.	2-Year (%)	5-Year (%)	2-Year (%)	5-Year (%)
T1	8	100	100	100	100
T2	33	79	74	86	81
Reprinted with permission of ref. (50).					

CONCLUSION

Radiation therapy is highly effective in controlling most early stage squamous cell carcinomas of the head and neck. Treatment should be aimed at maximizing the chance for cure with an acceptable low risk of late complications. Innovative treatment techniques often allow for sparing of adjacent normal tissue, as well as the contralateral salivary glands While beyond the scope of this chapter, newer strategies incorporating recent technological advances further refine the radiotherapist's ability to maximize the therapeutic ratio, such as intensity modulated radiotherapy (IMRT). The next decade will likely witness a substantial shift in treatment algorithms to reflect such advances, with a resultant decrease in the incidence of late sequelae, possibly coupled with an improvement in local control.

REFERENCES

1. Marcus RB, Jr., Million RR, Mitchell TP. A preloaded, custom-designed implantation device for stage T1-T2 carcinoma of the floor of mouth. Int J Radiat Oncol Biol Phys 1980;6:111-113.

2. Ellingwood KE, Million RR, Mitchell TP. A preloaded radium needle implant device for maintenance of needle spacing. Cancer 1976;37:2858-2860.

3. Parsons JT, Palta JR, Mendenhall WM, Bova FJ, Million RR. Head and neck cancer. Levitt SH, Khan FM, Potish RA, Perez CA, editors. Levitt and Tapley's Technological Basis of Radiation Therapy: Clinical Applications, 3 ed. Baltimore: Lippincott Williams & Wilkins; 1999:269-299.

4. Gardner KE, Parsons JT, Mendenhall WM, Million RR, Cassisi NJ. Time-dose relationships for local tumor control and complications following irradiation of squamous cell carcinoma of the base of tongue. Int J Radiat Oncol Biol Phys 1987;13:507-510.

5.   Mendenhall WM, Million RR, Bova FJ. Analysis of time-dose factors in clinically positive neck nodes treated with irradiation alone in squamous cell carcinoma of the head and neck. Int J Radiat Oncol Biol Phys 1984;10:639-643.

6.   Amdur RJ, Parsons JT, Mendenhall WM, Million RR, Cassisi NJ. Split-course versus continuous-course irradiation in the postoperative setting for squamous cell carcinoma of the head and neck. Int J Radiat Oncol Biol Phys 1989;17:279-285.

7.   Parsons JT, Bova FJ, Million RR. A re-evaluation of split-course technique for squamous cell carcinoma of the head and neck. Int J Radiat Oncol Biol Phys 1980;6:1645-1652.

8.   Mendenhall WM, Cassisi NJ. Therapeutic principles in the management of head and neck tumors (in press). Souhami RL, Tannock I, Hohenberger P, Horiot J-C, editors. Oxford Textbook of Oncology, 2 ed. Oxford, England : Oxford University Press; 2000.

9.   Mendenhall WM, Amdur RJ, Siemann DW, Parsons JT. Altered fractionation in definitive Irradiation of squamous cell carcinoma of the head and neck. Curr Opin Oncol 2000;12:207-214.

10.   Mendenhall WM, Parsons JT. Altered fractionation in radiation therapy for squamous-cell carcinoma of the head and neck. Cancer Invest 1998;16:594-603.

11.   Mendenhall WM, Parsons JT, Million RR. Radiation therapy in the management of head and neck cancer. Meyerhoff WL, Rice DH, editors. Otolaryngology--Head and Neck Surgery, 1st ed. Philadelphia: W.B. Saunders; 1992:1011-1025.

12.   American Joint Committee on Cancer. Manual for Staging of Cancer. 2nd ed. Philadelphia: J.B. Lippincott Company; 1983:37-42.

13.   American Joint Committee on Cancer. AJCC Cancer Staging Handbook. 5 ed. Philadelphia: Lippincott-Raven Publishers; 1998:25-61.

14.   Parsons JT, McCarty PJ, Rao PV, Mendenhall WM, Million RR. On the definition of local control (Editorial). Int J Radiat Oncol Biol Phys 1990;18:705-706.

15.   Mendenhall WM, Million RR. Elective neck irradiation for squamous cell carcinoma of the head and neck: Analysis of time-dose factors and causes of failure. Int J Radiat Oncol Biol Phys 1986;12:741-746.

16.   Barkley HT, Jr., Fletcher GH, Jesse RH, Lindberg RD. Management of cervical lymph node metastases in squamous cell carcinoma of the tonsillar fossa, base of tongue, supraglottic larynx, and hypopharynx. Am J Surg 1972;124:462-467.

17.   Mendenhall WM, Million RR, Cassisi NJ. Elective neck irradiation in squamous-cell carcinoma of the head and neck. Head Neck Surg 1980;3:15-20.

18.   Parsons JT, Mendenhall WM, Million RR. Radiotherapy of tumors of the oral cavity. Thawley SE, Panje WR, Batsakis JG, Lindberg RD, editors. Comprehensive Management of Head and Neck Tumors, 2 ed. Philadelphia: W.B. Saunders Company; 1999:695-719.

19.   Fein DA, Mendenhall WM, Parsons JT, McCarty PJ, Stringer SP, Million RR, Cassisi NJ. Carcinoma of the oral tongue: A comparison of results and complications of treatment with radiotherapy and/or surgery. Head Neck 1994;16:358-365.

20.   Mendenhall WM, Parsons JT, Stringer SP, Cassisi NJ, Million RR. T2 oral tongue carcinoma treated with radiotherapy: Analysis of local control and complications. Radiother Oncol 1989;16:275-281.

21.   Benk V, Mazeron JJ, Grimard L, Crook J, Haddad E, Piedbois P, Calitchi E, Raynal M, Martin M, Le Bourgeois JP. Comparison of curietherapy versus external irradiation combined with curietherapy in stage II squamous cell carcinomas of the mobile tongue. Radiother Oncol 1990;18:339-347.

22.   Fu KK, Chan EK, Phillips TL, Ray JW. Time, dose and volume factors in interstitial Radium I mplants of carcinoma of the oral tongue. Radiology 1976;119:209-213.

23.   Pernot M, Malissard L, Aletti P, Hoffstetter S, Forcard JJ, Bey P. Iridium-192 brachytherapy in the management of 147 T2N0 oral tongue carcinomas treated with irradiation alone: Comparison of two treatment techniques. Radiother Oncol 1992;23:223-118.

24.   Wendt CD, Peters LJ, Delclos L, Ang KK, Morrison WH, Maor MH, Robbins KT, Byers RM, Carlson LS, Oswald MJ. Primary radiotherapy in the treatment of stage I and II oral tongue cancers: Importance of the proportion of therapy delivered with interstitial therapy. Int J Radiat Oncol Biol Phys 1990;18:1287-1292.

25. Lees AW. The treatment of carcinoma of the anterior two-thirds of the tongue by radiotherapy. Int J Radiat Oncol Biol Phys 1976;1:849-858.

26. Fu KK, Ray JW, Chan EK, Phillips TL. External and interstitial radiation therapy of carcinoma of the oral tongue. A review of 32 years' experience. Am J Roentgenol 1976;126:107-115.

27. Horiuchi J, Okuyama T, Shibuya H, Takeda M. Results of brachytherapy for cancer of the tongue with special emphasis on local prognosis. Int J Radiat Oncol Biol Phys 1982;8:829-835.

28. Leung TW, Lee AW, Chan DK. Definitive radiotherapy for carcinoma of the oral tongue. Acta Oncol 1993;32:559-564.

29. Million RR, Cassisi NJ, Mancuso AA. Oral cavity. Million RR, Cassisi NJ, editors. Management of Head and Neck Cancer: A Multidisciplinary Approach, 2 ed. Philadelphia: J.B. Lippincott Company; 1994:321-400.

30. Rodgers LW, Stringer SP, Mendenhall WM, Parsons JT, Cassisi NJ, Million RR. Management of squamous cell carcinoma of the floor of the mouth. Head Neck 1993;15:16-19.

31. Fein DA, Lee WR, Amos WR, Hinerman RW, Parsons JT, Mendenhall WM, Stringer SP, Cassisi NJ, Million RR. Oropharyngeal carcinoma treated with radiotherapy: A 30-year experience. Int J Radiat Oncol Biol Phys 1996;34:289-296.

32. Mendenhall WM, Amdur RJ, Stringer SP, Villaret DB, Cassisi NJ. Radiation therapy for squamous cell carcinoma of the tonsillar region: A preferred alternative to surgery? J Clin Oncol 2000;18:2219-2225.

33. Parsons JT, Mendenhall WM, Moore GJ, Million RR. Radiotherapy of tumors of the oropharynx. Thawley SE, Panje WR, Batsakis JG, Lindberg RD, editors. Comprehensive Management of Head and Neck Tumors, 2 ed. Philadelphia: W.B. Saunders Company; 1999:861-875.

34. Erkal HS, Serin M, Amdur RJ, Villaret DB , Stringer SP, Mendenhall WM. Squamous cell carcinomas of the soft palate treated with radiation therapy alone or followed by planned neck dissection (in press). Int J Radiat Oncol Biol Phys 2001;49.

35. Mendenhall WM, Stringer SP, Amdur RJ, Hinerman RW, Moore-Higgs GJ, Cassisi NJ. Is radiation therapy a preferred alternative to surgery for squamous cell carcinoma of the base of tongue? J Clin Oncol 2000;18:35-42.

36. Steiner W. Results of curative laser microsurgery of laryngeal carcinomas. Am J Otolaryngol 1993;14:116-121.

37. Zeitels SM, Koufman JA, Davis RK, Vaughan CW. Endoscopic treatment of surpaglottic and hypopharynx cancer. Laryngoscope 1994;104:71-78.

38. Davis RK, Kelly SM, Hayes J. Endoscopic CO_2 laser excisional biopsy of early supraglottic cancer. Laryngoscope 1991;101 :680-683.

39. Million RR, Cassisi NJ, Mancuso AA, Stringer SP, Mendenhall WM, Parsons JT. Management of the neck for squamous cell carcinoma. Million RR, Cassisi NJ, editors. Management of Head and Neck Cancer: A Multidisciplinary Approach, 2 ed. Philadelphia: J.B. Lippincott Company; 1994:75-142.

40. Hinerman RW, Mendenhall WM, Amdur RJ, Stringer SP, Villaret DB, Robbins KT. Carcinoma of the supraglottic larynx: Treatment results with radiotherapy alone or with planned neck dissection (Submitted). Int J Radiat Oncol Biol Phys 2001.

41. Mendenhall WM, Amdur RJ, Morris CG, Hinerman RW. T1-T2 N0 squamous cell carcinoma of the glottic larynx treated with radiation therapy. J Clin Oncol 2001.

42. Spector JG, Sessions DG, Chao KS, Hanson JM, Simpson JR, Perez CA. Management of stage II (T2N0M0) glottic carcinoma by radiotherapy and conservation surgery. Head Neck 1999;21:116-123.

43. Million RR, Cassisi NJ, Mancuso AA. Larynx. Million RR, Cassisi NJ, editors. Management of Head and Neck Cancer: A Multidisciplinary Approach, 2 ed. Philadelphia: J. B. Lippincott Company; 1994:431-497.

44.   Mendenhall WM, Parsons JT, Million RR, Fletcher GH. T1-T2 squamous cell carcinoma of the
         glottic larynx treated with radiation therapy: Relationship of dose-fractionation factors to local
         control and complications. Int J Radiat Oncol Biol Phys 1988;15:1267-1273.
45.   Hoffman HT, Karnell LH, Shah JP, Ariyan S, Brown GS, Fee WE, Glass AG, Goepfert H,
         Ossoff RH, Fremgen AM. Hypopharyngeal cancer patient care evaluation. Laryngoscope
         1997;107:1005-1017.
46.   Million RR, Cassisi NJ, Mancuso AA. Hypopharynx: Pharyngeal walls, pyriform sinus,
         postcricoid pharynx. Million RR, Cassisi NJ, editors. Management of Head and Neck Cancer:
         A Multidisciplinary Approach, 2 ed. Philadelphia: J.B. Lippincott Company; 1994:505-532.
47.   Amdur RJ, Mendenhall WM, Stringer SP, Villaret DB, Cassisi NJ. Organ preservation with
         radiotherapy for T1-T2 carcinoma of the pyriform sinus. Head Neck 2001;23:353-362.
48.   Mendenhall WM, Parsons JT, Cassisi NJ, Million RR. Squamous cell carcinoma of the
         pyriform sinus treated with radical radiation therapy. Radiother Oncol 1987;9:201-208.
49.   Mendenhall WM, Parsons JT, Mancuso AA, Cassisi NJ, Million RR. Squamous cell carcinoma
         of the pharyngeal wall treated with irradiation. Radiother Oncol 1988;11:205-212.
50.   Fein DA, Mendenhall WM, Parsons JT, Stringer SP, Cassisi NJ, Million RR. Pharyngeal wall
         carcinoma treated with radiotherapy: impact of treatment technique and fractionation. Int J
         Radiat Oncol Biol Phys 1993;26:751-757.

Chapter 6

ADVANCED HEAD AND NECK CANCER-SURGERY AND RECONSTRUCTION

Brandon G. Bentz, MD and Dennis H. Kraus, MD
Memorial Sloan-Kettering Cancer Center

INTRODUCTION

Traditional treatment of early head and neck cancer is surgery or radiation therapy as a single modality, while advanced (Stage III and IV) disease is treated more often with a combination of surgery and radiation therapy. Despite using this combined modality therapy, over the past three decades little improvement in overall and disease specific survival has been realized. The addition of chemotherapy to these established treatment strategies has begun to improve survival, and has fundamentally changed the way in which clinicians approach patients with head and neck cancer [1]. Yet, optimism for this improved survival must be tempered by the fact that very little prospective randomized data has demonstrated improvement in overall survival with this addition of chemotherapy [2]. Therefore, surgical therapy with reconstruction continues to play a central role for advanced stage head and neck cancer cases [3].

Because of the rapid evolution of therapeutic strategies, roles of individual treatment modalities and their interrelationships must be constantly reevaluated in order to provide each patient with the most optimal treatment approach to a given clinical problem. Within this chapter we will outline the role of surgical resection and reconstruction for advanced aerodigestive tract squamous cell carcinomas, advanced carcinomas of the salivary gland, paranasal sinuses, temporal bone, and skin. We will briefly describe the typical presenting signs and symptoms of these various tumors, discuss etiologies, consider the natural history of these tumors, and utilize this to describe the indications and contraindications for primary surgery versus surgical salvage. General details of some of the various surgical procedures will also be reviewed, and finally we will compare and contrast the difficulties of surgical salvage, and treatments for combined modality therapy failures.

AERODIGESTIVE TRACT SQUAMOUS CELL CARCINOMAS

Presentation

The overwhelming majority of cases of head and neck cancer involve mucosal squamous cell carcinoma of the upper aerodigestive tract. Presenting symptoms depend largely on the location of the primary lesion, which may impact on timely diagnosis and subsequent treatment. In example, primaries of the larynx present early with hoarseness and dysphagia, thus potentiating early detection and a favorable prognosis. On the other hand, pyriform sinus primaries have less conspicuous presenting signs and symptoms. This causes later diagnosis and negatively impacts prognosis. Therefore, a high index of suspicion and diligence in pursuit of possible subtle presentations can bring about early detection and a favorable outcome.

Nasopharyngeal carcinomas may present with very minor symptoms. Most commonly these tumors present as a unilateral or bilateral painless neck mass due to the tendency for early lymphatic metastasis [4]. Nasal symptoms may include unilateral nasal obstruction, blood stained nasal secretions, or epistaxis. Aural symptoms from Eustachian tube orifice blockage include hearing loss, tinnitus, otalgia, and/or a middle ear effusion. The incidence of cranial nerve dysfunction is about 20% [5], and may involve cranial nerves III, IV, VI, or IX to XII. Other less frequent symptoms are trismus and headaches.

Oral cavity squamous cell carcinomas most frequently present with a non-healing mucosal ulceration or area of induration, ill-fitting dentures, loosening of the teeth, trismus, or weight loss. A hyperkeratotic or an inflamed plaque may represent a premalignant lesion. Erosion increases the likelihood of representing a frank carcinoma [6]. Pain may also accompany these lesions. Because the presentation of a lesion in this area is conspicuous, oral cavity squamous cell carcinoma primaries tend to present earlier in their disease course.

The site of the oropharyngeal primary significantly influences the presentation of these lesions. Early presenting symptoms include a sore throat, referred otalgia, or a foreign body sensation. Later symptoms may include odynophagia, dysphagia, a muffled voice, trismus, hemoptysis, weight loss, or adenopathy [7]. Symptoms of persistent odynophagia or unexpected otalgia should raise concern. Overall, these tumors tend to present later in the course of disease progression and therefore carry a worse prognosis.

In contrast, laryngeal lesions tend to present earlier than prior areas discussed, and thus carry a better prognosis. In example, glottic carcinomas present very early as hoarseness. Other symptoms of glottic carcinomas include dysphagia or a globus sensation. In contrast, supraglottic or subglottic primaries may develop with only vague complaints of dysphagia or a mass sensation in the throat. These primaries tend to present later in the course of their disease, with a negative impact on prognosis.

Hypopharyngeal squamous cell carcinomas are notorious for presenting at a very late stage of disease. This is due to the fact that the presenting symptoms such as dysphagia occur secondary to massive disease. Furthermore, areas of the pyriform sinus, post-cricoid region, and posterior wall are not readily examined even with the use of flexible endoscopic examination. Other symptoms, such as weight loss or referred otalgia may be falsely attributed to other etiologies.

Etiology

The etiologic agents primarily responsible for the development of upper aerodigestive tract squamous cell carcinomas are alcohol and tobacco exposure. Overwhelming evidence supports the increased risk associated with tobacco use, accounting for a six-fold increase in risk of developing this disease [8]. Alcohol is considered an independent direct carcinogen, with squamous cell carcinoma being six times more common in drinkers than non-drinkers [9]. Other more controversial risk factors include viral exposure, of which human papilloma virus types 16 and 18 are thought to be related to the development of this disease [10]. Other less definite associations include chronic mucosal irritation [11], nutritional deficiencies [12], and immunosuppression [13]. Women with Plummer-Vinson Syndrome (Patterson-Kelley Syndrome) are at increased risk of developing post-cricoid and mobile tongue carcinomas [14], perhaps due to chronic mucosal inflammation or nutritional deficiencies.

Owing to the different patient population, nasopharyngeal squamous cell carcinomas (NPC) have a somewhat different spectrum of etiologies. Etiologic agents for NPC include nitrosamine exposure [15], salted smoked fish ingestion [4, 16], as well as EBV infections [17, 18]. The overwhelmingly high incidence in patients with southeastern Chinese ancestry suggests a genetic predisposition [19]. Evaluation must consider these risk factors.

Medical Work-up

Confirmation of clinical suspicion starts with a thorough history and physical exam. Epithelial malignancies usually present as a raised, indurated, and often ulcerated lesion of the mucosal lining. The lesion may be adherent to adjacent structures such as the skin or mandible, carrying with it prognostic as well as therapeutic implications. The size of the lesion should be estimated by inspection and palpation, and the metastatic status of the neck should be evaluated by deep palpation of all neck regions. Associated secondary signs of the malignancy should be sought. In example, a serous middle ear effusion may strongly suggest a nasopharyngeal carcinoma [20]. Lastly, the entire upper aerodigestive tract should be inspected by direct flexible fiberoptic examination in order to evaluate the extent of the primary lesion as well as evaluation for the presence of synchronous primary lesions that can occur in up to 15% of patients [21].

Radiographic evaluation should be done on all patients suspected of an upper aerodigestive tract squamous cell carcinoma. The aim of these radiographic exams is to gain information about the depth of invasion, as well as the metastatic disease status of the neck. This is necessary, since physical examination has been quoted to have only a 60% sensitivity for metastatic lymphadenopathy [22].

Indications/Contraindications for Surgical Therapy

Indications and contraindications for primary versus salvage surgery are evolving for advanced stage head and neck cancer, and are subsite-specific. Therefore, we will review these subsite-specific indications and contraindications of primary surgery with or without adjuvant therapy, and discuss the role of salvage surgery for those instances in which primary surgery is not indicated. We will then discuss the individual techniques, the difficulties of salvage after primary therapy by other modalities, and finally the reconstructive options for therapeutic failures followed by surgical salvage.

Nasopharyngeal Carcinoma (NPC)

Because the nasopharynx represents an area not easily accessible to surgical approach, the propensity for NPC to infiltrate surrounding tissues, and the inherent radiosensitivity of these tumors, surgical intervention is not used as primary therapy [23]. Furthermore, chemotherapy is increasingly demonstrating utility in the primary treatment setting [24]. Therefore, surgical interventions are reserved predominantly for salvage after failures from other modalities.

Regional recurrence or persistent disease after primary radiation therapy for NPC is not uncommon [25], and can be treated with a second course of radical external beam radiotherapy, brachytherapy, or surgical resection. Indications for surgical salvage include: 1) extension into the parapharyngeal space, 2) size that exceeds that which can be adequately controlled by brachytherapy, or 3) recurrence after brachytherapy [23]. Various approaches to the nasopharynx have been described; varying widely in the exposure provided and associated morbidities. Skull base approaches are associated with the morbidities of meningitis and encephalocele [26] due to subarachnoid space exposure and nasal cavity bacterial colonization. Transantral (through the maxillary sinus) or transnasal (through the nose) anterior approaches do not provide adequate exposure, especially laterally, for complete tumor removal [27]. Even the additional downfracturing of the palate after transverse maxillary osteotomies provides little added exposure to the lateral walls of the nasopharynx [28, 29]. The lateral approach to the nasopharynx has its supporters, but requires a radical mastoidectomy and exposure of the infratemporal fossa. This places the internal carotid artery, the Vth cranial nerve, and the floor of the middle cranial fossa within the field of dissection [30]. Other approaches, including the transpalatal, transmaxillary, and transcervical approaches [31], appear to be only indicated for small, centrally located recurrences, but the operative morbidity is low in the absence of carotid artery exposure [23]. Lastly, an anterolateral "maxillary swing" [32, 33] appears to provide adequate exposure, with minimal operative morbidity. Associated morbidities reported are palatal fistulas and trismus. Postoperative cosmesis is acceptable.

Another consideration for nasopharyngeal carcinoma post-irradiation failures is how to manage those tumors that fail in the neck. Studies utilizing serial sections of radical neck dissections for recurrent neck disease after chemoradiotherapy failure demonstrated that these recurrences had a higher likelihood of complete nodal involvement with extracapsular spread, multiple lymph nodes, and infiltration into adjacent structures. Therefore, surgical salvage should include a comprehensive radical neck dissection with sacrifice of the sternocleidomastoid, internal jugular vein, and spinal accessory nerve [34].

Oropharynx

Of all subsites of the upper aerodigestive tract, treatment strategies for primaries of the larynx and oropharynx have undergone the most change over the past 10 to 15 years. Prior to the advent of chemotherapeutic protocols, the primary mode of therapy for squamous cell carcinoma of the oropharynx had been irradiation or preoperative radiation therapy followed by surgery. These treatment approaches yielded only small improvements in cure rates [35]. More recent improvements in radiation therapy techniques [36], surgical resection [3], and the introduction of chemotherapy [37], as well as improved diagnostic awareness has started to positively impact prognosis.   Today, therapeutic approaches to the oropharynx are primary surgery, primary radiation therapy, and various combinations of chemoradiotherapy [38].

The role of primary surgical therapy with or without adjuvant radiation therapy varies with the oropharyngeal subsite involved. Primary surgery for advanced base of tongue squamous cell carcinoma have been reported to yield 5-year survival rates of 64% for Stage 3 and 59% for Stage 4 disease [3]. These data include the use of post-operative radiation therapy and neck dissection, either therapeutic or selective, for clinically N0 neck disease. Also, bilateral neck dissections should be strongly considered since the incidence of contralateral disease is high for primaries of this centrally located site [3, 39, 40].

Yet, high rates of cancer control and survival come at a price. Patients who undergo resection of more than half of their tongue base develop significant dysarthria, and are at least temporarily dependent upon a feeding tube for nutritional support.   Significant long-term morbidities include aspiration, dysarthria, life-long feeding tube placement, and cosmetic disfigurement [41]. Surgical mortality also varies between 0 and 4% [3, 40, 42-44].

For tonsillar lesions, indications for primary surgical resection are deep invasion without a significant exophytic component, or stage III and IV disease [45]. Surgical management of stage III or IV tonsillar lesions may lead to increased morbidity [45]. Planned combined surgery and radiation therapy has been shown to improve cure rate for T4 lesions by as much as 20% [46, 47]. Some have argued that the use of hyperfractionation schemes of radiation therapy alone can also significantly improve disease-specific survival for T4 lesions, but this appears to be less efficacious than combined therapy [48].

For carcinoma of the soft palate, excellent results can be achieved for T1 to T3 lesions with the use of radiation therapy alone, but the local control rate for T4 lesions drops off to less than 50% [45]. Therefore, patients with T4 cancer of the soft palate should be considered for combined surgery plus post-operative radiation therapy. Reconstruction most often includes prosthetic obturation [49].

Oropharyngeal wall lesions are usually large, requiring removal of a significant amount of pharyngeal wall with the potential for leaving the carotid artery exposed or causing significant cranial nerve dysfunction. Therefore, these tumors traditionally were treated with primary radiation therapy. Around the 1980's, advances in surgical reconstruction with the use of free-flap technology made resection of advanced pharyngeal wall carcinomas much less distasteful. Studies have demonstrated that improved survival can be accomplished with the combination of surgical resection and postoperative radiation therapy for pharyngeal wall primaries [50, 51]. Frequently, the ipsilateral neck will need to have a lymphatic dissection. Yet, pharyngeal resection carries with it significant morbidities including the loss of pharyngeal sensory and motor function leading to an increased risk of aspiration. In older patients, age-related loss of pulmonary reserve and other co-morbid disease may warrant a concomitant laryngectomy for aspiration protection when a significant amount of pharynx is to be resected [52]. Yet, preservation of the larynx is possible in selected patients [53]. Although surgery is an option, we are increasingly utilizing chemoradiotherapy for all patients with advanced squamous cell carcinoma of the oropharynx.

Oral Cavity

The choice of therapy for advanced oral cavity squamous carcinomas depends upon the site and size of the primary, the patient's physical, social, and personal status, and the physician's experience and skill. Advanced oral cavity squamous cell carcinomas are most often treated with a combination of surgery and radiation therapy [54]. In general, as oral cavity cancers increase in size, the potential for post-operative difficulties with swallowing and speech increases [55]. Additionally, there is much debate over the timing of radiation therapy. No prospective, randomized studies have been able to demonstrate a clear advantage of post-operative when compared to preoperative radiation therapy. Certain reports tend to show a benefit in loco-regional control with postoperative radiation therapy, but this does not translate into improvement in overall survival [56].

Lesions of the oral tongue usually require at least a partial glossectomy via mandibulotomy, a marginal, or segmental mandibulectomy approach for surgical resection followed by radiation therapy [57]. The resultant speech and swallowing morbidities of surgical resection are enhanced by the use of adjuvant radiation therapy. Reconstruction can be achieved with primary closure, local, regional, or distant flaps.

The best survival results for advanced lip carcinomas are seen with a combination of surgery and adjuvant radiation therapy [58]. Surgical resection of the lip must consider the size of the resultant defect in order to plan optimal reconstruction. Defects up to 70% may be closed primarily, but one must remember that the larger the defect the higher the likelihood of microstomia. Other more complex advancement and rotation flaps may be used in defects between one-half and two-thirds of the lip. Defects of near-total or total resections may be closed with advancement flaps, nasolabial flaps, regional flaps, and/or free microvascularized flaps [59].

Buccal mucosal carcinomas are usually managed with combined therapy, but often these patients present in such advanced stages that they are deemed inoperable. Studies have demonstrated that up to 50% of T4 cancers of the buccal mucosa are inoperable based on extensive fungation with edema, satellite nodules, pterygoid muscle involvement, severe trismus, and fixed metastatic nodes [60]. Post-treatment trismus may signify post-irradiation pterygoid muscle fibrosis or tumor invasion.

Due to the close proximity of buccal carcinomas to the mandible and maxilla, resection of normal mandibular or maxillary bone as a margin is often necessary. Excellent local control can be achieved [60]. Clinical or radiographic evidence of bony involvement requires comprehensive surgical resection.

Cancer of the floor of mouth often abuts the mandible, and therefore mandibular resection is often required. Additionally, these tumors may invade the sublingual gland and intrinsic muscles of the tongue [61], and therefore these structures must be addressed in an en-bloc resection. Several studies have documented improved locoregional control with the addition of postoperative radiation therapy to primary surgery for cancers of this subsite [62, 63].

Surgery for stage III and IV retromolar trigone lesions often includes a segmental mandibulectomy. Major resections for bulky lesions may include adjacent soft palate and/or oropharynx. Some defects can be closed primarily, but most often lateral defects are repaired with a skin graft, myocutaneous, or free flap. Lateral resections do not cause significant speech and swallowing morbidity, and obviate the need for mandibular reconstruction [8].

Assessment of alveolar ridge carcinomas must carefully evaluate the status of the mandibular cortex and mental nerve. Periosteum provides a barrier to invasion, but radiation therapy may remove the periosteal layer and thus make the extent of cancer less predictable. Invasion may occur through an old tooth socket or microperforations of the occlusal surface of the mandible. Larger lesions may invade directly through the cortex itself [64]. Any direct bone involvement requires mandibulectomy [8].

Advanced hard palate carcinomas require partial or total maxillectomy. After removal of the tumor, maxillary sinus mucosal defects can be lined with a skin graft. This allows for ease of inspection, close follow-up, and early recurrence detection. Palatal defects are closed with regional flaps or dental prostheses. Total palatal defects can be reconstructed with temporalis muscle flaps or free flaps with good results.

Larynx

Management of advanced stage glottic cancers is one of the more controversial topics of head and neck surgery today. Primary surgical therapy usually means a total laryngectomy that carries with it the associated issues of alaryngeal speech, stomal care, and social isolation. The advent of combined chemoradiotherapy protocols for organ preservation has added another level of complexity to treatment planning. Adding to the controversy is that selected patients with T3 and T4 glottic carcinomas can be cured with radiation therapy alone [65]. It appears that tumors not invading the vocal process of the arytenoids, unilateral in location, not obstructing the airway, or have a volume of less than 3.5 cm^3 fall into a "favorable" category for radiation therapy alone [66, 67]. Overall, it appears across a number of studies that the success of salvage with preservation of the larynx after initial radiation therapy approximates 50-60% [68, 69].

Five-year local control rates of 80-95% can be expected after total laryngectomy for T3 and T4 glottic carcinomas [70, 71]. Yet, this does not often translate into a similar increase in 5-year overall survival since many of these patients will eventually die of regional and distant disease failure [72]. Therefore, for local control, the total laryngectomy remains the gold standard for surgical intervention in patients with advanced glottic carcinomas.

An increasing number of studies are demonstrating that the addition of adjuvant radiation therapy to surgical interventions appears to improve locoregional control for advanced glottic carcinomas [73]. Although studies that compare surgery alone with surgery followed by radiation therapy directly are rare, most would agree that postoperative radiation therapy is indicated for those tumors with significant subglottic extension, involvement of the adjacent hypopharynx or tongue base, extralaryngeal or perineural spread, or concomitant neck disease which requires adjuvant radiation therapy [74].

Conservation surgery for very highly selected T3 glottic carcinomas have been advocated by several authors. What these groups have found is that the vertical hemilaryngectomy will achieve an adequate disease-free survival in these selected patients [75-77]. Ultimately, the decision about the use of conservation surgery lies in the mechanism of vocal cord fixation. Only direct invasion of the thyroarytenoid muscle as a cause for vocal cord paralysis allows for vertical hemilaryngectomy [76].

Surgical intervention for advanced stage supraglottic squamous cell carcinomas appears indicated for T3 tumors or larger. Local control for T3 cancers of the supraglottis treated with radiation therapy alone is approximately 60%, whereas T4 cancers treated similarly achieve only about a 40-50% local control rate [78-80]. Local control for surgery alone has been very poorly studied due to the overwhelming tendency to add postoperative radiation therapy for treatment of these tumors [74], but certain studies have demonstrated at least a 50-100% cure rate for T3 and T4 supraglottic carcinomas treated with surgery alone or surgery plus radiation therapy [81-83].

Only very selected T3 supraglottic tumors are eligible for a supraglottic laryngectomy. Those that are deemed T3 by preepiglottic space extension alone are well suited for this procedure. Also, tumors that extend onto the medial wall of the pyriform sinus are good candidates for supraglottic laryngectomy with inclusion of a portion of the pyriform sinus. Cancers that are T4 by extension onto the base of tongue or hyoid bone are also resectable by an extended supraglottic laryngectomy [74]. Resection of a portion of the pharynx may precipitate difficulties with swallowing, and therefore these patients may be better served with a total laryngectomy. An example of such patient is seen in Figure 1. This patient demonstrated a large supraglottic carcinoma with pre-epiglottic space involvement, extralaryngeal extension [Figure 1a.], pyriform sinus and skin involvement. Resection included a laryngopharyngectomy [Figure 1b.] with reconstruction including a jejunal free flap [Figure 1c.] and deltopectoral flap for skin coverage [Figure 1d].

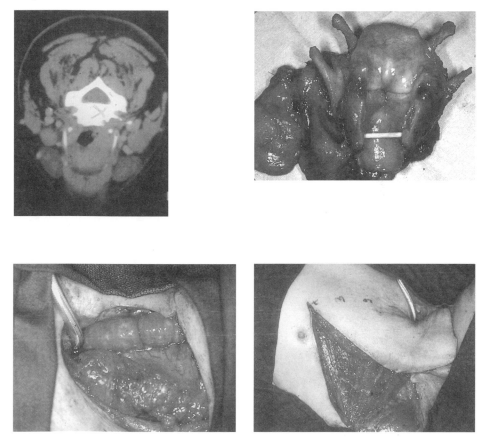

Figures 1a-1d. **Example of an advanced supraglottic treated with primary surgery. This patient had a large supraglottic carcinoma with pre-epiglottic space involvement, extralaryngeal extension (1a.), pyriform sinus and skin involvement. The patient underwent laryngopharyngectomy (1b) with reconstruction including a free flap (1c.) and deltopectoral flap (1d).**

An alternative treatment strategy primarily for T3 supraglottic carcinoma patients is radical radiation therapy with surgical salvage. Overall, this approach compares favorably with the results achieved by primary surgery with or without postoperative radiation therapy, but a higher percentage retain their larynges [78, 84, 85].

The addition of chemotherapy to radiation therapy for advanced laryngeal carcinomas has increased the awareness of organ preservation as an outcome goal. Figure 2 demonstrates a patient with a large glottic carcinoma [Figure 2a] in which the CT scan demonstrates significant subglottic extension [Figure 2b]. Figure 2c shows the 3-dimensional reconstruction of the lesion. Following combined chemotherapy/radiation therapy treatment, the patient was left with a large synechia of the subglottis [Figure 2d.]. Yet, the patient continues to have a functional larynx [Figure 2e. demonstrates a view of the adducted larynx on fiberoptic laryngoscopy], and he continues to work as a trial lawyer.

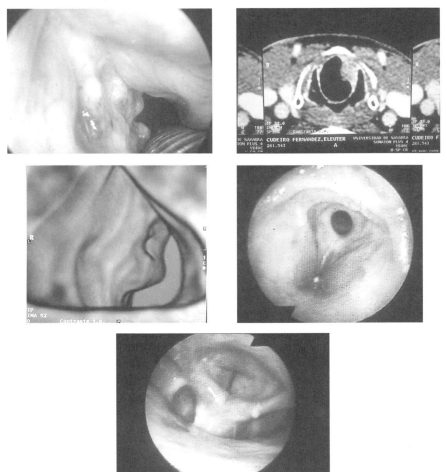

Figure 2a- 2e. **Example of an advanced laryngeal cancer treated with organ preservation with chemotherapy and radiation (2a). Significant sublglottic extension is noted in 2b. Fig 2c shows 3-dimensional reconstruction. A large subglottic synechia (2d) did not interfere with laryngeal function (2e).**

Utilization of radical radiotherapy with surgical salvage must take into account the increase in postoperative complications with total laryngectomy after radiotherapy [86, 87]. Fistula rates average about 40% for these cases compared with 5-10% for primary laryngectomy [88]. Others argue that primary radiation causes an inability to detect recurrent cancer leading to a decreased overall survival [89], an increased rate of distant metastases due to radiation-induced alterations in lymphatic drainage [90], and a philosophical stance of treating the neck and primary with a single treatment modality.

Subglottic carcinomas are so rare that no large series have examined treatments for advanced stage disease. Overall these tumors present late, and therefore the results of any treatment strategy are relatively poor. A number of small series recommend total laryngectomy with or without neck dissections along with post-operative radiation therapy for advanced lesions [91, 92].

Complications of surgical treatment for advanced laryngeal carcinomas depend upon the type of procedure performed and the general health of the patient. Complications from vertical hemilaryngectomy include aspiration, delayed decannulation, and diminished vocal quality. Total laryngectomy complications include wound infection, fistula formation, and pharyngeal stenosis. As would be expected, all these complications occur at a higher frequency with the use of radiation therapy prior to surgical resection [93]. Free tissue transfer may obviate these complications. Stenosis of the tracheostoma is a relatively common complication that has been reported to vary from 4-42% [94, 95]. Factors contributing to stomal stenosis include radiation therapy use, previous tracheotomy, inadequate removal of surrounding soft tissues, transection of tracheal rings, concomitant tracheoesophageal puncture for voice restoration, fistula formation, pectoralis flap reconstruction, and tracheostomal infection [96].

Surgical management of neck metastasis is closely linked to the primary subsite of the larynx. The highest incidence of clinically evident or occult nodal metastasis is seen in carcinomas of the supraglottis, with lateral neck nodes being most at risk. Nodal metastasis to the submandibular and submental nodes occurs in only 5% [97, 98]. Carcinoma of the glottic larynx carries much less of a risk of nodal metastasis, but lateral neck nodes are still the most at-risk nodal group [97]. Bilateral and contralateral nodal metastasis is rare in glottic carcinomas except for tumors with extensive supraglottic or subglottic extension. Lastly, very little is written about the metastatic behavior of subglottic laryngeal carcinomas, but overall estimates approximate 20%. Some reports suggest about a 65% incidence of paratracheal lymphatic metastasis from subglottic carcinomas [99]. Taken together, therapeutic neck dissections are indicated for any clinically positive nodal disease. Prophylactic neck dissections are indicated for any supraglottic or subglottic carcinomas, and for high T stage glottic carcinomas. Therapeutic neck dissections should always be undertaken for clinically evident nodal disease.

SALIVARY CARCINOMAS

Clinical Presentation

Cancers of the salivary glands most often present as an asymptomatic, slow-growing, solitary mass. Pain is reported in 10-29% of patients with cancer of the parotid gland, while only 6.5% of cancers of submandibular origin present with pain [100]. Episodic pain suggests that the mass is more likely to be of inflammatory or obstructive in etiology rather than neoplastic. Constant pain is more suggestive of a malignant than a benign process [101]. The duration of symptoms tend to be much shorter in patients with cancer. Other signs to suggest a malignant process include facial nerve dysfunction (in 10-15% of parotid malignancies) [102], or fixation to adjacent structures. Minor salivary gland carcinomas can present as an ulceration of the mucosa that resembles a squamous cell carcinoma. Needle biopsy makes the definitive diagnosis.

Etiology

The etiology of salivary gland carcinomas remains poorly understood. Alcohol and tobacco, etiologic agents that figure prominently in aerodigestive tract carcinogenesis, does not appear to play a significant role in the athogenesis of salivary gland carcinomas. Some studies have demonstrated an association with the development of breast cancer, but other studies refute this association [103]. Additional hypothesized etiologies include low-dose radiation [104], since survivors of the atomic bomb at Nagasaki or Hiroshima are associated with an increased incidence of salivary tumors. Occupational exposure to wood dust and the furniture industry has been linked with an increased incidence of minor salivary gland neoplasms, particularly adenocarcinoma of the sinonasal tract [105].

Natural History

The natural history of malignant salivary gland tumors is one of progressive growth, invasion of surrounding structures with functional compromise, and eventual lymphatic metastasis. Other than dysfunction of the VII nerve, V, IX, X or XII nerves can rarely be involved. Parotid carcinomas can traverse the stylomandibular tunnel and cause considerable lateral pharyngeal wall distortion from deep lobe/parapharyngeal space involvement [106].

Salivary cancers can present in a variety of histopathological types [See Table 1]. Those subtypes that demonstrate a higher metastatic rate (i.e. high-grade mucoepidermoid carcinoma, adenocarcinoma, undifferentiated carcinoma, and squamous cell carcinoma) may warrant a prophylactic selective neck dissection [107]. Cancers of low histological grade (low grade mucoepidermoid carcinoma, acinic cell carcinoma) do not necessitate a neck dissection unless clinical evidence of metastatic disease exists [108]. Surrounding lymph nodes can be inspected and palpated during excision of the primary lesion, with suspicious lymph nodes sent for frozen section diagnosis [109]. Frozen section specimens that are positive require neck dissection. If concern exists over the adequacy of surgical resection or the stage or grade of the primary tumor, post-operative radiation therapy can include prophylactic neck irradiation [110].

Table 1.
Malignant Salivary Gland Tumors
Carcinoma Ex-Pleomorphic Adenoma
Mucoepidermoid Carcinoma
       High, Intermediate, Low Grade
Adenoid Cystic Carcinoma
Acinic Cell Carcinoma
Adenocarcinoma
       Mucus Producing, Salivary Duct
Oncocytic Carcinoma
Clear Cell Carcinoma
Epithelial/Myoepithelial Carcinoma
Squamous Cell Carcinoma
Undifferentiated Carcinoma
Metastatic Lesions
Miscellaneous Lesions

Clinical and Radiographic Evaluation

The clinical evaluation of a patient with a salivary gland carcinoma starts with a thorough head and neck examination. Submandibular gland lesions are palpated bimanually to assess the extent of the tumor as well as invasion of adjacent structures. Bulging of the lateral wall of the oropharynx suggests a deep lobe parotid tumor that has extended through the stylomandibular tunnel. The palate and mucosa are examined for subtle submucosal masses that suggest a minor salivary gland lesion. Trismus is seen with involvement of the pterygoid musculature. The neck is also palpated for pathologically enlarged lymph nodes, especially in those tumors with a high propensity for lymphatic metastasis such as high-grade mucoepidermoid carcinoma. Skin tethering is a relatively rare finding, but is thought to be a negative prognostic sign [111].

Radiographic evaluation is required for adequate assessment of the extent of invasion into surrounding structures. For this purpose, the CT scan and/or the MRI may be utilized. The CT scan provides better delineation of bony structures, whereas the MRI will offer better definition of soft tissue invasion, including intracranial extension. Some reports espouse the superiority of MRI analysis for salivary carcinomas [112]. Clinical judgment should guide the use of radiographic analysis.

Surgery for Advanced Salivary Carcinomas

The standard surgical therapy for advanced malignant salivary tumors remains resection of the involved gland and invaded adjacent structures [108]. The smallest procedure to be performed for a parotid tumor, benign or malignant, is a superficial parotidectomy. This procedure entails the removal of all parotid tissue superficial to the plane of the facial nerve as it traverses the parenchyma of the parotid gland. The overwhelming majority of submandibular gland tumors are successfully removed with a submandibular gland and submandibular triangle excision. Extensive tumors may require resection of adjacent masseter, sternocleidomastoid or pterygoid muscles, mandible or mastoid, skin, and/or nerves [113]. Immediate reconstruction of the facial nerve after resection provides the most optimum functional outcomes. The techniques of reconstruction used often depend upon the tissue resected and the tissue remaining.

As mentioned earlier, parapharyngeal space involvement may present as a mass in the lateral pharyngeal wall. As the tumor expands, other signs and symptoms may arise (Horner's syndrome, jugular foramen syndrome, and/or middle ear effusion) and are highly suggestive of a malignant tumor.

CT scans and MRI are both essential to evaluate these tumors [114]. The transparotid-transcervical approach is most commonly used to surgically access these tumors [115]. Extension into the infratemporal fossa may be addressed by extending the preauricular incision into a bicoronal incision. Osteotomy of the zygoma with downward transposition of the temporalis muscle allows access to the infratemporal region. Removal of the styloid process and dislocation or osteotomy of the mandible may allow for even more exposure.

Resection of a margin of normal tissue is usually essential to an adequate surgical intervention. With salivary carcinomas this may not always be possible since they may literally lie on top of vital structures, such as the VII nerve, without direct involvement of that structure. The surgeon must rely heavily on clinical judgment as well as radiological assessment when planning the extent of surgical resection. The decision to sacrifice the facial nerve or resect other vital structures should not be made on frozen section biopsy since permanent section diagnoses is found to change in a significant number of cases [116]. Only intraoperative evidence of direct nerve involvement warrants facial nerve sacrifice [117].

If the facial nerve is to be resected due to surgical evidence of tumor involvement, frozen section confirmation of negative nerve margins can be obtained. This may require tracing the nerve into the mastoid via a mastoidectomy. If the cancer is locally invasive, all other structures that are involved with tumor should be resected including the skin, muscle, mandible, temporal bone, and deep lobe of the parotid. After sacrifice of an involved nerve, repair options must be considered.

ADVANCED PARANASAL SINUS CARCINOMAS

Advanced carcinomas of the sinonasal tract represents a complex and difficult problem, not only from the standpoint of the anatomical proximity to vital structures, but also with respect to the wide variety of pathological entities that are found in this area [Table 2]. Despite these challenges, technical advances in diagnosis, imaging, and surgical resection has fostered optimism over improvement in disease-free and overall survival for these patients.

Table 2.
Sinonasal Tract Malignant Tumors
Epithelial
        Squamous Cell Carcinoma
            Differentiated
            Basaloid squamous
            Adenosquamous
        Nonsquamous cell carcinoma
            Adenoid cystic carcinoma
            Mucoepidermoid carcinoma
            Adenocarcinoma
            Neuroendocrine carcinoma
            Hyalinizing clear cell carcinoma
      Melanoma
      Olfactory neuroblastoma
      Sinonasal undifferentiated carcinoma (SNUC)
Nonepithelial
      Chondrosarcoma
      Osteogenic sarcoma
      Soft tissue sarcoma
          Fibrosarcoma
          Malignant fibrous histiocytoma
          Hemangiopericytoma
          Angiosarcoma
          Kaposi's sarcoma
          Rhabdomyosarconma
    Lymphoproliferative
          Lymphoma
          Polymorphic reticulosis
          Plasmacytoma
      Metastatic

Etiology

Although the causes of sinonasal neoplasms remain unknown, certain epidemiological associations have been established. In general, sinus cancer is found to be more prevalent in developing countries heavily involved with chemical industries [118]. Workers in the heavy metal industries exposed to nickel, chromium, and radium demonstrate an increased incidence of these carcinomas. One study found that nickel workers involved in electrolytic work for more than 15 years were found to have a 250-fold increased incidence of sinus carcinoma [119]. This study found that biopsies taken from the middle turbinate of these patients demonstrated evidence of dysplasia in 21% of the workers. This figure is similar to another study examining nickel workers middle turbinate, demonstrating a 17% incidence of dysplastic changes [120]. All these were found to be independent from smoking history.

Another study demonstrated a 1000 times increased incidence of adenocarcinoma of the ethmoid sinus in patients with a history of woodworking when compared to the general population [121]. This increased incidence was found to approximate the incidence of lung carcinoma. An additional study examining woodworkers in the United States found that hard or softwood dust possibly synergize with smoking to increase the incidence of sinonasal carcinoma [122].

Another risk factor was radium dial painters who are at increased risk of osteosarcomas, including facial bones. Exposure to leather and boot industry products, especially those involved in the tanning process are at increased risk of sinonasal epithelial malignancies [123]. Other industrial exposures that increase the risk of developing these malignancies are mineral or isopropyl oils, lacquer paints, soldering and welding chemicals [122]. Unproven, but speculated risk factors include chronic infection, tobacco, alcohol, and previous irradiation [124].

Physical Examination

The most important aspect of diagnosis that improves survival is early detection, and subsequent early treatment. Signs and symptoms of early sinonasal tumors are subtle and nonspecific with early lesions often being completely asymptomatic. Extension of tumor into adjacent structures becomes the presenting complaint. Therefore, a high index of suspicion will pay off for these patients.

Unilateral nasal or sinus complaints require investigation. Any unilateral polyposis on anterior rhinoscopy requires biopsy [125]. Additionally, epistaxis or anosmia should have a thorough investigation. Extension to adjacent structures may be indicated by proptosis, diplopia, and/or limitation of ocular mobility. Extension into the anterior cranial fossa may be indicated by anosmia. Cranial nerve dysfunction also indicates tumor extension beyond the confines of the nasal/paranasal region. Extension anteriorly through the anterior face of the maxilla or inferiorly through the palate will lead to facial or oral cavity swelling.

Imaging

Imaging of the paranasal sinuses is indicated whenever there is a clinical suspicion of a neoplastic process. Bony destruction and soft tissue invasion suggest an aggressive process, usually a malignant neoplasm. Imaging allows for the evaluation of location, size, extent, and invasiveness of the primary tumor as well as the presence or absence of regional or distant metastasis. Such information is crucial for preoperative and/or therapeutic considerations. Lastly, the advantages and disadvantages of each of the imaging modalities should be weighed prior to utilization.

Neoplasms of the paranasal sinuses should initially be evaluated by CT scan [124]. The main advantage of the CT scan is delineation of bony architecture and contrast enhanced tumor definition. The MRI is unsurpassed in the delineation of soft tissue details both intracranially and into the surrounding soft tissue spaces. Obliteration of fat planes such as the pterygopalatine fossa, the infratemporal fossa, and other cervical compartments usually indicates invasion of tumor through these boundaries. Dural involvement or perineural spread can be identified with a high-quality MRI [124]. Even more important is the ability of the MRI to distinguish tumor from retained sinus secretions, therefore avoiding overestimation of the extent of disease [126]. Lastly, angiography is seldom required since the advent of magnetic resonance angiography (MRA). Yet traditional angiography may be beneficial in such vascular neoplasms as the juvenile nasal angiofibroma, to delineate invasion into major arteries such as the internal carotid, for preoperative embolization, or to evaluate collateral cerebral circulation if resection and/or ligation of intracerebral blood supply is considered.

Finally, biopsy is required to make a definitive pathological diagnosis [124]. This not only confirms the clinical diagnosis, but also guides the choice of therapeutic options. Approaches to obtain a biopsy can be endoscopic or less often via an open approach. If the diagnosis of lymphoma is entertained, fresh tissue should be sent in saline rather than fixed in formalin. Further, if a vascular tumor is suspected, biopsy should be deferred until angiography and possible embolization is performed [127]. Rarely, an intracranial communication such as a meningocele, an encephalocele, or a nasal glioma is suspected and should be confirmed by imaging prior to biopsy. This avoids the attendant risk of CSF leak and subsequent meningitis.

Treatment of Advanced Stage Disease

Surgical extirpation with or without adjunctive radiation remains the mainstay of treatment for these challenging tumors. This approach provides the best chance for control or cure of these diseases. Surgery is indicated whenever the tumor can be safely resected with acceptable morbidity and in the absence of distant metastasis [128, 129]. The development of new craniofacial approaches has extended the indications for surgery to include skull base involvement [130, 131]. Furthermore, advances in reconstruction, including microvascular free flaps, pericranial flaps, and prosthetic rehabilitation has provided less morbidity and better rehabilitation following extensive resection efforts [132].

The presence of distant metastasis, extensive intracranial extension, bilateral cavernous sinus extension, and/or involvement of both orbits are relative contraindications to surgical intervention. However, in very selected cases, surgery may offer palliation even in the presence of extensive disease [124].

Surgery for Advanced Disease

The discussion of surgical therapy for sinonasal tumors must differentiate surgical approaches from surgical resection. Approaches describe incisions and elevation of tissues to expose the extent of the tumor for adequate removal. The extent of the resection is the structures removed during surgery in an attempt to obtain negative margins. Approaches include endoscopic, lateral rhinotomy, transoral or tranpalatal, midfacial degloving, the Weber-Fergusson approach, and combined craniofacial approaches. The extent of resection may include a medial maxillectomy, inferior or total maxillectomy, orbital exenteration, or various anterior and antero-lateral skull base resections. The surgeon must determine the extent of resection prior to the operation so that planned adequate reconstruction of such vital structures as the orbital floor, the velopharynx, and the skull base can be undertaken [132].

The medial maxillectomy removes the lateral nasal wall and the medial maxillary segment up to the infraorbital nerve. Usually, a complete sphenoethmoidectomy is performed. The most common indication for this procedure is an inverting papilloma of the lateral nasal wall, but this procedure can also provide exposure for removal of other malignant and non-malignant sinonasal lesions. Approaches to this type of resection most often entail a lateral rhinotomy incision, but a midfacial degloving approach is also used [133].

The inferior maxillectomy involves resection of the inferior maxillary sinus below the plane of the infraorbital nerve. The most common indication for this procedure is a tumor of the maxillary alveolar process without extension into the antrum [134]. Lesions of the hard palate that spare the antrum can also be treated with this procedure. Sublabial and palatal incision may be used, or a midfacial degloving incision that crosses the midline can also be used. Reconstruction of the maxillary or palatal defect is most simply done by an obturator prosthesis, which can be incorporated into a denture. This allows for ease of follow-up examination and cleaning of the antral cavity [49]. The defect cavity can be lined with a split-thickness or full-thickness skin graft or a free tissue transfer such as a radial forearm flap.

A total maxillectomy is indicated for the treatment of antral carcinomas [135]. Decision about sacrifice of the facial skin or orbital contents is determined by radiographic, clinical or intraoperative involvement of the subcutaneous and periorbital tissues respectively. Ethmoidal air cells are totally removed during this procedure, and a wide sphenoidotomy is performed. The periorbital region, pterygoid musculature, and cheek flap are lined with a split thickness skin graft to facilitate close follow-up examination for tumor recurrence. Obturation is achieved by a preformed prosthesis that is wired to the remaining contralateral maxilla and dentition [136].

Determination whether orbital exenteration is required must be carefully considered since removal of the eye carries considerable emotional burden for the patient [137]. The reported indications for orbital exenteration include invasion of the periorbita, infraorbital or posterior ethmoid nerves, or orbital apex [138]. Yet, most common opinion regarding the removal of orbital contents is that it is indicated only for frank invasion of the orbital fat or musculature. Currently, bony invasion by itself does not constitute an indication for removing the orbital contents. But, the preoperative decision for exenteration should be included in clinically evident orbital invasion such as proptosis, diplopia, decreased visual acuity, and restricted ocular mobility. In the absence of clinical signs, the determination of invasion rests in radiographic diagnosis. The CT scan is not absolutely reliable for determining orbital invasion. Differentiating orbital invasion from tumor that lies just adjacent to the periorbita is difficult, and cannot always reliably be determined other than by intraoperative inspection. The MRI is thought to be better in distinguishing soft tissue invasion from adjacent non-invasive tumor, but this still does not reach the accuracy of intraoperative determination.

An important and often overlooked aspect of determining the need for exenteration is consideration of the potential loss of function of that eye after adjunctive treatment. Studies have demonstrated up to 79% functional loss of the conserved ipsilateral eye after postoperative radiation therapy [139], but this complication may vary with the radiation techniques utilized and probably will improve with the advent of intensity modulated radiation therapy (IMRT) [140]. Another functional consideration is the extent of resection of the orbital floor and the techniques of reconstruction to be used prior to radiation [132]. If only a split-thickness skin graft is utilized to reconstruct this vital bony support mechanism, less than 20% will enjoy significant function from that eye. There are those surgeons that believe that if the floor is resected, the orbit should be exenterated [137]. Yet other surgeons believe that meaningful ocular function can be achieved with reconstruction using bony or synthetic material [132].

Skull base resections can be performed via a cranio-facial, a basal subfrontal, or antero-lateral cranial base approach. En bloc resection of the anterior cranial base in sinonasal malignancies is indicated for tumors involving the cribiform plate [131]. By definition, this is done for almost all cases of esthesioneuroblastomas or most carcinomas of the ethmoid sinuses approaching the anterior skull base [124]. The dura of the anterior cranial fossa acts as a barrier which delays brain invasion. Dural resection often provides an adequate oncologic margin of normal tissues. In some cases though, limited frontal lobe involvement may be addressed with an anterior craniofacial approach.

The basal-subfrontal approach to sinonasal tumors provides a relatively wide angle of visualization in the area of the sphenoid sinus and upper clivus with only limited retraction of the frontal lobes. This approach has been described and popularized by Derome and Sekhar [141, 142]. In principle, a bicoronal flap elevation allows for a bifrontal craniotomy and removal of the intervening segment of the superior orbital ridges and the nasion between the orbital roofs bilaterally. This allows for clear visualization of the sphenoid sinus and the carotid arteries on both sides.

The anterolateral approach is most commonly utilized for paramedian disease of the lateral aspect of the orbit, sphenoid or maxillary sinuses, pterygoids, infratemporal fossa, or any other that demonstrates a preferential growth pattern laterally [143]. The anterolateral approach combines features of the craniofacial and basal subfrontal with features of the lateral approaches often used by neuro-otologic surgeons. The principle goal of the anterolateral approach is to achieve an unobstructed view of the midline and lateral skull base, and thus is used primarily to extirpate lesions that cannot be reached through the craniofacial or basal subfrontal approach alone.

The goals of reconstruction of the surgical defects are as follows: 1) oronasal separation, 2) cranionasal separation, 3) eye and cheek support, 4) dental restoration, and 5) restoration of facial defects, and these goals may be achieved by prosthetic rehabilitatation, surgical construction, or both [124]. Prosthetic obturator rehabilitation is utilized most effectively for oronasal separation. Preoperative prosthodontic evaluation allows for obturator design prior to resection with the advantage of immediate rehabilitation, early postoperative speech and oral feeding. Retention is usually achieved by wiring the prosthesis to the remaining maxilla and dentition.

Surgical reconstruction is needed whenever the cranial and nasal cavities are in communication [144]. Watertight separation is mandatory to reduce the risk of CSF leaks, with the attendant complication of meningitis. Dural closure can be achieved by suture closure and/or dural patching with fascia lata, pericranium, or temporalis grafts. Vascularized galeal-pericranial flaps are the most frequently used to reconstruct the cranial floor. Lumbar subarachnoid drainage for several days postoperatively helps reduce CSF pressure and allows dural closures to heal. Occasionally, larger defects require bulky reconstructions of the cavity and reduction of dead space. Vascularized tissues via regional flaps, such as the temporalis muscle, can be utilized. If this muscle bulk is inadequate, microvascularized free flaps are utilized. Free-tissue transfer may provide adequate vascularized tissue [145]. Figure 3 is an example of a craniofacial resection for an ethmoidal squamous cell carcinoma demonstrated in the left ethmoid sinus on coronal CT scan [Figure 3a]. The MRI demonstrates extension to just underneath the cribiform plate [Figure 3b.]. Through a bicoronal approach, a galeal-pericranial flap was elevated [Figure 3c.], and concomitant facial incisions allow for access from below [Figure 3d.]. The resection is seen through the anterior cranial base defect in Figure 3e., and the specimen is viewed in Figure 3f.. On long-term follow-up, the cosmetic results of this surgical resection are very acceptable [Figure 3g.].

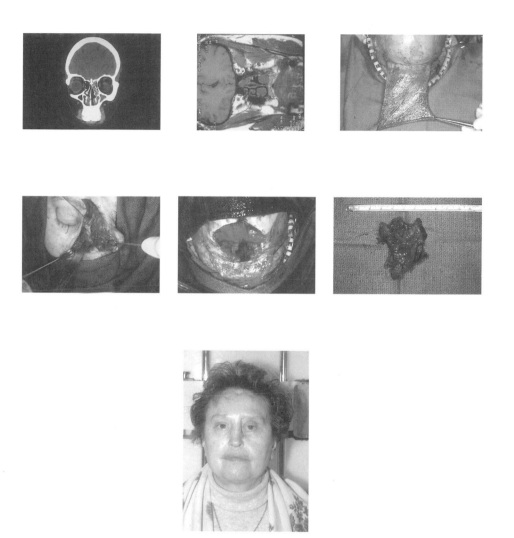

Figures 3a-3g. **Example of a craniofacial resection for an ethmoidal carcinoma. Fig 3a shows coronal view, MRI (3b) shows extension to just below cribiform plate. Through a bicoronal approach, a galeal-pericranial flap was elevated (3c) and concomitant facial incisions allowed for access from below (3d). The resection is seen through the anterior cranial defect in (3e), and specimen in (3f). (fig 3g) shows long-term follow-up.**

ADVANCED TEMPORAL BONE CARCINOMAS

External Auditory Canal Carcinomas

The most common carcinomas of the external auditory canal (EAC) are basal and squamous cell carcinomas. These tumors arise most frequently from excessive solar exposure. Other malignant tumors of this area include malignant melanoma, cerumin gland and adenoid cystic carcinomas, and rhabdomyosarcomas [146].

Squamous cell carcinoma is the most frequent pathology of the pinna and external canal [147]. Overall, fair-skinned patients with actinic skin changes are the most likely to develop squamous cell carcinoma of the external ear. Men are more likely to develop this disease than women, probably having to do with the higher prevalance of outdoor jobs [146].

All too often squamous cell carcinoma of the external auditory canal is diagnosed late in the course of disease. Patients have often been treated for otitis externa for some time before the diagnosis of carcinoma is made. The survival rate for external ear squamous cell carcinomas remain low, somewhere around 50%, which is most likely attributable to this late diagnosis [148]. Grossly, squamous cell carcinoma presents as an ulcerated lesion that is prone to bleed, and demonstrates very indiscrete margins. Erosion into or fixation to the cartilage suggests an aggressive lesion.

Patients with canal carcinoma often present with pruritis and pain. Foul discharge from the ear, hearing loss, and facial nerve weakness or paralysis may also be found. Persistent otitis externa that does not resolve with conservative measures should raise the suspicion of malignancy.

The etiology of this disease is uncertain, however, sun or ultraviolet radiation is thought to play a role. Chronic infection of the canal may be an additional etiological agent [149], but the role of chronic inflammation remains to be clearly defined. Infiltration of the anterior canal wall into the parotid gland, or posterior auricular cartilage over the mastoid is frequently encountered since the canal offers little resistance to invasion [146]. Tumors of the bony canal tend to invade the middle ear, the cartilaginous, or membranous canal, or both.

Basal carcinoma is not as common on the pinna or external auditory canal as it is for the rest of the head and neck skin [146]. The most common sites for basal cell carcinoma of the auricle are postauricular and preauricular areas. Much like squamous cell carcinomas, basal cell carcinoma is more common in men than in women, and is more commonly seen in fair skinned individuals.

The presentation of basal cell carcinomas can be either a nodular lesion or a plaque-like area of skin. These lesions tend to be firm and thick, and are most often nontender. They may crust and bleed and can be confused with benign dermal lesions.

Treatment of basal cell carcinoma predominantly involves local intervention. More aggressive tumors may extend along embryonic fusion planes and neurovascular adventitia. Except in the most aggressive cases, cervical lymphatic metastasis is rare.

Another tumor that is seen in this region is adenoid cystic carcinoma. These tumors are derived from the cerumin secretory coils of the external auditory canal or from locally invasive adenoid cystic carcinomas of the parotid gland that invades the canal wall [150]. An additional carcinoma of the external canal is the ceruminous gland adenocarcinoma. This is a malignant glandular tumor found in the external auditory canal that demonstrates apocrine secretory differentiation. Little is known about this tumor, since it is poorly described in the literature [146].

Diagnostic Imaging

The diagnosis of auricular tumors is usually made by physical examination and biopsy. One must have a high index of suspicion of cancer in a patient with otitis externa and either granulation tissue within the canal or erosion of the skin of the canal. Tumors in this area become painful after the periosteum has been invaded. Biopsy should be performed after the canal is thoroughly cleaned and inspected.

Diagnostic imaging is more important in the evaluation of cancer of the EAC than tumors of the pinna since CT allows for accurate assessment of the bony extent of the tumor [151]. For more extensive disease, the MRI may additionally evaluate the extent of intracranial or soft tissue invasion [152].

Surgical Treatment for Advanced External Ear Carcinomas

Large lesions that involve the cartilage and posterior auricular sulcus require a total auriculectomy [153]. There has been some debate about the usefulness of radiation therapy in cancers of the auricle [154], but the risk of chondronecrosis may obviate potential benefits of radiation in advanced disease. Whenever possible, the superior aspect of the auricle should be left intact to aid with support of eyeglass wearing, and the tragus may be utilized to camouflage the anterior aspect of a prosthesis. Osteointegrated implants may also serve to anchor a prosthesis that would then accommodate eyeglasses [146].

Radiation therapy alone has not proven to be an effective method of treating EAC carcinomas, in that most tumors recur rapidly [155-158]. Despite the overall concern for the use of radiation therapy alone for advanced EAC carcinomas, all studies were retrospective in nature and prospective studies are needed to definitively resolve this controversy. Recent data supports the en bloc resection of tumors of the external auditory canal rather than piecemeal resection as had been advocated in the past. Parsons and Lewis advocated the removal of the middle ear, mastoid, external canal, parotid, root of the zygoma, and temporomandibular joint [159]. Others have championed the subtotal temporal bone resection, contending that the radical mastoidectomy has unacceptable rate of associated morbidity [150]. Currently, the adage of "radical early" seems to be an appropriate compromise [146]. In example, Figures 4a. and b. demonstrate an axial and coronal CT scan respectively of a patient with an external ear basal cell carcinoma. This patient required a lateral temporal bone resection [Figure 4c., incisions mapped out on the operating room table, and 4d., resection of involved tissues]. Reconstruction was performed with a rectus free flap Figure 4e. Certain studies have demonstrated that patients who undergo en bloc resection followed by radiation therapy had better survival rates than piecemeal resections [158].

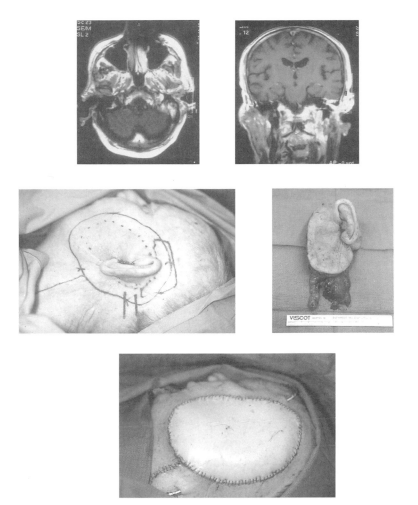

Figures 4a-4e. **Example of external ear cancer requiring temporal bone resection. Fig 4a. and 4b demonstrate axial and coronal CT of a patient with an external basal cell carcinoma. 4c shows incisions mapped out in the operating room, and 4d resection of the involved tissues. A rectus free flap reconstruction was used.**

Middle Ear and Temporal Bone Tumors

Primary tumors of the temporal bone are exceedingly rare, the majority (86%) being squamous cell carcinoma [160]. Adenoid cystic carcinoma may arise as a consequence of neural spread to the skull base and temporal bone [146]. The prognosis for these patients is dismal, and a high recurrence rate is associated with skip lesions along nerves and failure to recognize the extent of neural involvement at the time of primary surgical resection. Metastasis is rare for this type of carcinoma, and is usually found late in the disease course [161]. Treatment requires radical surgery followed by radiation therapy. Other malignant tumors seen in the temporal bone are basal cell carcinoma, melanoma, and mucoepidermoid carcinomas.

Rhabdomyosarcoma occurs most frequently in the pediatric population, and 10% of all rhabdomyosarcomas occur in the ear [162]. Easily resectable tumors may be surgically removed followed by adjuvant chemotherapy. Alternatively, these tumors can be treated with radiation and chemotherapy. Either approach produces high survival rates (90%). Less easily resectable tumors are treated with combined radiation therapy and chemotherapy. These tumors carry a poorer (57%) survival rate.

Secondary tumors of the temporal bone include tumors that invade from contiguous sites such as the nasopharynx or the clivus, as well as metastatic tumors. These types of temporal bone tumors are not within the scope of this chapter and the reader is referred to several excellent reviews [163-169].

Clinical Presentation

Primary tumors of the temporal bone are usually diagnosed at an advanced stage [146]. Due to the numerous areas of entrance and exit of blood vessels, nerves, the Eustachian tube, and muscles, tumors may grow without bony erosion, while invasion into most surrounding structures is associated with a poor prognosis.

Typically, malignant tumors of the temporal bone present with a chronically draining ear. Diagnosis in this area is often based on symptomatic presentation as the tumor begins to erode through bone or affect vital surrounding structures. There is often an insidious onset of conductive hearing loss and aural fullness, sometimes accompanied by bleeding, pain, and swelling. Neurological dysfunction of the VII, VI, V, IV, and IX through XII nerves may give an indication about the direction of tumor spread.

After meticulous cleaning of the ear canal, examination includes assessing the posterior canal wall for erosion, the presence of granulation tissue, or other suspicious findings. Any suspicious soft tissue lesions not readily identifiable should undergo a fine-needle aspiration biopsy. The posterior auricular area is inspected for swelling or skin changes. Assessment of the nasopharynx should be undertaken via direct or indirect means. A full cranial nerve examination should also be undertaken. Lastly, the neck is palpated for gross lymphadenopathy.

A high-resolution CT scan is the best method for evaluation of the temporal bone. MRI scanning delineates the total extent of intracranial disease [170].

Treatment

Surgical resection followed by radiation therapy for large tumors or positive margins appears to be the best option [146]. Of course, the rarity of these tumors makes prospective evaluation of treatment options impossible.

Several different surgical options for removal of temporal bone carcinomas exists; but for advanced disease the subtotal temporal bone resection in selected cases and more often total temporal bone resection is required [146]. Subtotal temporal bone resection includes the removal of the bony and cartilaginous canal, malleus, incus, and the otic capsule. The total temporal bone resection removes the entire temporal bone including the above structures and the petrous apex. Whatever the surgical procedure, cancers of the temporal bone require an en bloc resection. Data from Lewis and Page demonstrate a poor outcome seen with piecemeal resection of temporal bone cancers [171]. More recently, data from Prasad and Janeka demonstrate that cancers restricted to the external auditory canal can be resected with a lateral or subtotal mastoidectomy with comparable results [172]. Unfortunately, patients with dural involvement do not benefit from surgical resection, and chemotherapy and/or radiation therapy is then considered.

Reconstruction of these defects includes pedicled myocutaneous flaps, such as the pectoralis major myocutaneous flap, latissimus dorsi, or trapezius flaps. Another reconstructive option for these defects is musculocutaneous free flaps, such as the rectus abdominus, or latissimus dorsi flaps [145]. Whatever the reconstruction considered, the most important consideration is that exposed bone be covered with vascularized muscle and skin.

CANCER OF THE SKIN

Introduction

Cancer of the skin is the most common form of malignancy, with the head and neck region being the most frequent site of involvement. In white males, ninety percent of all skin cancers occur in the head and neck region, while 85% of all skin cancers among white females occur in the head and neck [173]. Of patients with skin cancer, 25% have more than one lesion at the time of diagnosis. One in five Americans will develop a skin cancer at some time in their lives. Approximately 60% of all cancers of the skin are basal cell carcinoma, with 30% being squamous cell carcinoma, and the other 10% being a mixture of more rare tumors [174].

Considering the high prevalence of skin cancer, the ease of early diagnosis and infrequent metastatic spread a high cure should be expected. Exposure to sunlight is the predominant predisposing factor [175, 176], and therefore treatment must be accompanied by avoidance to further sun exposure, protection with appropriate sunscreens and treatment of premalignant lesions such as actinic keratoses. Patients at high risk include those with fair skin, sun exposure, or occupations requiring them to work in the outdoors.

Ultraviolet light is by far the most important cause of skin cancer. Certain populations, such as the Celts, have skin types that lack natural protective mechanisms. Migration of cancer prone people to areas of high sun intensity, such as Australia, has increased their susceptibility. Studies have also demonstrated that wind exposure and drying of the skin enhances ultraviolet injury [175]. Other causes of skin cancer include soot exposure for chimney sweeps, exposure to tar, tar products, and pitch, polycyclic aromatic hydrocarbons, and creosote just to name a few [177]. Multiple less well-defined factors thought to increase the formation of non-melanomatous skin cancers are viral exposure in squamous cell carcinoma, and increased susceptibility to carcinogens and/or a decreased immunological response with aging [178]. Whatever the underlying combination of risk factors, the major message is that protection from the damaging effects of sun exposure must be the primary preventative measure.

Basal Cell Carcinoma

Basal cell carcinoma (BCCa) is the most common type of skin cancer and has numerous clinical variations [177]. The tumor may be flat and eczematous, with a propensity for radial growth without a vertical component, or threadlike waxy border may herald a superficial multicentric variant. Nodular BCCa are usually pinkish to red in character owing to the dilated blood vessels over a translucent tumor surface. Pigmented basal cell carcinomas may resemble melanoma or a pigmented nevus, and at times may ulcerate producing a deeply infiltrative lesion. Perhaps the most deceptive type of basal cell carcinoma is the morpheaform type. These lesions are macular, whitish, having an indistinct margin, and may go unnoticed for long periods of time without alarming the patient or the physician [179].

Genetically, basal cell carcinomas have been associated with the basal cell nevus syndrome. This autosomal dominant condition is associated with multiple basal cell carcinomas, especially located on the head and neck, which occur at a very early age. Other anomalies associated with this condition are cysts of the jaw [180].

Location also can influence the biological behavior of the lesion, with any morphological type of basal cell carcinoma located in an embryological fusion plane generally considered to be more aggressive by virtue of invasion of multiple tissue planes and higher rates of recurrence after therapy [181].

Although metastasis is extremely rare, this possibility must be entertained when faced with a lesion that is multiply recurrent or treatment has been delayed for years [182]. In these instances, spread to regional lymphatics, lungs or bone may occur.

Surgical Treatment for Advanced Basal Cell Carcinoma

The increased health awareness of our society today has resulted in fewer delays in diagnosis from complacency, ignorance, or fear [177]. Appropriate treatment for basal cell carcinoma should achieve approximately a 90% cure rate. Due to this trend, most advanced basal cell carcinomas seen today are from failures of initial therapies.

Curettage excision with electrodessication, cryosurgery, and topical chemotherapy are not usually appropriate for advanced or recurrent BCCa lesions. More likely these lesions will be treated by Moh's micrographic surgery, conventional surgical excision, or irradiation either alone or in combination. Irradiation is not within the scope of this chapter and will not be discussed herein.

Moh's micrographic surgery is a descendent of the original surgical procedure of Moh's chemosurgery [183]. In the original procedure, tumors were treated with a topical fixative, zinc chloride, prior to dissection and microscopic margin evaluation. Present day technique involved fresh tumor resection, and margin examination as frozen sections [184].

Moh's micrographic surgery is performed under local anesthetic with or without conscious sedation. The main bulk of the tumor is excised in a fashion that allows for careful orientation, inking and correlation of the margin to the patient's in-situ margin. All margins are evaluated closely, including the deep one, for microscopic residual tumor. A detailed diagram of the surgical site, including the areas of inking, aids in orientation. If a positive margin is identified, the procedure of resection and frozen section evaluation is repeated until the margin is negative. The experienced Moh's surgeon can easily do excision of a basal cell carcinoma along multiple tissue planes including extension along the periosteum, blood vessels, or nerves.

Simple surgical excision for basal cell carcinomas is usually indicated for recurrences after previous irradiation, for bone or cartilage involvement, or for discreet lesions that can be handled more readily with surgery than irradiation [185]. Surgical management for advanced basal cell carcinomas requires meticulous attention to surgical technique to prevent failure. For lesions with a distinct border, a surgical margin of 1 cm may be adequate. Lesions in which the border cannot be accurately delineated require wider resection margins. The deep margin should be as wide as the lateral margins. Cartilage or bone invasion creates a special problem. Full thickness excision of the involved cartilage is necessary, and the extent of bone resection is dictated by the extent of involvement [177]. Periosteal resection may be the only thing required if bone is not grossly involved. Occasionally, adjuvant radiation therapy may be used, especially if the surgical procedure does not yield negative margins.

Although reconstructive and cosmetic considerations should not alter the oncologic approach to patients with basal cell carcinoma, they must be considered in any post-ablative defect. Wounds vary according to the size of the defect, the area that it encompasses, the surrounding as well as the distant potential areas of donor tissue for reconstruction, the depth of the wound and the various layers of tissue sacrificed. Patient factors to be considered include the age, overall patient's health including the social habits such as smoking, expectations, and the occupational pressures on the patient after surgery.

A list of possible wound closure techniques is seen in Table 3. Immediate reconstruction would be the most favorable approach, but secondary intention can result in very acceptable cosmesis. Wounds in which immediate closure is desirable must consider the pros and cons of each procedure. Special considerations must be taken for bone, cartilage, periosteal, and/or perichondrial defects. Split thickness skin grafts will not take on tissues offering little vascular support such as bone, and therefore regional and microvascular flap coverage must then be considered.

Table 3.
Techniques for Closure of Skin Cancer Excision Defects

Second Intention Healing	Flaps	
Partial Closure		Advancement
Primary Closure		Rotation
Grafting		Transposition
Full-thickness		Island
Split-thickness		Free Flap
Delayed		Combination

Squamous Cell Carcinoma

Cutaneous squamous cell carcinoma (SCCa) is the second most common skin malignancy, second only to BCCa in incidence. Exposure to sunlight is a risk factor, as it is for BCCa.

As with BCCa, multiple variations in clinical presentation exist [177]. The typical cutaneous SCCa presents as an opaque nodule that may be ulcerated. Actinic keratosis is generally thought of as a premalignant condition that predisposes the patient to development of SCCa [186]. Another type of presentation is the cutaneous horn, which appears as a hornlike projection from the skin that may show invasion at the base of the lesion. Papillomatous proliferation with indistinct solid infiltrating margins and a slowly forming central ulceration may occur. The raw, crusted area easily bleeds with minimal trauma. In general, persistent lesions that bleed warrant a biopsy for histologic diagnosis. At times, SCCa may show minimal tendency for vertical growth and will spread superficially in an eczematous fashion. This usually represents a carcinoma in situ, which is termed Bowen's disease or bowenoid keratosis.

Surgical Treatment of Advanced Cutaneous Squamous Cell Carcinoma

The advanced SCCa's of the skin are usually a result of neglect on the part of the patient or his or her physician, and local recurrences and locoregional or distant metastasis occurs even after seemingly adequate treatment.

The treatment of advanced skin SCCa involves many principles applicable to basal cell carcinomas. However, much more consideration for regional lymphatics must be entertained [187]. The primary lesion in many cases may be treated with Moh's micrographic surgery, routine surgical excision, or irradiation with similar results (as long as bone or cartilage is not involved).

Moh's micrographic surgery offers excellent cosmetic results, sparing the most normal tissue possible. Surgical resection on the other hand requires a wide lateral margin (1-2 cm) and an adequate deep margin. Frozen section control of the margin status is important for ensuring adequate resection, but does not assure surgical cure.

Variables associated with a higher risk of metastasis from cutaneous SCCa have been identified [188, 189]. These include recurrence, tumor thickness of greater than 6 mm, size greater than 2 cm, poorly differentiated histology, an immunocompromised host, the anatomic site of the primary such as the ear, temple, dorsum of the hand, and lip, perineural invasion, and rapid growth.

Metastasis to regional lymph nodes is influenced by the location of the primary lesion [177]. Lesions of the scalp, forehead, temple, and auricle may metastasize to the paraparotid or intraparotid lymph nodes as well as the deep jugular lymph node chain. Lesions located elsewhere on the skin of the head and neck region usually metastasize to the submandibular and deep cervical nodes. Regional metastasis may also become apparent some time after adequate treatment of the primary lesion.

Because the incidence of metastasis is low, prophylactic neck dissection is usually not indicated. However, clinically positive lymph node metastasis should undergo a neck dissection and/or a superficial parotidectomy depending upon the location of the primary lesion.

Other Epithelial Carcinomas

A number of more rare epithelial carcinomas exist, and the exact strategy of management for the advanced cases of these tumors has not been well defined. Basosquamous cell carcinomas appear to behave similar to BCCa, and therefore should be treated similarly [177].

Keratoacanthoma represents a cancer of very low malignant potential [190]. It is exceedingly rare that these tumors would present as late stage disease, and therefore no consensus on the exact means with which to approach such a scenario is established.

Carcinomas of the skin appendages represent a set of other rare skin tumors for which treatment must be individualized. Sebaceous gland carcinomas occur most frequently on the eyelids, and behave more aggressively when originating from this site than from other sites of the head and neck [177]. Metastasis is more frequent from this site as well. Eccrine and apocrine gland carcinomas occur in the head and neck region, and represent locally aggressive tumors with low metastatic potential [191]. Treatment is usually surgical excision.

Other more rare tumors that will only be mentioned include microcystic adenexal carcinomas, various sarcomas including dermatofibrosarcoma protruberans, atypical fibroxanthoma, and malignant fibrous histiocytoma, angiosarcomas, hemangiopericytoma, neuroendocrine tumors such as neurofibrosarcoma and Merkel cell carcinomas, as well as a variety of miscellaneous tumors. The interested reader is referred to several references for more information about these rare tumors [192-196].

Melanoma

The incidence of melanoma is increasing at an alarming rate [197, 198]. Almost a fourfold increase in the incidence of melanoma has been seen from 1975 to 1995 [199]. This increased incidence may in part be due to an increased awareness of the disease on the part of patients and physicians alike, or increasing sun exposure. It is interesting to note that the mortality from melanoma has also increased, but not nearly at the same rate as the incidence [200]. Undoubtedly, this is due to the higher rate of diagnosis at earlier stages accompanied by its high curability at these early stages.

Approximately 10 to 25% of all melanomas originate in the head and neck region [201, 202]. The distribution of head and neck melanomas according to sites is listed in *Table 4*. Cutaneous melanoma of the face originates most commonly on the cheek, whereas the occipital scalp is another fairly common site of occurrence. Other sites include the external ear and the supero-lateral aspect of the neck. Mucosal melanomas are extremely rare, and originate most frequently on the hard palate or nasal mucosa [203].

Table 4. Distribution of Melanomas of the Head and Neck According to Site

Location	Aggregate Percentage
Facial skin	46.2%
Neck	19.6%
Scalp	17.7%
External ear	11.5%
Nose	1.6%
Mucosa	1.6%
Eyelids	1.0%
Unknown	0.8%

Although the etiology of melanoma is not definitively determined, numerous associations points to the fact that the most important risk factor is intermittent sun exposure, particularly during childhood [204, 205]. Severe sunburn during childhood appears to be especially harmful, whereas chronic sun exposure related to outdoor occupations does not appear to increase the risk of melanoma and may even be protective [206].

Race is another risk factor. The incidence of melanoma among of whites is approximately 12 times higher than that of blacks, and 7 times higher than in Hispanics [207]. Among white patients, the risk of developing melanoma increases in people of fair complexion, blue or green eyes, and blond or red hair [205, 208, 209]. It appears that the most important pigmentary risk factor a propensity to sunburn or an inability to tan [210].

Several pre-existing pigmented lesions are additional risk factors for the development of melanoma. Lesions suspected of being a precursor to cutaneous malignant melanomas are: a) certain congenital nevi, b) dysplastic nevi, and c) melanotic freckle of Hutchinson [211, 212].

Immunosuppression increases the risk of developing malignant melanoma [213-215]. A higher incidence of melanoma has been reported among renal transplant recipients and in patients with lymphoma and leukemia. Interestingly, most of the melanomas that occur in this patient population develop in dysplastic nevi. Therefore, any suspicious mole in an immunosuppressed patient must be kept under close observation and excised without delay if change is noted.

The role of pregnancy in the etiology of malignant melanoma, and the prognostic implications of melanoma in this situation, remain to be settled. Several meta-analyses have failed to demonstrate a true relationship between pregnancy and the development of melanoma [216, 217]. Other risk factors that increase the patient's risk of melanoma development include prior melanomas and relatives with melanomas [208, 218, 219].

Clinical Evaluation

The clinical presentation of melanoma is too varied to be pathognomonic, however, certain clinical features are suggestive of a malignancy in a pigmented lesion [200]. These characteristics are: 1) asymmetry, referring to the irregular shape and surface of most melanomas, 2) border irregularity, 3) color variegation, from white to pink or light brown to dark blue or black, and 4) diameter greater than 6 mm in a pigmented lesion. Lesions with these characteristics should raise the suspicion of malignancy. In addition, any recent change in the size or color of a mole, the occurrence of bleeding, or the development of satellite lesions should focus attention on the need for a biopsy.

Excisional, rather than an incisional, biopsy is preferred whenever possible to allow for complete histopathologic examination. When full excision is not possible, either because of the size of the lesion or its location, an incisional biopsy may be necessary to establish a diagnosis prior to therapeutic planning. The center or ulcerated portion of the lesion must be avoided, since it may contain a large area of necrotic devitalized tissue that may not yield a diagnosis. Properly done elliptical incision or a punch biopsy will provide representative tissue. Curettage or shave biopsies are inappropriate, since they do not allow for the measurement of thickness of invasion. Additionally, needle biopsies and incisional biopsies of suspected nodal metastasis are also discouraged.

Accurate determination of the status of the regional lymphatics is crucial in the management and anticipated prognosis for these patients. Besides a thorough examination of the neck, the examiner must evaluate the preauricular, retroauricular, suboccipital, parotid, and buccinator regions [220]. In patients with melanoma that is located in the lateral and posterior aspects of the lower portion of the neck, it is important to examine the status of the axillary lymph nodes. Distant metastasis screening includes a chest radiograph, and liver function tests particularly alkaline phosphatase.

Over the past 25 years, several clinical and histological parameters have been identified as useful indicators of biological behavior of melanomas and are therefore utilized by clinicians to make therapeutic decisions and anticipate prognosis. It has become evident that stage II disease patients demonstrate a risk of associated nodal metastasis of about 60%, but the risk of distant metastasis is only 15% [200]. In some studies, elective lymph node dissection appears to have a beneficial effect on survival for this group of melanoma patients [221]. Furthermore, melanomas greater than 4.0 mm thick are associated with a high risk of occult nodal (62%) and distant (72%) metastasis. Consequently, prognosis for these patients is poor and neck dissection does not appear to alter overall outcome [200]. Other factors influencing the prognosis of patients with melanoma is ulceration [221-223], and location of the primary [221, 223]. Scalp location appears to be an independent risk for local recurrence and survival independent of tumor thickness.

Stage III melanoma represents palpable lymph node metastasis, and the principle prognostic factor is tumor burden. An indicator of tumor burden is the number of lymph nodes involved by tumor or the presence of extranodal extension of tumor [224]. Thickness of the primary tumor has no predictive prognostic value in patients with lymphatic metastasis [225], probably owing to the overshadowing influence of metastatic disease.

Surgical Treatment for Advanced Stage Melanoma

For tumors of intermediate-thickness (1-4 mm), surgical resection with a 2 cm margin is appropriate [226]. Yet because the studies that prove this systematically excluded patients with head and neck melanomas, this can only be used as a rough guide. In the head and neck region, the surgeon is faced many times with areas in which a 2 cm margin is not possible without sacrificing vital structures not clinically involved, and therefore judgment is required.

The majority of lesions of the cheek and face are adequately excised with a 1.5 to 2.0-cm margin of normal skin. The defect often has to be closed with local or regional skin flaps or a full-thickness skin graft. Melanomas of the pinna are often adequately removed with a partial resection of the pinna. With extensive, recurrent, or centrally located lesions the entire pinna must be excised. As with squamous cell carcinoma of the external ear, a small area of the root of the helix is left to aid in the use of glasses. In this case a full-thickness skin graft gives adequate cosmetic rehabilitation [227].

Most melanomas of the skin of the nose are adequately excised with resection of skin and subcutaneous tissues of the affected area, preserving the underlying perichondrium or periosteum. A full thickness graft can be used to cover the surgical defect. With a large defect, it is preferable to excise the skin and subcutaneous tissues of an aesthetic subunit of the nose and replace it with a full-thickness skin graft. The cosmetic results of this operation are usually very good. A partial or total resection of the nose is necessary with advanced or recurrent cases [228]. Prosthetic rehabilitation offers the best cosmetic result for this type of excision.

Melanomas of the neck and scalp are usually excised with a wider margin of normal skin (3-5 cm). These larger defects are better repaired with a split-thickness skin graft, except when the excision of the lesion of the neck is combined with a nodal dissection. In such cases, the cervical flaps can usually be fashioned and mobilized to close the defect.

At present there is not enough evidence to recommend Moh's micrographic surgery as an alternative to conventional resection for cutaneous melanoma [229]. It is certainly the case that no studies to date have examined its role in advanced or recurrent melanomas. Certain aspects of the evaluation of margins are difficult. An example is that freeze artifact during frozen section diagnosis can obscure interpretation. Therefore, there is no place at this time for Moh's with advanced melanoma.

Treatment of the neck with cutaneous melanoma is highly dependent upon the thickness of the primary, being that the incidence of lymphatic metastasis increases in direct proportion to the thickness of the lesion [220]. When metastatic lymph nodes become large enough to be clinically palpable, unquestionably the treatment should include a neck dissection. The choice of treatment is much more controversial when nodal metastasis is not palpable but are likely to be present based on the thickness of the primary lesion. Several recent prospective non-randomized studies have demonstrated that patients with intermediate thickness melanomas did benefit from elective lymphatic dissection [230, 231]. The enthusiasm for these results must be tempered in light of more recent findings of larger groups of patients with intermediate thickness melanoma of the head and neck that found that the advantage of elective lymph node dissection seen on univariate analysis was lost on multivariate analysis [223, 232].

Increasing the treatment complexity of melanoma is the addition of lymphoscintigraphy, which can be used pre-operatively in evaluating patients considered for elective lymph node dissection to: a) map the lymphatic drainage for a given melanoma [233], b) to identify the sentinel lymph-node, which when biopsied and examined histologically allows for a more extensive lymph node dissection, and/or 3) determine patients who are candidates for adjuvant therapy. An example is seen in Figure 5. This patient demonstrated a melanoma of intermediate depth on the right side of the neck [Figure 5a.] Lymphscintigraphy mapped the sentinel node to the contralateral lower neck [Figure 5b.]. In situ dissection of this sentinel lymph node demonstrated an afferent lymphatic channel and lymph node that stained positive with blue dye [Figure 5c.], and Figure 5d. demonstrates the final dissected node.

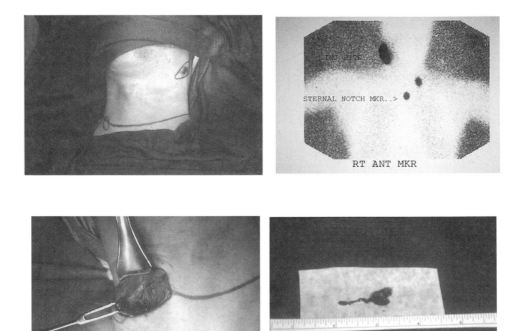

Figures 5a-5d. **Sentinel lymph node m,apping for head and neck melanoma. 5a shows an intermediate thickness melanoma of the right neck. Lymphoscintigraphy mapped the sentinel node to the contralateral lower neck (5b). 5c shows staining of the afferent lymphatic channel and lymph node with blue dye, and 5d shows the final dissected lymph node.**

CONCLUSIONS

It is evident from this discussion that the surgery and reconstruction plays an important role in the management of advance stage head and neck cancer. Surgical excision, appropriate reconstruction, and adjuvant therapies offer these unfortunate patients the best chance for meaningful survival. Yet, the role of surgical management of these advanced lesions must be continuously reevaluated to continue to refine the interactive nature of surgery with chemotherapy and radiation therapy protocols for organ preservation. Therefore, the complementary roles of each of these treatment modalities used for the patient faced with an advanced head and neck cancer will continue to evolve for years to come.

REFERENCES

1. Pfister, D.G., et al., Current status of larynx preservation with multimodality therapy. Oncology (Huntingt), 1992. 6(3): p. 33-8, 43; discussion 44, 47.
2. Shah, J.P., Chemotherapy in head and neck cancer: an unfulfilled promise and a continued challenge. J Surg Oncol, 1994. 55(2): p. 69-70.
3. Kraus, D.H., et al., Surgical management of squamous cell carcinoma of the base of the tongue. Am J Surg, 1993. 166(4): p. 384-8.
4. Ho, J.H., An epidemiologic and clinical study of nasopharyngeal carcinoma. Int J Radiat Oncol Biol Phys, 1978. 4(3-4): p. 182-98.
5. Neel, H.B., 3rd, A prospective evaluation of patients with nasopharyngeal carcinoma: an overview. J Otolaryngol, 1986. 15(3): p. 137-44.
6. Silverman, S., Jr., M. Gorsky, and F. Lozada, Oral leukoplakia and malignant transformation. A follow-up study of 257 patients. Cancer, 1984. 53(3): p. 563-8.
7. Steinberg C.M., Oropharyngeal Cancer, in Head and Neck Surgery-Otolaryngology, Bailey B.J., J.T. Johnson, H.C. Pillsbury, R.I, Kohut, and M.E. Tardy, Editors. 1993, JB Lippincott: Philadelphia. p. 1274-1275.
8. Alvi A., E.N. Myers, and J.T. Johnson, Cancer of the Oral Cavity, in Cancer of the Head and Neck, 3rd edition, Myers E.N., and J.Y. Suen, Editors. 1996, WB Saunders Co.: Philadelphia. p. 321-360.
9. Mashberg, A., L. Garfinkel, and S. Harris, Alcohol as a primary risk factor in oral squamous carcinoma. CA Cancer J Clin, 1981. 31(3): p. 146-55.
10. Shibata, D.K., N. Arnheim, and W.J. Martin, Detection of human papilloma virus in paraffin-embedded tissue using the polymerase chain reaction. J Exp Med, 1988. 167(1): p. 225-30.
11. Yarkut, E., [Mucosal cancer due to denture irritation]. Istanbul Univ Dishekim Fak Derg, 1968. 2(1): p. 28-31.
12. Prasad, A.S., et al., Nutritional and zinc status of head and neck cancer patients: an interpretive review. J Am Coll Nutr, 1998. 17(5): p. 409-18.
13. Singh, B., et al., Upper aerodigestive tract squamous cell carcinoma. The human immunodeficiency virus connection. Arch Otolaryngol Head Neck Surg, 1996. 122(6): p. 639-43.

14.   Rashid, Z., A. Kumar, and M. Komar, Plummer-Vinson syndrome and postcricoid carcinoma: late complications of unrecognized celiac disease. Am J Gastroenterol, 1999. 94(7): p. 1991.
15.   Fong, Y.Y. and W.C. Chan, Bacterial production of di-methyl nitrosamine in salted fish. Nature, 1973. 243(5407): p. 421-2.
16.   Yu, M.C., et al., Cantonese-style salted fish as a cause of nasopharyngeal carcinoma: report of a case-control study in Hong Kong. Cancer Res, 1986. 46(2): p. 956-61.
17.   zur Hausen, H., et al., EBV DNA in biopsies of Burkitt tumours and anaplastic carcinomas of the nasopharynx. Nature, 1970. 228(276): p. 1056-8.
18.   Henle, G. and W. Henle, Epstein-Barr virus-specific IgA serum antibodies as an outstanding feature of nasopharyngeal carcinoma. Int J Cancer, 1976. 17(1): p. 1-7.
19.   Buell, P., The effect of migration on the risk of nasopharyngeal cancer among Chinese. Cancer Res, 1974. 34(5): p. 1189-91.
20.   Weiss, M.H., et al., Otitis media with effusion in head and neck cancer patients. Laryngoscope, 1994. 104(1 Pt 1): p. 5-7.
21.   Shaha, A.R., et al., Synchronicity, multicentricity, and metachronicity of head and neck cancer. Head Neck Surg, 1988. 10(4): p. 225-8.
22.   Knappe, M., M. Louw, and R.T. Gregor, Ultrasonography-guided fine-needle aspiration for the assessment of cervical metastases. Arch Otolaryngol Head Neck Surg, 2000. 126(9): p. 1091-6.
23.   Wei WI, S.J. Sham, Cancer of the nasopharynx, in Cancer of the Head and Neck, Myers E.N., and J.Y. Suen, Editors. 1996, WB Saunders: Philadelphia. p. 277-293.
24.   Harrison, L.B., D.G. Pfister, and G.J. Bosl, Chemotherapy as part of the initial treatment for nasopharyngeal cancer. Oncology (Huntingt), 1991. 5(2): p. 67-70;discussion 70-1,74,79 passim.
25.   Mesic, J.B., G.H. Fletcher, and H. Goepfert, Megavoltage irradiation of epithelial tumors of the nasopharynx. Int J Radiat Oncol Biol Phys, 1981. 7(4): p. 447-53.
26.   Derome, P.J., The transbasal approach to tumors invading the base of skull, in Operative Neurosurgical Techniques, S.W. Schmidek HH, Editor. 1982, Grune & Stratton: New York.
27.   Wilson, C.P., Observations on the surgery of the nasopharynx. Annals of Otology, Rhinology, and Laryngology, 1957. 66: p. 5-40.
28.   Uttley, D., A. Moore, and D.J. Archer, Surgical management of midline skull-base tumors: a new approach. J Neurosurg, 1989. 71(5 Pt 1): p. 705-10.
29.   Belmont, J.R., The Le Fort I osteotomy approach for nasopharyngeal and nasal fossa tumors. Arch Otolaryngol Head Neck Surg, 1988. 114(7): p. 751-4.
30.   Fisch, U., The infratemporal fossa approach for nasopharyngeal tumors. Laryngoscope, 1983. 93(1): p. 36-44.
31.   Fee, W.E., Jr., J.B. Roberson, Jr., and D.R. Goffinet, Long-term survival after surgical resection for recurrent nasopharyngeal cancer after radiotherapy failure. Arch Otolaryngol Head Neck Surg, 1991. 117(11): p. 1233-6.
32.   Wei, W.I., K.H. Lam, and J.S. Sham, New approach to the nasopharynx: the maxillary swing approach. Head Neck, 1991. 13(3): p. 200-7.
33.   Wei, W.I., et al., Maxillary swing approach for resection of tumors in and around the nasopharynx. Arch Otolaryngol Head Neck Surg, 1995. 121(6): p. 638-42.
34.   Wei, W.I., et al., Pathological basis of surgery in the management of postradiotherapy cervical metastasis in nasopharyngeal carcinoma. Arch Otolaryngol Head Neck Surg, 1992. 118(9): p. 923-9; discussion 930.
35.   Hussey, D.H., H.B. Latourette, and W.R. Panje, Head and neck cancer: an analysis of the incidence, patterns of treatment, and survival at the University of Iowa. Ann Otol Rhinol Laryngol Suppl, 1991. 152: p. 2-16.
36.   Zelefsky, M.J., et al., Combined chemotherapy and radiotherapy versus surgery and postoperative radiotherapy for advanced hypopharyngeal cancer. Head Neck, 1996. 18(5): p. 405-11.

37. Harrison, L.B., et al., A prospective phase II trial of concomitant chemotherapy and radiotherapy with delayed accelerated fractionation in unresectable tumors of the head and neck. Head Neck, 1998. 20(6): p. 497-503.

38. Pfister, D.G., et al., Organ-function preservation in advanced oropharynx cancer: results with induction chemotherapy and radiation. J Clin Oncol, 1995. 13(3): p. 671-80.

39. Zelefsky, M.J., L.B. Harrison, and J.G. Armstrong, Long-term treatment results of postoperative radiation therapy for advanced stage oropharyngeal carcinoma. Cancer, 1992. 70(10): p. 2388-95.

40. Weber, R.S., et al., Treatment selection for carcinoma of the base of the tongue. Am J Surg, 1990. 160(4): p. 415-9.

41. Civantos, F. and B.L. Wenig, Transhyoid resection of tongue base and tonsil tumors. Otolaryngol Head Neck Surg, 1994. 111(1): p. 59-62.

42. Foote, R.L., et al., Base of tongue carcinoma: patterns of failure and predictors of recurrence after surgery alone. Head Neck, 1993. 15(4): p. 300-7.

43. Jaulerry, C., et al., Results of radiation therapy in carcinoma of the base of the tongue. The Curie Institute experience with about 166 cases. Cancer, 1991. 67(6): p. 1532-8.

44. Rollo, J., et al., Squamous carcinoma of the base of the tongue: a clinicopathologic study of 81 cases. Cancer, 1981. 47(2): p. 333-42.

45. Civantos, F., Goodwin WJ Jr., Cancer of the Oropharynx, in Cancer of the Head and Neck, Myers E.N., and J.Y. Suen, Editors. 1996, W.B. Saunders: Phildelphia. p. 361-380.

46. Givens, C.D., Jr., M.E. Johns, and R.W. Cantrell, Carcinoma of the tonsil. Analysis of 162 cases. Arch Otolaryngol, 1981. 107(12): p. 730-4.

47. Perez, C.A., et al., Carcinoma of the tonsillar fossa: a nonrandomized comparison of irradiation alone or combined with surgery: long-term results. Head Neck, 1991. 13(4): p. 282-90.

48. Lee, W.R., et al., Carcinoma of the tonsillar region: a multivariate analysis of 243 patients treated with radical radiotherapy. Head Neck, 1993. 15(4): p. 283-8.

49. Kornblith, A.B., et al., Quality of life of maxillectomy patients using an obturator prosthesis. Head Neck, 1996. 18(4): p. 323-34.

50. Spiro, R.H., et al., Squamous carcinoma of the posterior pharyngeal wall. Am J Surg, 1990. 160(4): p. 420-3.

51. Marks, J.E., P.G. Smith, and D.G. Sessions, Pharyngeal wall cancer. A reappraisal after comparison of treatment methods. Arch Otolaryngol, 1985. 111(2): p. 79-85.

52. Martini, D.V., et al., Swallowing and pharyngeal function in postoperative pharyngeal cancer patients. Ear Nose Throat J, 1997. 76(7): p. 450-3, 456.

53. Steinhart, H., J. Constantinidis, and H. Iro, [Larynx preserving surgery in carcinomas of the posterior hypopharyngeal wall by reconstruction with a free flap]. Hno, 1998. 46(2): p. 135-9.

54. Vikram, B., et al., Failure at the primary site following multimodality treatment in advanced head and neck cancer. Head Neck Surg, 1984. 6(3): p. 720-3.

55. Sultan, M.R. and J.J. Coleman, 3rd, Oncologic and functional considerations of total glossectomy. Am J Surg, 1989. 158(4): p. 297-302.

56. Kramer, S., et al., Combined radiation therapy and surgery in the management of advanced head and neck cancer: final report of study 73-03 of the Radiation Therapy Oncology Group. Head Neck Surg, 1987. 10(1): p. 19-30.

57. Franceschi, D., et al., Improved survival in the treatment of squamous carcinoma of the oral tongue. Am J Surg, 1993. 166(4): p. 360-5.

58. Harrison, L.B., Applications of brachytherapy in head and neck cancer. Semin Surg Oncol, 1997. 13(3): p. 177-84.
59. Freedman, A.M. and D.A. Hidalgo, Full-thickness cheek and lip reconstruction with the radial forearm free flap. Ann Plast Surg, 1990. 25(4): p. 287-94.
60. Pradhan, S.A. and M.R. Rajpal, Marginal mandibulectomy in the management of squamous cancer of the oral cavity. Indian J Cancer, 1987. 24(3): p. 167-71.
61. Steinhart, H. and O. Kleinsasser, Growth and spread of squamous cell carcinoma of the floor of the mouth. Eur Arch Otorhinolaryngol, 1993. 250(6): p. 358-61.
62. Shons, A.R., F. Magallanes, and D. McQuarrie, The results of aggressive regional operation in the treatment of cancer of the floor of the mouth. Surgery, 1984. 96(1): p. 29-34.
63. Aygun, C., et al., Carcinoma of the floor of the mouth: a 20-year experience. Int J Radiat Oncol Biol Phys, 1984. 10(5): p. 619-26.
64. McGregor, A.D. and D.G. MacDonald, Routes of entry of squamous cell carcinoma to the mandible. Head Neck Surg, 1988. 10(5): p. 294-301.
65. Mendenhall, W.M., T3-4 squamous cell carcinoma of the larynx treated with radiation therapy alone. Semin Radiat Oncol, 1998. 8(4): p. 262-9.
66. Million, R.R., The larynx ... so to speak: everything I wanted to know about laryngeal cancer I learned in the last 32 years. Int J Radiat Oncol Biol Phys, 1992. 23(4): p. 691-704.
67. Parsons, J.T., et al., Radiotherapy Alone for Moderately Advanced Laryngeal Cancer (T2-T3). Semin Radiat Oncol, 1992. 2(3): p. 158-162.
68. Lundgren, J.A., et al., T3N0M0 glottic carcinoma--a failure analysis. Clin Otolaryngol, 1988. 13(6): p. 455-65.
69. Mendenhall, W.M., et al., Stage T3 squamous cell carcinoma of the glottic larynx: a comparison of laryngectomy and irradiation. Int J Radiat Oncol Biol Phys, 1992. 23(4): p. 725-32.
70. Johnson, J.T., et al., Outcome of open surgical therapy for glottic carcinoma. Ann Otol Rhinol Laryngol, 1993. 102(10): p. 752-5.
71. DeSanto, L.W., T3 glottic cancer: options and consequences of the options. Laryngoscope, 1984. 94(10): p. 1311-5.
72. Razack, M.S., et al., Management of advanced glottic carcinomas. Am J Surg, 1989. 158(4): p. 318-20.
73. Yuen, A., et al., Management of stage T3 and T4 glottic carcinomas. Am J Surg, 1984. 148(4): p. 467-72.
74. Sinard R.J., J.L. Netterville, C.G. Garrett, and R.H. Ossoff, Cancer of the Larynx, in Cancer of the Head and Neck, E.N. Myers, and J.Y. Suen, Editors. 1996, WB Saunders: Philadelphia. p. 381-422.
75. Biller, H.F. and W. Lawson, Partial laryngectomy for vocal cord cancer with marked limitation or fixation of the vocal cord. Laryngoscope, 1986. 96(1): p. 61-4.
76. Lesinski, S.G., W.C. Bauer, and J.H. Ogura, Hemilaryngectomy for T3 (fixed cord) epidermoid carcinoma of larynx. Laryngoscope, 1976. 86(10): p. 1563-71.
77. Som, M.L., Cordal cancer with extension to vocal process. Laryngoscope, 1975. 85(8): p. 1298-307.
78. Harwood, A.R., et al., Supraglottic laryngeal carcinoma: an analysis of dose-time-volume factors in 410 patients. Int J Radiat Oncol Biol Phys, 1983. 9(3): p. 311-9.
79. Mendenhall, W.M., R.R. Million, and N.J. Cassisi, Squamous cell carcinoma of the supraglottic larynx treated with radical irradiation: analysis of treatment parameters and results. Int J Radiat Oncol Biol Phys, 1984. 10(12): p. 2223-30.
80. Robson, N.L., V.H. Oswal, and L.M. Flood, Radiation therapy of laryngeal cancer: a twenty year experience. J Laryngol Otol, 1990. 104(9): p. 699-703.
81. Som, M.L., Conservation surgery for carcinoma of the supraglottis. J Laryngol Otol, 1970. 84(7): p. 655-78.

82.   Bocca, E., O. Pignataro, and C. Oldini, Supraglottic laryngectomy: 30 years of experience. Ann Otol Rhinol Laryngol, 1983. 92(1 Pt 1): p. 14-8.
83.   DeSanto, L.W., Cancer of the supraglottic larynx: a review of 260 patients. Otolaryngol Head Neck Surg, 1985. 93(6): p. 705-11.
84.   Spaulding, C.A., et al., Radiotherapeutic management of cancer of the supraglottis. Cancer, 1986. 57(7): p. 1292-8.
85.   Karim, A.B., et al., Radiation therapy for advanced (T3T4N0-N3M0) laryngeal carcinoma: the need for a change of strategy: a radiotherapeutic viewpoint. Int J Radiat Oncol Biol Phys, 1987. 13(11): p. 1625-33.
86.   Crellin, R.P., et al., Salvage laryngectomy after radical radiotherapy for laryngeal carcinoma. Clin Otolaryngol, 1992. 17(5): p. 449-51.
87.   McCombe, A.W. and A.S. Jones, Radiotherapy and complications of laryngectomy. J Laryngol Otol, 1993. 107(2): p. 130-2.
88.   Kraus, D.H., et al., Salvage laryngectomy for unsuccessful larynx preservation therapy. Ann Otol Rhinol Laryngol, 1995. 104(12): p. 936-41.
89.   Croll, G.A., et al., Primary radiotherapy with surgery in reserve for advanced laryngeal carcinoma. Results and complications. Eur J Surg Oncol, 1989. 15(4): p. 350-6.
90.   Slotman, G.J., et al., The incidence of metastases after multimodal therapy for cancer of the head and neck. Cancer, 1984. 54(9): p. 2009-14.
91.   Shaha, A.R. and J.P. Shah, Carcinoma of the subglottic larynx. Am J Surg, 1982. 144(4): p. 456-8.
92.   Sessions, D.G., J.H. Ogura, and M.P. Fried, Carcinoma of the subglottic area. Laryngoscope, 1975. 85(9): p. 1417-23.
93.   Natvig, K., M. Boysen, and J. Tausjo, Fistulae following laryngectomy in patients treated with irradiation. J Laryngol Otol, 1993. 107(12): p. 1136-9.
94.   Panje, W.R. and V.V. Kitt, Tracheal stoma reconstruction. Arch Otolaryngol, 1985. 111(3): p. 190-2.
95.   Yonkers, A.J. and G.A. Mercurio, Jr., Tracheostomal stenosis following total laryngectomy. Otolaryngol Clin North Am, 1983. 16(2): p. 391-405.
96.   Kuo, M., et al., Tracheostomal stenosis after total laryngectomy: an analysis of predisposing clinical factors. Laryngoscope, 1994. 104(1 Pt 1): p. 59-63.
97.   Shah, J.P., Patterns of cervical lymph node metastasis from squamous carcinomas of the upper aerodigestive tract. Am J Surg, 1990. 160(4): p. 405-9.
98.   Candela, F.C., et al., Patterns of cervical node metastases from squamous carcinoma of the larynx. Arch Otolaryngol Head Neck Surg, 1990. 116(4): p. 432-5.
99.   Harrison, D.F., The pathology and management of subglottic cancer. Ann Otol Rhinol Laryngol, 1971. 80(1): p. 6-12.
100.   Alvi A.A., E.N. Myers, and R.L. Carrau, Malignant tumors of the salivary glands, in Cancer of the Head and Neck, Myers E.N., and J.Y. Suen, Editors. 1996, WB Saunders: Philadelphia. p. 525-561.
101.   Shemen, L.J., A.G. Huvos, and R.H. Spiro, Squamous cell carcinoma of salivary gland origin. Head Neck Surg, 1987. 9(4): p. 235-40.
102.   Eneroth, C.M., Facial nerve paralysis. A criterion of malignancy in parotid tumors. Arch Otolaryngol, 1972. 95(4): p. 300-4.
103.   Johns, M.E., et al., Multiple primary neoplasms in patients with salivary gland or thyroid gland tumors. Laryngoscope, 1986. 96(7): p. 718-21.
104.   Preston-Martin, S., et al., Prior exposure to medical and dental x-rays related to tumors of the parotid gland. J Natl Cancer Inst, 1988. 80(12): p. 943-9.
105.   Klintenberg, C., et al., Adenocarcinoma of the ethmoid sinuses. A review of 28 cases with special reference to wood dust exposure. Cancer, 1984. 54(3): p. 482-8.

106.   Moraitis, D., et al., Pleomorphic adenoma causing acute airway obstruction. J Laryngol Otol, 2000. 114(8): p. 634-6.

107.   Spiro, R.H., Management of malignant tumors of the salivary glands. Oncology (Huntingt), 1998. 12(5): p. 671-80; discussion 683.

108.   Spiro, R.H., The management of salivary neoplasms: an overview. Auris Nasus Larynx, 1985. 12(Suppl 2): p. S122-7.

109.   Eisele D.W., and M.E. Johns, Salivary gland neoplasms, in Head & Neck Surgery-Otolaryngology, Bailey B.J., J.T. Johnson, H.C. Pillsbury, R.I, Kohut, and M.E. Tardy, Editors. 1993, JB Lippincott: Philadelphia. p. 1125-1147.

110.   Spiro, R.H., Changing trends in the management of salivary tumors. Semin Surg Oncol, 1995. 11(3): p. 240-5.

111.   Hanna E. Y., and J.Y. Suen., Neoplasms of the Salivary Gland, in Otolaryngology-Head and Neck Surgery, Cummings C.W., J.M. Fredrickson, L.A. Harker, C.J. Krause, M.A. Richardson, and D.E. Schuller, Editors. 1993, Mosby-Year Book: St. Louis.

112.   Leverstein, H., J.A. Castelijns, and G.B. Snow, The value of magnetic resonance imaging in the differential diagnosis of parapharyngeal space tumours. Clin Otolaryngol, 1995. 20(5): p. 428-33.

113.   Weber, R.S., et al., Submandibular gland tumors. Adverse histologic factors and therapeutic implications. Arch Otolaryngol Head Neck Surg, 1990. 116(9): p. 1055-60.

114.   Som, P.M., et al., Common tumors of the parapharyngeal space: refined imaging diagnosis. Radiology, 1988. 169(1): p. 81-5.

115.   Nanson, E.M., The surgery of the deep lobe of the parotid salivary gland. Surg Gynecol Obstet, 1966. 122(4): p. 811-6.

116.   Heller, K.S., J.N. Attie, and S. Dubner, Accuracy of frozen section in the evaluation of salivary tumors. Am J Surg, 1993. 166(4): p. 424-7.

117.   Woods, J.E., The facial nerve in parotid malignancy. Am J Surg, 1983. 146(4): p. 493-6.

118.   Roush, G.C., Epidemiology of cancer of the nose and paranasal sinuses: current concepts. Head Neck Surg, 1979. 2(1): p. 3-11.

119.   Barton, R.T., Nickel carcinogenesis of the respiratory tract. J Otolaryngol, 1977. 6(5): p. 412-22.

120.   Torjussen, W. and L.A. Solberg, Histological findings in the nasal mucosa of nickel workers. A preliminary report. Acta Otolaryngol, 1976. 82(3-4): p. 266-7.

121.   Acheson, E.D., et al., Nasal cancer in woodworkers in the furniture industry. Br Med J, 1968. 2(605): p. 587-96.

122.   Hernberg, S., et al., Nasal and sinonasal cancer. Connection with occupational exposures in Denmark, Finland and Sweden. Scand J Work Environ Health, 1983. 9(4): p. 315-26.

123.   Acheson, E.D., E.C. Pippard, and P.D. Winter, Nasal cancer in the Northamptonshire boot and shoe industry: is it declining? Br J Cancer, 1982. 46(6): p. 940-6.

124.   Stern SJ, Hanna E., Cancer of the nasal cavity and paranasal sinuses, in Cancer of the Head and Neck, Myers E.N., and J.Y. Suen, Editors. 1996, W.B. Saunders, Co.: Philadelphia. p. 205-233.

125.   Lareo, A.C., et al., History of previous nasal diseases and sinonasal cancer: a case-control study. Laryngoscope, 1992. 102(4): p. 439-42.

126.   Lanzieri, C.F., et al., Use of gadolinium-enhanced MR imaging for differentiating mucoceles from neoplasms in the paranasal sinuses. Radiology, 1991. 178(2): p. 425-8.

127.   Herve, S., et al., Management of sinonasal hemangiopericytomas. Rhinology, 1999. 37(4): p. 153-8.

128.   Beale, F.A. and P.G. Garrett, Cancer of the paranasal sinuses with particular reference to maxillary sinus cancer. J Otolaryngol, 1983. 12(6): p. 377-82.

129.   Lindeman, P., U. Eklund, and B. Petruson, Survival after surgical treatment in maxillary neoplasms of epithelial origin. J Laryngol Otol, 1987. 101(6): p. 564-8.

130.   Janecka, I.P., et al., Treatment of paranasal sinus cancer with cranial base surgery: results. Laryngoscope, 1994. 104(5 Pt 1): p. 553-5.

131.   Shah, J.P., et al., Craniofacial resections for tumors involving the base of the skull. Am J Surg, 1987. 154(4): p. 352-8.

132.   Cordeiro, P.G., et al., Reconstruction of total maxillectomy defects with preservation of the orbital contents. Plast Reconstr Surg, 1998. 102(6): p. 1874-84; discussion 1885-7.

133.   Maniglia, A.J. and D.A. Phillips, Midfacial degloving for the management of nasal, sinus, and skull-base neoplasms. Otolaryngol Clin North Am, 1995. 28(6): p. 1127-43.

134.   Pearson, B.W., The surgical anatomy of maxillectomy. Surg Clin North Am, 1977. 57(4): p. 701-21.

135.   Kondo, M., et al., Prognostic factors influencing relapse of squamous cell carcinoma of the maxillary sinus. Cancer, 1985. 55(1): p. 190-6.

136.   Wang, R.R., Sectional prosthesis for total maxillectomy patients: a clinical report. J Prosthet Dent, 1997. 78(3): p. 241-4.

137.   Stern, S.J., et al., Orbital preservation in maxillectomy. Otolaryngol Head Neck Surg, 1993. 109(1): p. 111-5.

138.   Kennedy, R.E., Indications and surgical techniques for orbital exenteration. Ophthalmology, 1979. 86(5): p. 967-73.

139.   Jiang, G.L., et al., Maxillary sinus carcinomas: natural history and results of postoperative radiotherapy. Radiother Oncol, 1991. 21(3): p. 193-200.

140.   Claus, F., et al., Postoperative radiotherapy of paranasal sinus tumours: a challenge for intensity modulated radiotherapy. Acta Otorhinolaryngol Belg, 1999. 53(3): p. 263-9.

141.   Derome P.J., Transbasal approach to tumors invading the base of skull, in Operative Neurosurgical Techniques, S.W. Schmidek HH, Editor. 1982, Grune & Stratton: Orlando, FL. p. 357.

142.   Sekhar, L.N., I.P. Janecka, and N.F. Jones, Subtemporal-infratemporal and basal subfrontal approach to extensive cranial base tumours. Acta Neurochir, 1988. 92(1-4): p. 83-92.

143.   Nuss D.W., and I.P. Janeka, Cranial base tumors, in Cancer of the Head and Neck, Myers E.N., and J.Y. Suen, Editors. 1996, W.B. Saunders: Philadelphia, PA. p. 234-275.

144.   Chang, D.W. and G.L. Robb, Microvascular reconstruction of the skull base. Semin Surg Oncol, 2000. 19(3): p. 211-7.

145.   Disa, J.J., V.M. Rodriguez, and P.G. Cordeiro, Reconstruction of lateral skull base oncological defects: the role of free tissue transfer. Ann Plast Surg, 1998. 41(6): p. 633-9.

146.   Ross D.A., C.T. Sasaki, Cancer of the ear and temporal bone, in Cancer of the Head and Neck, Myers E.N., and J.Y. Suen, Editors. 1996, W.B. Saunders Co.: Philadelphia, PA. p. 586-597.

147.   Shockley, W.W. and F.J. Stucker, Jr., Squamous cell carcinoma of the external ear: a review of 75 cases. Otolaryngol Head Neck Surg, 1987. 97(3): p. 308-12.

148.   Zhang, B., et al., Squamous cell carcinoma of temporal bone: reported on 33 patients. Head Neck, 1999. 21(5): p. 461-6.

149.   Savic, D.L. and D.R. Djeric, Malignant tumours of the middle ear. Clin Otolaryngol, 1991. 16(1): p. 87-9.

150. Pulec, J.L., Glandular tumors of the external auditory canal. Laryngoscope, 1977. 87(10 Pt 1): p. 1601-12.
151. Arriaga, M., et al., The role of preoperative CT scans in staging external auditory meatus carcinoma: radiologic-pathologic correlation study. Otolaryngol Head Neck Surg, 1991. 105(1): p. 6-11.
152. Leonetti, J.P., et al., Invasion patterns of advanced temporal bone malignancies. Am J Otol, 1996. 17(3): p. 438-42.
153. Chen, D., et al., Prosthetic auricular reconstruction. Otolaryngol Head Neck Surg, 1983. 91(5): p. 556-8.
154. Gal, T.J., et al., Auricular carcinoma with temporal bone invasion: outcome analysis. Otolaryngol Head Neck Surg, 1999. 121(1): p. 62-5.
155. Wagenfeld, D.J., et al., Primary carcinoma involving the temporal bone: analysis of twenty-five cases. Laryngoscope, 1980. 90(6 Pt 1): p. 912-9.
156. Sinha, P.P. and H.I. Aziz, Treatment of carcinoma of the middle ear. Radiology, 1978. 126(2): p. 485-7.
157. Lederman, M., C.H. Jones, and R.F. Mould, Cancer of the middle ear; technique of radiation treatment. Br J Radiol, 1965. 38(456): p. 895-905.
158. Arena, S. and M. Keen, Carcinoma of the middle ear and temporal bone. Am J Otol, 1988. 9(5): p. 351-6.
159. Urbach, F., Geographical pathology of skin cancer, in The Biologic Effects of Ultraviolet Radiation, Urbach, F., Editor. 1969, Pergamon Press: Oxford, England. p. 635.
160. Kinney, S.E., Clinical Evaluation and Treatment of Ear Tumors, in Comprehensive Management of Head and Neck Tumors, Thawley, S.E., W.R. Panje, J.G. Batsakis, and R.D. Lindberg, Editors. 1999, W.B. Saunders Co.: Philadelphia, PA. p. 395.
161. Gulmen, S. and J.T. Crosson, Adenoid cystic carcinoma of the external auditory canal. Eye Ear Nose Throat Mon, 1975. 54(7): p. 274-6.
162. Wiener, E.S., Head and neck rhabdomyosarcoma. Semin Pediatr Surg, 1994. 3(3): p. 203-6.
163. Gates, G.A., The lateral facial approach to the nasopharynx and infratemporal fossa. Otolaryngol Head Neck Surg, 1988. 99(3): p. 321-5.
164. Goel, A., Extended lateral subtemporal approach for petroclival meningiomas: report of experience with 24 cases. Br J Neurosurg, 1999. 13(3): p. 270-5.
165. Kawase, T., R. Shiobara, and S. Toya, Middle fossa transpetrosal-transtentorial approaches for petroclival meningiomas. Selective pyramid resection and radicality. Acta Neurochir, 1994. 129(3-4): p. 113-20.
166. Mori, K., et al., Craniopharyngiomas with unusual topography and associated with vascular pathology. Acta Neurochir, 1980. 53(1-2): p. 53-68.
167. Gloria-Cruz, T.I., et al., Metastases to temporal bones from primary nonsystemic malignant neoplasms. Arch Otolaryngol Head Neck Surg, 2000. 126(2): p. 209-14.
168. Chao, C.K., et al., Treatment, outcomes, and prognostic factors of ear cancer. J Formos Med Assoc, 1999. 98(5): p. 314-8.
169. Streitmann, M.J. and A. Sismanis, Metastatic carcinoma of the temporal bone. Am J Otol, 1996. 17(5): p. 780-3.
170. Castillo, M. and H.C. Pillsbury, 3rd, Rhabdomyosarcoma of the middle ear: imaging features in two children. AJNR Am J Neuroradiol, 1993. 14(3): p. 730-3.
171. Lewis, J.S. and R. Page, Radical surgery for malignant tumors of the ear. Arch Otolaryngol, 1966. 83(2): p. 114-9.
172. Prasad, S. and I.P. Janecka, Efficacy of surgical treatments for squamous cell carcinoma of the temporal bone: a literature review. Otolaryngol Head Neck Surg, 1994. 110(3): p. 270-80.
173. MacDonald EJ, J.M., Murphy A, Regional patterns in morbidity from melanomas in Texas. Cancer Bull, 1971. 23: p. 51.

174. Miller, D.L. and M.A. Weinstock, Nonmelanoma skin cancer in the United States: incidence. J Am Acad Dermatol, 1994. 30(5 Pt 1): p. 774-8.

175. Owens, D.W., et al., Influence of humidity on ultraviolet injury. J Invest Dermatol, 1975. 64(4): p. 250-2.

176. Unna P.G., The Histopathology of the Diseases of the Skin. 1986, New York, NY: Macmillan.

177. Dinehart S.M., and G.T. Jansen, Cancer of the skin, in Cancer of the Head and Neck, Myers E.N., and J.Y. Suen, Editors. 1996, W.B. Saunders Co.: Philadelphia, PA. p. 143-159.

178. Kripke, M.L., Immunology and photocarcinogenesis. New light on an old problem. J Am Acad Dermatol, 1986. 14(1): p. 149-55.

179. Barsky, D. and W.J. Vasileff, Extensive morphea-form basal cell carcinoma invasion of the iris and the orbital contents. Henry Ford Hosp Med J, 1987. 35(1): p. 71-3.

180. Runger, T.M., et al., Repair of directly and indirectly UV-induced DNA lesions and of DNA double-strand breaks in cells from skin cancer-prone patients with the disorders dysplastic nevus syndrome or basal cell nevus syndrome. Recent Results Cancer Res, 1997. 143: p. 337-51.

181. Granstrom, G., F. Aldenborg, and P.H. Jeppsson, Influence of embryonal fusion lines for recurrence of basal cell carcinomas in the head and neck. Otolaryngol Head Neck Surg, 1986. 95(1): p. 76-82.

182. Davies, R., et al., Metastatic basal cell carcinoma of the eyelid. Report of a case. Arch Ophthalmol, 1995. 113(5): p. 634-7.

183. Mohs F.E., Chemosurgery in microscopically controlled method of cancer excision. Arch Surg, 1941. 42: p. 279.

184. Tromovitch, T.A. and S.J. Stegeman, Microscopically controlled excision of skin tumors. Arch Dermatol, 1974. 110(2): p. 231-2.

185. Jackson, R. and R.H. Adams, Horrifying basal cell carcinoma: a study of 33 cases and a comparison with 435 non-horror cases and a report on four metastatic cases. J Surg Oncol, 1973. 5(5): p. 431-63.

186. Glogau, R.G., The risk of progression to invasive disease. J Am Acad Dermatol, 2000. 42(1 Pt 2): p. 23-4.

187. Kraus, D.H., J.F. Carew, and L.B. Harrison, Regional lymph node metastasis from cutaneous squamous cell carcinoma. Arch Otolaryngol Head Neck Surg, 1998. 124(5): p. 582-7.

188. Dinehart, S.M. and S.V. Pollack, Metastases from squamous cell carcinoma of the skin and lip. An analysis of twenty-seven cases. J Am Acad Dermatol, 1989. 21(2 Pt 1): p. 241-8.

189. Johnson, T.M., et al., Squamous cell carcinoma of the skin (excluding lip and oral mucosa). J Am Acad Dermatol, 1992. 26(3 Pt 2): p. 467-84.

190. AG, F., Kerato-acanthoma. Aust J Dermatol, 1954. 2: p. 144.

191. Massa, M.C. and M. Medenica, Cutaneous adnexal tumors and cysts: a review. Part II--Tumors with apocrine and eccrine glandular differentiation and miscellaneous cutaneous cysts. Pathol Annu, 1987. 22(Pt 1): p. 225-76.

192. Patel, S.G., A.R. Shaha, and J.P. Shah, Soft tissue sarcomas of the head and neck: an update. Am J Otolaryngol, 2001. 22(1): p. 2-18.

193. Lydiatt, W.M., A.R. Shaha, and J.P. Shah, Angiosarcoma of the head and neck. Am J Surg, 1994. 168(5): p. 451-4.

194. Batsakis, J.G. and R.B. Brannon, Dermal analogue tumours of major salivary glands. J Laryngol Otol, 1981. 95(2): p. 155-64.

195.   Boutilier, R., et al., Merkel cell carcinoma: squamous and atypical fibroxanthoma-like differentiation in successive local tumor recurrences. Am J Dermatopathol, 2001. 23(1): p. 46-9.

196.   Anderson, P.J., A.R. McPhaden, and R.J. Ratcliffe, Atypical fibroxanthoma of the scalp. Head Neck, 2001. 23(5): p. 399-403.

197.   McGregor, S.E., et al., Cutaneous malignant melanoma in Alberta: 1967-1976. Cancer, 1983. 52(4): p. 755-61.

198.   Pathak, D.R., et al., Malignant melanoma of the skin in New Mexico 1969-1977. Cancer, 1982. 50(7): p. 1440-6.

199.   Silverberg, E., C.C. Boring, and T.S. Squires, Cancer statistics, 1990. CA Cancer J Clin, 1990. 40(1): p. 9-26.

200.   Medina J.E., and V. Canfield, Malignant melanoma of the head and neck, in Cancer of the Head and Neck, Myers E.N., and J.Y. Suen, Editors. 1996, W.B. Saunders Co.: Philadelphia, PA. p. 160-183.

201.   Wilmes, E. and J. Bujia, Recommendations for therapy of head and neck cutaneous melanoma. Am J Otolaryngol, 1993. 14(4): p. 267-70.

202.   Balch, C.M., et al., Management of cutaneous melanoma in the United States. Surg Gynecol Obstet, 1984. 158(4): p. 311-8.

203.   Batsakis, J.G., et al., The pathology of head and neck tumors: mucosal melanomas, part 13. Head Neck Surg, 1982. 4(5): p. 404-18.

204.   Gallagher, R.P., J.M. Elwood, and G.B. Hill, Risk factors for cutaneous malignant melanoma: the Western Canada Melanoma Study. Recent Results Cancer Res, 1986. 102: p. 38-55.

205.   Green, A., et al., Risk factors for cutaneous melanoma in Queensland. Recent Results Cancer Res, 1986. 102: p. 76-97.

206.   Osterlind, A., Epidemiology on malignant melanoma in Europe. Acta Oncol, 1992. 31(8): p. 903-8.

207.   Horm J.W., et al., SEER program: Cancer incidence and mortality in the United States 1973-1981.US Dept. of Health and Human Services publication no. (NIH) 85-1837. 1984, National Cancer Institute: Bethesda, MD.

208.   Holman, C.D. and B.K. Armstrong, Pigmentary traits, ethnic origin, benign nevi, and family history as risk factors for cutaneous malignant melanoma. J Natl Cancer Inst, 1984. 72(2): p. 257-66.

209.   Scotto, J. and T.R. Fears, The association of solar ultraviolet and skin melanoma incidence among caucasians in the United States. Cancer Invest, 1987. 5(4): p. 275-83.

210.   Osterlind, A., Malignant melanoma in Denmark. Occurrence and risk factors. Acta Oncol, 1990. 29(7): p. 833-54.

211.   Consensus conference, Precursors to malignant melanoma. JAMA, 1984. 251: p. 1864.

212.   Arnolt, K.A., Precursors to malignant melanoma: congenital and dysplastic nevi. Jama, 1984. 251(14): p. 1882-3.

213.   Tucker, M.A., et al., Cutaneous malignant melanoma after Hodgkin's disease. Ann Intern Med, 1985. 102(1): p. 37-41.

214.   Greene, M.H. and J. Wilson, Second cancer following lymphatic and hematopoietic cancers in Connecticut, 1935-82. Natl Cancer Inst Monogr, 1985. 68: p. 191-217.

215.   Greene, M.H., T.I. Young, and W.H. Clark, Jr., Malignant melanoma in renal-transplant recipients. Lancet, 1981. 1(8231): p. 1196-9.

216.   Holly, E.A., Cutaneous melanoma and oral contraceptives: a review of case-control and cohort studies. Recent Results Cancer Res, 1986. 102: p. 108-17.

217.   Driscoll, M.S., C.M. Grin-Jorgensen, and J.M. Grant-Kels, Does pregnancy influence the prognosis of malignant melanoma? J Am Acad Dermatol, 1993. 29(4): p. 619-30.

218. Tucker, M.A., J.D. Boice, Jr., and D.A. Hoffman, Second cancer following cutaneous melanoma and cancers of the brain, thyroid, connective tissue, bone, and eye in Connecticut, 1935-82. Natl Cancer Inst Monogr, 1985. 68: p. 161-89.

219. Rhodes, A.R., et al., Risk factors for cutaneous melanoma. A practical method of recognizing predisposed individuals. JAMA, 1987. 258(21): p. 3146-54.

220. Shah, J.P., et al., Patterns of regional lymph node metastases from cutaneous melanomas of the head and neck. Am J Surg, 1991. 162(4): p. 320-3.

221. Urist, M.M., et al., Head and neck melanoma in 534 clinical Stage I patients. A prognostic factors analysis and results of surgical treatment. Ann Surg, 1984. 200(6): p. 769-75.

222. Ringborg, U., et al., Cutaneous malignant melanoma of the head and neck. Analysis of treatment results and prognostic factors in 581 patients: a report from the Swedish Melanoma Study Group. Cancer, 1993. 71(3): p. 751-8.

223. O'Brien, C.J., et al., Experience with 998 cutaneous melanomas of the head and neck over 30 years. Am J Surg, 1991. 162(4): p. 310-4.

224. Singletary, S.E., et al., Prognostic factors in patients with regional cervical nodal metastases from cutaneous malignant melanoma. Am J Surg, 1986. 152(4): p. 371-5.

225. Balch, C.M., et al., A multifactorial analysis of melanoma: III. Prognostic factors in melanoma patients with lymph node metastases (stage II). Ann Surg, 1981. 193(3): p. 377-88.

226. Balch, C.M., et al., Efficacy of 2-cm surgical margins for intermediate-thickness melanomas (1 to 4 mm). Results of a multi-institutional randomized surgical trial. Ann Surg, 1993. 218(3): p. 262-7; discussion 267-9.

227. Byers, R.M., et al., Malignant melanoma of the external ear. Review of 102 cases. Am J Surg, 1980. 140(4): p. 518-21.

228. Byers, R.M., L. Smith, and R. DeWitty, Malignant melanoma of the skin of the nose. Am J Otolaryngol, 1982. 3(3): p. 202-3.

229. National Institute of Health Consensus Development Conference Statement on Diagnosis and Treatment of Early Melanoma. Am J Dermatopathol, 1993. 15: p. 34-43.

230. Milton, G.W., et al., Prophylactic lymph node dissection in clinical stage I cutaneous malignant melanoma: results of surgical treatment in 1319 patients. Br J Surg, 1982. 69(2): p. 108-11.

231. Balch, C.M., Surgical management of regional lymph nodes in cutaneous melanoma. J Am Acad Dermatol, 1980. 3(5): p. 511-24.

232. Fisher, S.R., Cutaneous malignant melanoma of the head and neck. Laryngoscope, 1989. 99(8 Pt 1): p. 822-36.

233. Berman, C.G., et al., Lymphoscintigraphy in malignant melanoma. Ann Plast Surg, 1992. 28(1): p. 29-32.

Chapter 7

MODIFIED FRACTIONATED RADIOTHERAPY IN HEAD AND NECK SQUAMOUS CELL CARCINOMA (HNSCC) & RE-IRRADIATION IN RECURRENT HEAD AND NECK CARCINOMAS

De Crevoisier R.M.D., Bourhis J., Eschwège F.M.D.
Institut Gustave Roussy

In the past decades, two new developments have appeared in the field of radiotherapy (RT) for HNSCC. The first approach concerns the modification of fractionation in order to improve the anti-tumor effect, while maintaining acceptable normal tissues reactions. The second approach concerns the use of re-irradiation in patients with inoperable local-regional relapses occurring in a previously irradiated area. A review of these two techniques and their potential interest in HNSCC is presented.

MODIFIED FRACTIONATION

Rational for a modified fractionation

Ionizing radiation has been used for more than one century in the management of head and neck squamous cell carcinomas. The clinical experience accumulated throughout this time has led to the use in routine practice of so called conventional radiotherapy delivering 2 Gy per fraction, 5 times per week, up to total dose of 60 to 70 Gy. Several ways have been tested to improve the anti-tumor effect of radiotherapy in HNSCC including radio-chemotherapy combinations, radiosensitizers, and modified fractionation. Although the conventional radiotherapy offered an acceptable compromise between efficacy and tolerance, a considerable interest was focused in the early 1980s on the possibility of improving the therapeutic index of radiotherapy when using modified fractionated radiotherapy. Two types of modified fractionation have been developed including hyperfractionated and more recently accelerated radiotherapy. This recent progress has been made possible due to a better understanding of the parameters of fractionation (total dose, dose per fraction, interval, and overall time) involved in determining acute normal tissues reactions (mucositis, epithelitis) as well as late effects (fibrosis, necrosis). Decreasing the dose per fraction (<1.2 Gy) can protect the late responding normal tissues more than tumor cells, leading to a differential effect which allows one to deliver a total dose higher than the conventional dose in the same overall time and constitutes the basis of hyperfractionated schedules. Modified fractionated RT aims to increase the "dose intensity" of radiotherapy by delivering a total dose as high as possible in an overall time as short as possible. This increased dose intensity of radiotherapy has been obtained either by increasing the total dose (hyperfractionation) and/or decreasing the overall time (acceleration) as compared to conventional radiotherapy. Several regimens have used a combination of both accelerated and hyperfractionated radiotherapy.

Randomized studies comparing conventional Radiotherapy and modified fractionated radiotherapy

Modified fractionated radiotherapy has been tested in more than 20 randomized studies in HNSCC patients showing in most cases a benefit in terms of local tumor control, with limited impact on overall survival. Interestingly the reference arm was in most studies conventional radiotherapy delivering 66-70 Gy over 6.5 to 7 weeks, whereas these studies can be classified in 3 groups according the total dose and the overall treatment time used in the experimental arm :

• Total dose higher and same overall time than the reference arm : hyperfractionated radiotherapy (1-7).

• Total dose the same but overall time shorter than the reference arm : moderately accelerated radiotherapy (8, 9, 10, 12, 13, 14, 17, 20).
• Total dose reduced and overall time much shorter than the reference arm : very accelerated radiotherapy (11, 15, 16, 18, 19).

• Total dose higher and same overall time compared to the reference arm : hyperfractionated radiotherapy

Some randomized studies of modified fractionation have tested a « pure hyperfractionated regimen ». The primary change was to decrease the dose per fraction (< 1.2 Gy) giving 2 fractions per day along with a sufficiently large interval between fraction (> 4-6 hours). Lowering the dose per fraction can reduce the probability of late effects and consequently allowed to increase markedly the total dose without increasing deleterious effect.

Several randomized studies have been performed comparing such hyperfractionated radiotherapy to conventional radiotherapy (3-7) including the EORTC 22791 study reported by J.C. Horiot (3). This study included 356 patients with a T2-T3 N0-1 oropharyngeal cancer and showed that hyperfractionation (1.15 Gy twice daily) allowed one to deliver a total dose of 80.5 Gy in 7 weeks as compared to 70 Gy in 7 weeks in the reference arm. The results of the study showed a significant improvement in tumor control probability at 5 years with a significant survival benefit but without increased late effects. Interestingly the benefit associated with hyperfractionated radiotherapy was essentially found in the largest tumors (T3) whereas no benefit was seen in T2 patients.

The benefit of hyperfractionated radiotherapy on local tumor control probability was also reported in 3 other randomized studies which tested a comparable regimen to conventional radiotherapy (4, 5, 7), whereas none of them showed a significant benefit in overall survival. The most recent of these studies was the RTOG 90-03 trial (7) which tested in a large 4 arm study (> 1113 patients) a regimen very close to the EORTC (81.6 Gy / 7 weeks) and showed also a significant benefit (9%) in tumor control probability. In this group, Cummings in Toronto (6) reported an additional study performed in the Princess Margaret Hospital and compared their reference arm consisting of 51 Gy / 4 weeks delivering 5 times 2.5 Gy / week to an experimental hyperfractionated arm consisting of 58 Gy in 4 weeks, with 1.25 Gy, 2 times per day. An improvement in tumor control probability was observed in favor of the hyperfractionated arm along with a trend towards better survival.

Total dose the same but overall time shorter than the reference arm : moderately accelerated radiotherapy

In this situation, the total dose is not increased but maintained as compared to conventional radiotherapy, whereas the overall duration of radiotherapy in markedly reduced to overcome tumor cell repopulation during the whole course of radiotherapy. Several randomized studies have been performed, including the EORTC 22-851 (9-10) and a large Danish trial (DAHANCA) (14). More recently two Polish studies have been reported including a trial using a regimen very similar to the DAHANCA in patients with T1-3 larynx carcinoma (20). In this group was also reported recently the results of the RTOG 90-03 (concomitant boost) and a study from MD Anderson performed in post-operative patients (13). The primary change in these studies was to reduce the overall time by 1 (DANANCA, Hilniak, RTOG 90-03) or 2 weeks (EORTC, CAIR), either by treating 1 or 2 extra fractions per week (6 or 7 days in stead of 5 days / week, DAHANCA and Polish trials) or by accelerating at the end of the course of radiotherapy (concomitant boost in RTOG 90-03 and MD Anderson studies). In most of these trials the total dose was the same as the reference arm (68-72 Gy), whereas the dose per fraction was either the same (2 Gy) or slightly less (between 1.5 Gy-2 Gy) than the reference arm.

The EORTC (9-10) included between 1985 and 1995, 512 patients with a T2-4 N0-3 HNSCC. The patients were randomized between 70 Gy / 7 weeks versus accelerated regimen delivering 3 x 1.6 Gy / day separated by an interval of 3-4 hours. In the accelerated arm a first sequence of 28.8 Gy was delivered followed by a split of 12-14 days. The cumulative total dose was 72 Gy/5 weeks. There was a significant increase of acute toxicity in the accelerated arm and more importantly of late effects. Indeed the probability of severe late effect free survival at 3 years (grade 3-4) was 85% in the conventional arm versus 63% in the accelerated arm (p < 0.001). With a median follow-up of 4.5 years, the local-regional control rate was 46% versus 59%, in favor of the accelerated arm (p = 0.02) with no improvement in survival. This study is one of the most important contributions to the field of modified fractionated radiotherapy in terms of understanding the effect of fractionation parameters on both acute and late effects. Indeed, as expected, a marked increase of acute toxicity was observed in the accelerated arm due to the 2 weeks reduction in the overall treatment time. However the marked increase of late effects was less expected and likely due to the conjunction of a high total dose (72 Gy), along with a relatively high dose per fraction (1.6 Gy) with too short intervals between fractions (3-4 hours). Using such a schedule, the amount of reparable but non repaired damage in normal tissues is probably too high and exposes patients to an increase probability of late effects

In this group of trials the DAHANCA 7 (14) tested moderately accelerated RT in a series of 791 patients with a T2-T4 of the pharynx, larynx and oral cavity. A conventional RT 66-68 Gy / 6.5 weeks was compared to the same total dose in 5.5 weeks. The hypoxic sensitizer Nimorazole was given in both arms. Acute toxicity was moderately increased, but no changes in late effects were seen and the tumor control was improved in the accelerated arm without significant survival benefit. A Polish trial (20) has used the same schedule in T1-3 larynx carcinoma showing the same trend whereas a second Polish trial (CAIR, 17) has tested a more accelerated schedule comparing 7 x 2 Gy versus 5 x 2 Gy per week with the same total dose in both arms and showed a major benefit in favor of the accelerated radiotherapy. However, the results of this study have to be considered with caution since they were obtained in a limited series of patients (100 pts).

More recently the RTOG 90-03 four-arm randomized study confirmed the benefit associated with moderately accelerated radiotherapy showing that the concomitant boost schedule (72 Gy in 6 weeks) led to a significant 9% increase in tumor control probability, without significant survival benefit.

Total dose reduced and overall time much shorter than the reference arm : Very Accelerated Radiotherapy

In this group several randomized studies have been performed including the large CHART trial (32), a very similar study from Austria (15), and 2 additional studies from the GORTEC (Groupe d'Oncologie Radiothérapie Tête et Cou) (16) and the TROG (Trans Tasmanian Radiotherapy Oncology Group) (18). In all these studies the total dose was markedly reduced in the accelerated arm, whereas the overall duration of radiotherapy was also markedly reduced leading a total duration of 1.5 to 4 weeks.

In the CHART performed between 1990 and 1995 (11), 918 HNSCC patients were randomized between 66 Gy in 6.5 weeks versus continuous accelerated hyperfractionated radiotherapy (CHART), delivering 54 Gy in 12 days (1.5 Gy x 3 times / day, 6 hours interval). Acute toxicity was moderately increased whereas late effects were less pronounced with the accelerated regimen. No significant benefit was observed in favor of accelerated radiotherapy although when considering only the T3-4 subgroup of patients (> 500 patients) accelerated radiotherapy was associated with a significant improvement of tumor control probability. The results of the CHART showing no significant benefit (except for large tumors) were confirmed by the study of Dobrowsky and also suggest that reducing the total dose has to be considered with caution in the context of modified fractionation. More recently, the TROG (371 patients) (18) has used an intermediate total dose of 59.5 Gy in 4 weeks and the GORTEC tested a higher total dose of 64 Gy in 3 weeks (16). This GORTEC 94-02 study (268 patients) showed a marked benefit of 24% at 2 years in tumor control probability in favor of accelerated arm, suggesting the importance of maintaining a sufficiently high total dose when using very accelerated RT. However maintaining a high total dose was also associated in the GORTEC experience with a marked increase of acute toxicity (90% of patients with confluent mucositis and feeding tube) whereas the late toxicity was not increased.

CONCLUSION

This clinical overview underlines the potential interest of increasing the dose intensity of radiotherapy by using modified fractionated RT in head and neck squamous cell carcinoma. The first randomized trial that showed a benefit in tumor control due to hyperfractionation was the EORTC 22791 study. These results were then confirmed by several other randomized studies. More recently acceleration of radiotherapy was tested showing that in most cases that this type of modified fractionation was also able to improve significantly tumor control probability. However most of these modified fractionation schedules failed to improve significantly overall survival. One of the drawbacks also is the absence of effect on distant metastases since these modifications of radiotherapy essentially aimed to improve local-regional control. Importantly several studies (EORTC 22791, CHART, Cummings, Hilniak, DAHANCA 6/7) have strongly suggested that the benefit associated with modified fractionation was much more pronounced in locally advanced HNSCC (T3-T4), as compared to early stages. In some studies such as the GORTEC 94-02, having including essentially T4 disease, the benefit appears to be relatively high (24% improvement in tumor control).

As we have seen in this review, a large variety of schedules have been tested, but it is not possible to draw conclusions regarding the optimal regimen to be used. These studies have also emphasized the importance of the total dose, dose per fraction and interval between fraction to avoid late toxicity.

Finally the feasibility of modified fractionated radiotherapy allows one to envisage combining RT with concurrent chemotherapy which has been done recently providing promising results in favor of the combined approach.

Re-Irradiation

The majority of patients with HNSCC present with locally advanced disease and surgery and/or radiotherapy can cure 30-60% of them. Most of the local relapses occur within the first 2 years after the primary treatment and at least 50% of patients who died from uncontrolled tumor have local and/or regional disease as a sole site of failure. In addition, about 30% of these patients will develop new primary tumors within 10 years (21). The treatment of patients with recurrent or second primary HNSCC in previously irradiated areas represents a major challenge. Salvage surgery may be effected successfully in a small proportion of selected patients. Chemotherapy may offer palliation but is not curative with response rates that range from 10% to 30% (22,23). Although re-irradiation is not currently considered a standard approach fore these patients, it may constitutes an alternative approach.

Curative radiotherapy often involves treating a volume of normal tissue to the limit of tolerance. The main concerns with re-irradiation are damage to previously irradiated normal tissues such as the spinal cord, and the extent to which these tissue can recover from previous radiation damage. At least, for re-treatment with curative intent a moderate increase in the risk of normal tissue complications might be considered as acceptable.

Several techniques of re-irradiation have been used including brachytherapy, and various techniques of external radiotherapy which are summarized in this review.

Brachytherapy

Brachytherapy has the theoretical advantage of delivering a relatively high dose of radiation in the tumor that falls off rapidly and can consequently sparc neighboring tissues.

A small proportion of patients with recurrent head and neck carcinoma can be salvaged by interstitial irradiation with acceptable morbidity (24). The main conditions for performing salvage brachytherapy are : (a) encompass the entire tumor volume with adequate margins, (b) delivery of a total dose in the tumor of at least 60 Gy using whenever possible a low dose rate (0.4-0.7 Gy/h), (c) well limited exophytic and/or moderately infiltrating tumors and (d) selection of the site : soft palate, nasopharynx, tonsillar fossa, and tongue. Depending on the series, 5 year overall survival rates are 19 to 27% (25-31). Various techniques of brachytherapy have been employed depending on the location of the tumor: intra-cavitary brachytherapy sources may be used in nasopharyngeal carcinoma and interstitial implants can be inserted directly into the tumor by using flexible afterloading plastic tubes and button techniques.

Brachytherapy has been used alone (26-34) or combined with external irradiation (27-34). Some authors have reported in a retrospective study better results when combining external re-irradiation plus brachytherapy versus external irradiation only (27). However a higher rate of severe complications (33%) was observed in patients treated with the combined treatment.

Several authors have used re-irradiation with brachytherapy alone in oropharyngeal carcinoma (26,27,29-32,35). In the series reported by Peiffert, no grade 3 or 4 complications were observed, which could be explained by a small target volume (small tumors), the use of a mandibular lead shielding and the use of low dose rate brachytherapy. Fontanesi et al showed that the dose rate had a significant impact on the occurrence of severe complications in a series of 23 patients re-irradiated with interstitial iridium-192 (31).

For selected patients with recurrent disease exclusively confined to the nasopharynx, gold grain implantation alone is an alternative technique, leading to a 5-year local control rate and 5-year overall survival rates of 63% and 54% in a series of 53 patients (33). Complications included headache, palatal fistula and mucosal necrosis occurred in 19% of the patients. There was no life-threatening complications. Finally another technique has been used in recurrent nasopharyngeal carcinoma combining of high-dose rate intra-cavitary brachytherapy and external beam radiation with encouraging results (36). In the cases of brachytherapy for recurrent nasopharynx carcinoma, because of the difficulty to delimitate precisely clinically the tumor, the use of dosimetry based on imaging (CT-scan or MRI) may lead to increase local control and minimize side effects.

In conclusion, low dose-rate brachytherapy delivering a dose of at least 60 Gy in the target volume provides a useful method for the re-treatment of selected patients with limited and accessible recurrent carcinoma in a previously irradiated area.

External re-irradiation

The analysis of the literature shows about 40 heterogeneous publications concerning external re-irradiation of head and neck carcinoma (27,36-63). These studies show that full dose re-irradiation is feasible with acceptable tolerance. Several rules have been applied to this type of irradiation, including the use of limited volume with minimal margins around the tumor and no prophylactic irradiation (nodes). In addition, the spiral cord is constantly spared and not re-irradiated. Acute toxicity observed during re-irradiation is generally not different than that observed during the first course of irradiation. The rate of acute grade 3 and grade 4 mucositis ranges from 30% to 47% (27,41-43,49,56). These variations can be related to the concomitant administration (or not) of chemotherapy. The frequency and severity of late effects after full-dose re-irradiation is not well established, since it has been reported only in a limited number of series. Fatal carotid hemorrhage was reported in a few series (43,49,56,61). Three studies reported deaths from cerebral necrosis following re-irradiation for recurrent nasopharyngeal carcinoma (61). The rates of mucosal necrosis and osteoradionecrosis range in the literature from 1% to 20% (37,42,43,45,52-55,57,59,60). The rate of trismus ranges in the series from 2% to 30%. Comparison of results concerning efficacy is difficult because of heterogeneity in the selection of patients, tumor types, therapeutic modalities and methods of evaluation following re-irradiation. The published series reported a 5-year survival rate from 13% to 93% (27,43,48,51,53,57,59,61). The higher 5-year survival rates concern the re-irradiation of small laryngeal carcinoma (43) and the majority are 15-20% corresponding to a median survival of 8-11 months. In our series of 169 patients re-irradiated for unresectable head and neck carcinoma, most of the long-term disease-free survivors were found in the subgroup of patients treated with radiotherapy with concomitant chemotherapy (Vokes protocol) (43). They received 4 to 7 cycles with 7-day rest periods between cycles. Each cycle delivered from day 1 to day 5, 2 Gy/d, hydroxyurea (1,5 g/d) and 5-FU (800 mg/m²/d). The median total dose of radiotherapy delivered was 60 Gy.

Independent prognostic factors for overall survival found in the literature were: age (40), histology (40), interval to recurrence (40,49,64), surface area and volume of the second irradiation (43). The total dose of re-irradiation (higher than 60 Gy) was also found to be associated with a better outcome (39,47,49,52,59,61), but may be due to the selection of the patients. In conclusion the analysis of the literature shows that full-dose re-irradiation alone or in combination with chemotherapy in patients with inoperable head and neck carcinoma is feasible to a total dose of at least 60 Gy. The incidence and severity of late toxicity is markedly increased as compared to that observed after the first irradiation. Median survival may reach 10-11 months which is higher than the survival rates achieved using palliative chemotherapy alone and a small proportion of patients are long term (> 5 years) disease-free survivors (13/169 in our series). The use of appropriate imaging and three-dimensional conformal radiotherapy technique and intensity modulation in the re-irradiation of head and neck carcinoma may extend the indication of treatment and improve local control by sparing critical organs.

There are very few series concerning the feasibility of full dose re-irradiation after salvage surgery of head and neck carcinoma (42,44,51,57). In 2 series, the quality of surgical resection was not specified and no safety data were provided (51,57). The selection of patients was comparable in 2 others series comprising 25 and 14 patients with a high risk of recurrence (positive surgical margin and/or lymph node involvement with capsular rupture) (42,44). The 2 year survival rates were relatively high, respectively 43% and

36%. In our series 16% of the patients had osteoradionecrosis (44), which was higher rate as compared to patients re-irradiated in the same institution without surgery, using the same radio-chemotherapy regimen.

Stereotactic re-irradiation and radio-surgery

Stereotactic radiation can deliver high dose of irradiation in a precise defined target that may be smaller than 4 cm, allowing an accurate limitation of the normal tissue to be re-irradiated. Clinical experiences of radiosurgery concern the re-treatment of recurrent nasopharyngeal carcinoma. The series are limited comprising very few patients (less than 4 patients) with short follow-up. Complete regression of tumor and symptomatic improvement are reported (65-68). Using a single high dose per fraction, neurological complications were also reported (66,67,69) leading to the use of a fractionated stereotactic radiotherapy (70). These preliminary results may suggest the potential interest of stereotactic radiation in appropriately selected patients with recurrent nasopharynx carcinoma.

In conclusion, this review of the literature shows that there is a small group of selected patients with recurrent unresectable disease who can be cured using salvage re-irradiation alone or combined with chemotherapy. Moderate to severe late complications were seen more frequently after re-irradiation than after a first irradiation but are still acceptable.

REFERENCES

1.   Sanchiz F., Milla A., Torner J., et al. Single fraction versus two fractions per day versus radio-chemotherapy in the treatment of HNSCC. Int. J. Radiat. Oncol. Biol. Phys. 1990 ; 19 : 1347-50.
2.   Marcial V.A., Pajak T.F., Chang C. et al. Hyperfractionated photon radiation therapy in the treatment of advanced squamous cell carcinoma of the oral cavity, pharynx, larynx, and sinuses, using radiation therapy as the only planned modality: (preliminary report) by the Radiation Therapy Oncology Group (RTOG). Int. J. Radiat. Oncol. Biol. Phys. 1987;13: 41-47.
3.   Horiot JC, LeFur R, N' Guyen T et al. Hyperfractionation versus conventional fractionation in oropharyngeal carcinoma: final analysis of a randomized trial of the EORTC cooperative group of radiotherapy. Radiother Oncol 1992; 25 : 231-241.
4.   Datta N.R., Dutta Choudhry A., Gupta S, Bose A.K.. Twice a day versus once a day radiation therapy in head and neck cancer . Int. J. Radiat. Oncol. Biol. Phys. 1989 ; 17 (suppl 1): 132.
5.   Pinto L.H.J., Canary P.C.V., Araujo C.M.M. et al. Prospective randomized trial comparing hyperfractionated versus conventional radiotherapy in stage III and IV oropharyngeal carcinoma. Int. J. Radiat. Oncol. Biol. Phys. 1991;21: 557-562.
6.   Cummings B, O'Sullivan B, Keane T et al. 5-year results of 4 week/twice daily radiation schedule – The Toronto Trial. Rad. Oncol. 2000; 56 (suppl. 1): S8.

7. Fu KK, Pajak TF, Trotti A, et al. A radiation therapy oncology group (RTOG) phase III randomized study to compare hyperfractionation and two variants of accelerated fractionation to standard fractionation radiotherapy for head and neck squamous cell carcinomas: first report of RTOG 9003. Int J Rad Oncol Biol Phys 2000, 48: 7-16.

8. Olmi P, Fallai C, Rossi F, Crispino S, Marsoni S, Torri V, Flann M. Conventional radiotherapy versus accelerated hyperfractionated radiotherapy versus conventional radiotherapy and concomitant chemotherapy in advanced oropharyngeal carcinoma: a randomized clinical trial. Proc. 4th International Conference on Head and Neck Cancer 1996 : 213.

9. Horiot JC, Bontemps P., van den Bogaert W. et al. Accelerated fractionation (AF) compared to conventional fractionation (CF) improves loco-regional control in the radiotherapy of advanced head and neck cancer: results of the EORTC 22851 randomized trial. Rad Oncol 1997;44: 111-121.

10. Bernier J, Horiot JC, Van den Bogaert, et al. EORTC update of the head and neck cancer altered fractionation phase III trials. Rad. Oncol. 2000; 56 (suppl. 1): S8.

11. Dische S, Saunders M, Barrett A, et al. A randomized multicentre trial of CHART vs conventional radiotherapy in head and neck cancer. Rad Oncol 1997;44: 123-136.

12. Jackson SM, Weir LM, Hay JH, Tsang VHY, Durham JS. A randomized trial of accelerated versus conventional radiotherapy in head and neck cancer. Rad. Oncol. 1997;43:39-46.

13. Ang KK, Trotti A, Garden AS, et al. Impact of risk factors and total time for combined surgery and radiotherapy on the outcome of patients with advanced head and neck cancer. Int J Rad Oncol Biol Phys 1999, 45 (suppl. 3): 199.

14. Grau C, Overgaard J, Hansen H et al. Acute and late normal tissue reactions following accelerated radiotherapy for head and neck cancer. Results from DAHANCA-7. Rad. Oncol. 2000; 56 (suppl. 1): S12.

15. Dobrowsky W, Naudé J. Continuous hyperfractionated accelerated radiotherapy with/without mitomycin C in head and neck cancer. Rad Oncol 2000;57:119-124.

16. Bourhis J, Lapeyre M, Rives M, Tortochaux J, Bourdin S, Lasaulnier F, et al. Very accelerated radiotherapy in HNSCC: results of the GORTEC 94-02 randomized trial. Proc Am Soc Clin Oncol 2000;19:412a.

17. Skaladowski K, Maciejewski B, Golen M, et al. Randomized clinical trial on 7-days continuous accelerated irradiation (CAIR) of head and neck cancer - report on 3-year tumor control and normal tissue toxicity. Rad. Oncol. 2000; 55: 101-110.

18. Denham J, Poulsen M, Lamb DS et al. The TROG 91.01 randomised controlled trial addressing the question of accelerated fractionation. Rad. Oncol. 2000; 56 (suppl. 1): S7.

19. Tandon N, Keshwar TS, Srivastava M, et al. Continuous hyperfractionated accelerated radiotherapy (CHART) in head and neck malignancies. XVth Asia Pacific Cancer Conference, December 1999, Chennai. Proceeding of XVth Asia Pacific Cancer Conference: 90.

20. Hliniak A, Gwiazdowska B, Szutkowski Z, et al. Radiotherapy of the laryngeal cancer. The estimation of the therapeutic gain and the enhancement of toxicity by the one-week shortening of the treatment time. Results of the randomized phase III multicenter trial. Rad Oncol 2000; 56 (suppl. 1): S5.

21. Lippman SM, Hong WK: Second malignant tumors in head and neck squamous cell carcinoma: the overshadowing threat for patients with early-stage disease. Int J Radiat Oncol Biol Phys 1989; 17:691-694.

22. Hong WK, Bromer R: Chemotherapy in head and neck cancer. N Engl J Med 1983; 308:75-79.

23. Liggett WJ, Forastiere AA: Chemotherapy advances in head and neck oncology. Semin Surg Oncol 1995; 11:265-271.

24.   Puthawala AA, Syed AM: Interstitial re-irradiation for recurrent and/or persistent head and neck cancers. Int J Radiat Oncol Biol Phys 1987; 13:1113-1114.
25.   Mazeron JJ, Langlois D, Glaubiger D, et al: Salvage irradiation of oropharyngeal cancers using iridium 192 wire implants: 5-year results of 70 cases. Int J Radiat Oncol Biol Phys 1987; 13:957-962.
26.   Housset M, Barrett JM, Brunel P, et al: Split course interstitial brachytherapy with a source shift: the results of a new technique for salvage irradiation in recurrent inoperable cervical lymphadenopathy greater than or equal to 4 cm diameter in 23 patients. Int J Radiat Oncol Biol Phys 1992; 22:1071-1074.
27.   Levendag PC, Meeuwis CA, Visser AG: Reirradiation of recurrent head and neck cancers: external and/or interstitial radiation therapy. Radiother Oncol 1992; 23:6-15.
28.   Lee DJ, Liberman FZ, Park RI, et al: Intraoperative I-125 seed implantation for extensive recurrent head and neck carcinomas. Radiology 1991; 178:879-882.
29.   Maulard C, Housset M, Delanian S, et al: Salvage split course brachytherapy for tonsil and soft palate carcinoma: treatment techniques and results. Laryngoscope 1994; 104:359-363.
30.   Langlois D, Hoffstetter S, Pernot M: Selection of patients for re-irradiation with local implants in carcinomas of oropharynx and tongue. Acta Oncol 1988; 27:571-573.
31.   Fontanesi J, Hetzler D, Ross J: Effect of dose rate on local control and complications in the reirradiation of head and neck tumors with interstitial iridium-192. Int J Radiat Oncol Biol Phys 1989; 17:365-369.
32.   Mazeron JJ: Interstitial re-irradiation for recurrent and/or persistent head and neck cancers. Int J Radiat Oncol Biol Phys 1987; 13:1261
33.   Kwong DL, Wei WI, Cheng AC, et al: Long term results of radioactive gold grain implantation for the treatment of persistent and recurrent nasopharyngeal carcinoma. Cancer 2001; 91:1105-1113.
34.   Lee AW, Foo W, Law SC, et al: Reirradiation for recurrent nasopharyngeal carcinoma: factors affecting the therapeutic ratio and ways for improvement. Int J Radiat Oncol Biol Phys 1997; 38:43-52.
35.   Peiffert D, Pernot M, Malissard L, et al: Salvage irradiation by brachytherapy of velotonsillar squamous cell carcinoma in a previously irradiated field: results in 73 cases. Int J Radiat Oncol Biol Phys 1994; 29:681-686.
36.   Leung TW, Tung SY, Sze WK, et al: Salvage radiation therapy for locally recurrent nasopharyngeal carcinoma. Int J Radiat Oncol Biol Phys 2000; 48:1331-1338.
37.   Haraf DJ, Vokes EE, Weichselbaum RR, et al: Concomitant chemoradiotherapy with cisplatin, 5-fluorouracil and hydroxyurea in poor-prognosis head and neck cancer. Laryngoscope 1992; 102:630-636.
38.   Schaefer U, Micke O, Schueller P, et al: Recurrent head and neck cancer: retreatment of previously irradiated areas with combined chemotherapy and radiation therapy-results of a prospective study. Radiology 2000; 216:371-376.
39.   Teo PM, Kwan WH, Chan AT, et al: How successful is high-dose (> or = 60 Gy) reirradiation using mainly external beams in salvaging local failures of nasopharyngeal carcinoma? Int J Radiat Oncol Biol Phys 1998; 40:897-913.
40.   Hwang JM, Fu KK, Phillips TL: Results and prognostic factors in the retreatment of locally recurrent nasopharyngeal carcinoma. Int J Radiat Oncol Biol Phys 1998; 41:1099-1111.
41.   Gandia D, Wibault P, Guillot T, et al: Simultaneous chemoradiotherapy as salvage treatment in locoregional recurrences of squamous head and neck cancer. Head Neck 1993; 15:8-15.
42.   Benchalal M, Bachaud JM, Francois P, et al: Hyperfractionation in the reirradiation of head and neck cancers. Result of a pilot study. Radiother Oncol 1995; 36:203-210.

43. De Crevoisier R, Bourhis J, Domenge C, et al: Full-dose reirradiation for unresectable head and neck carcinoma: experience at the Gustave-Roussy Institute in a series of 169 patients. J Clin Oncol 1998; 16:3556-3562.

44. De Crevoisier R, Domenge C, Wibault P, et al: Full dose reirradiation combined with chemotherapy after salvage surgery in head and neck carcinoma. Cancer 2001; 91:2071-2076.

45. McNeese MD, Fletcher GH: Retreatment of recurrent nasopharyngeal carcinoma. Radiology 1981; 138:191-193.

46. Wang CC: Radical re-irradiation for carcinoma arising from the previously irradiated larynx. Laryngoscope 1967; 77:2189-2195.

47. Wang CC: Re-irradiation of recurrent nasopharyngeal carcinoma--treatment techniques and results. Int J Radiat Oncol Biol Phys 1987; 13:953-956.

48. Wang CC, McIntyre J: Re-irradiation of laryngeal carcinoma--techniques and results. Int J Radiat Oncol Biol Phys 1993; 26:783-785.

49. Langlois D, Eschwege F, Kramar A, et al: Reirradiation of head and neck cancers. Presentation of 35 cases treated at the Gustave Roussy Institute. Radiother Oncol 1985; 3:27-33.

50. Tercilla OF, Schmidt-Ullrich R, Wazer DE: Reirradiation of head and neck neoplasms using twice-a-day scheduling. Strahlenther Onkol 1993; 169:285-290.

51. Pomp J, Levendag PC, van Putten WL: Reirradiation of recurrent tumors in the head and neck. Am J Clin Oncol 1988; 11:543-549.

52. Stevens KR, Britsch A, Moss WT: High-dose reirradiation of head and neck cancer with curative intent. Int J Radiat Oncol Biol Phys 1994; 29:687-698.

53. Yan JH, Hu YH, Gu XZ: Radiation therapy of recurrent nasopharyngeal carcinoma. Report on 219 patients. Acta Radiol Oncol 1983; 22:23-28.

54. Skolyszewski J, Korzeniowski S, Reinfuss M: The reirradiation of recurrences of head and neck cancer. Br J Radiol 1980; 53:462-465.

55. Orecchia R, Airoldi M, Sola B, et al: Results of chemotherapy plus external reirradiation in the treatment of locally advanced recurrences of nasopharyngeal carcinoma. Eur J Cancer B Oral Oncol 1992; 28B:109-111.

56. Weppelmann B, Wheeler RH, Peters GE, et al: Treatment of recurrent head and neck cancer with 5-fluorouracil, hydroxyurea, and reirradiation. Int J Radiat Oncol Biol Phys 1992; 22:1051-1056.

57. Emami B, Bignardi M, Spector GJ, et al: Reirradiation of recurrent head and neck cancers. Laryngoscope 1987; 97:85-88.

58. Lee AW, Law SC, Foo W, et al: Retrospective analysis of patients with nasopharyngeal carcinoma treated during 1976-1985: survival after local recurrence. Int J Radiat Oncol Biol Phys 1993; 26:773-782.

59. Pryzant RM, Wendt CD, Delclos L, et al: Re-treatment of nasopharyngeal carcinoma in 53 patients. Int J Radiat Oncol Biol Phys 1992; 22:941-947.

60. Haraf DJ, Vokes EE, Panje WR, et al: Survival and analysis of failure following hydroxyurea, 5-fluorouracil and concomitant radiation therapy in poor prognosis head and neck cancer. Am J Clin Oncol 1991; 14:419-426.

61. Haraf DJ, Weichselbaum RR, Vokes EE: Re-irradiation with concomitant chemotherapy of unresectable recurrent head and neck cancer: a potentially curable disease. Ann Oncol 1996; 7:913-918.

62. Cho JH, Kim GE, Cho KH, et al: Hyperfractionated re-irradiation using a 3-dimensional conformal technique for locally recurrent carcinoma of the nasopharynx; preliminary results. Yonsei Med J 2001; 42:55-64.

63.   Brockstein B, Haraf DJ, Stenson K, et al: A phase I-II study of concomitant chemoradiotherapy with paclitaxel (one-hour infusion), 5-fluorouracil and hydroxyurea with granulocyte colony stimulating factor support for patients with poor prognosis head and neck cancer. Ann Oncol 2000; 11:721-728.

64.   Wang CC: Decision making for re-irradiation of nasopharyngeal carcinoma. Int J Radiat Oncol Biol Phys 1993; 26:903

65.   Firlik KS, Kondziolka D, Lunsford LD, et al: Radiosurgery for recurrent cranial base cancer arising from the head and neck. Head Neck 1996; 18:160-165.

66.   Chua DT, Sham JS, Hung KN, et al: Stereotactic radiosurgery as a salvage treatment for locally persistent and recurrent nasopharyngeal carcinoma. Head Neck 1999; 21:620-626.

67.   Buatti JM, Friedman WA, Bova FJ, et al: Linac radiosurgery for locally recurrent nasopharyngeal carcinoma: rationale and technique. Head Neck 1995; 17:14-19.

68.   Miller RC, Foote RL, Coffey RJ, et al: The role of stereotactic radiosurgery in the treatment of malignant skull base tumors. Int J Radiat Oncol Biol Phys 1997; 39:977-981.

69.   Cmelak AJ, Cox RS, Adler JR, et al: Radiosurgery for skull base malignancies and nasopharyngeal carcinoma. Int J Radiat Oncol Biol Phys 1997; 37:997-1003.

70.   Ahn YC, Kim DY, Huh SJ, et al: Fractionated stereotactic radiation therapy for locally recurrent nasopharynx cancer: report of three cases. Head Neck 1999; 21:338-345.

Chapter 8

ORGAN PRESERVATION-INDUCTION CHEMOTHERAPY

A. Dimitrios Colevas, M.D.
Investigational Drug Branch, NCI/CTEP, Rockville, MD 20852

It is estimated that in the year 2001, 42000 persons will develop squamous cell carcinoma of the head and neck region (SCCHN), and a third to a half will die from their disease within 5 years of that diagnosis. [1] [2] Approximately one third of these tumors will arise from either the larynx or hypopharynx. The strongest predictor of survival for these patients is the extent of disease at diagnosis. Patients with limited disease confined to the larynx have an expected 5 year survival exceeding 80%, while patients with clinical involvement of regional lymph nodes can expect less than a 40% survival rate. The historical standard of care for patients with extensive loco-regional involvement by SCCHN, usually defined as AJCC stage T3-4 or N1-3, has been definitive surgery, often followed by adjuvant radiation therapy (refer to chapters 6 and 7 of this text).

Because of the risk of permanent disfigurement and loss of speech and swallowing function associated with surgical treatment of SCCHN, especially in the case of advanced disease of the larynx and pharynx, quality of life concerns have traditionally played a major role in the decision making process of patients and care providers. As recently as two decades ago the standard options for therapy were definitive surgery, with the almost certain risk of permanent loss of natural speech, significant compromise of swallowing and cough function, or initial radiation treatment as an attempt to control disease while keeping the local organs intact, and hopefully functional. Patients and providers explicitly accepted the trade-off between organ preservation and long-term survival. [3] The differences in survival between these two options were clinically relevant. For example, in the case of a patient with a T3 N0 larynx carcinoma, initial surgery could offer a 3 year survival of 60%, whereas radiation was believed to yield a survival rate of only 30-40%.

Over the past several decades there has been an effort on the part of SCCHN investigators to reduce the morbidity associated with definitive therapy of loco-regionally advanced SCCHN. Most of these efforts have been focused on patients with cancer of the larynx and hypopharynx, although many of the principles applied to these organ sites could be applied to cancers of the oral cavity and oropharynx as well.

Surgical research has included development of partial laryngectomy procedures, advanced reconstructive techniques, and limited neck dissection techniques. [4-6] Because of the highly selected nature of patients studied, it is difficult to extrapolate from the literature an expected loco-regional relapse rate and expected functional outcome.

Application of non-traditional radiation fractionation and use of conformal radiation therapy techniques have permitted a more effective anti-cancer application of radiation to the effected site while sparing normal tissues. [7-10] [11-13]

Chemotherapy was first applied against neoplasms of the head and neck in the 1940's. [14] In the ensuing half- century, hundreds of potentially anti-neoplastic compounds have been tested in humans with SCCHN. Methotrexate, bleomycin, 5-fluorouracil (5-FU) and hydroxyurea were initially used in the 1960's alone and in combination against SCCHN. [15] [16] [17,18] Cisplatin was initially found to have activity against SCCHN in 1974, and by the late 1970's was in use in combination with bleomycin and methotrexate in the induction setting prior to loco regional treatment. [19] [20-22] Subsequent to cisplatin, a plethora of agents have been shown to have significant activity against SCCHN. The most active include paclitaxel, docetaxel, carboplatin, ifosfamide and doxorubicin.

As a result of the initial excitement generated by high response rates to chemotherapy alone, investigators began to test a strategy of induction chemotherapy followed by either radiation, or surgery, or both. Very small early studies comparing chemotherapy followed by radiation to radiation alone in patients with loco regionally advanced disease established a theme which was to recur over the next 4 decades: the addition of chemotherapy was associated with a marked increase in complete response rates (67% versus 36%) but a lack of a difference in survival [23] [24]

Clinical investigators testing induction chemotherapy quickly noticed the prognostic significance of a robust anti-tumor response. A complete or near complete clinical response to the induction chemotherapy was noted to

be associated with improved locoregional control and overall survival. [25]
This association was noted both for patients who proceeded to definitive surgery following chemotherapy and those patients who subsequently underwent radiation treatment as their primary locoregional treatment modality. Several explanations for this phenomenon were put forward. In the case of surgery, it was thought that induction chemotherapy debulked the tumor , making definitive surgery feasible in cases where initially surgery was not considered an option. While surgery was an effective modality for tumor bulk reduction, in many cases it was clear that residual micro- metastatic disease in the tissues of the neck led to locoregional failures following "successful" surgeries. Those patients in whom chemotherapy effectively eradicated these foci of tumor would enjoy a longer survival and cure likelihood.

In the case of patients treated with definitive radiation, the association between chemotherapy response and improved outcome was thought to arise because either chemotherapy itself contributed to tumor kill or chemotherapy was a predictor for a tumor's sensitivity to radiation. [26]

Virtually all of the commonly used agents against SCCHN have been tested individually and in combination in the induction setting. A major impediment to the development of a standard induction chemotherapy regimen has been the failure to define either in the palliative or curative settings a regimen which is clearly superior to the rest with respect to overall survival. Data began accumulating in the late 1980's favoring the combination of high dose cisplatin and 5 day infusional 5-FU (PF) as the de facto standard induction regimen. Randomized trials of PF versus other single agents and combinations in the palliative setting failed to reproducibly and convincingly demonstrate a survival advantage over other combinations, but PF consistently edged out methotrexate based regimens and other platinum based combinations with respect to response rates [27-30,31]. The now standard regimen of cisplatin 100 mg/m2 on day one followed by a 5 day infusion of 5-FU 1000 mg/m2/d was also shown to be superior to combinations of platinum and 5-FU that utilized bolus 5-FU. [30,32 33]

A series of exploratory trials in the mid 1980's asked prospectively if a patient's response to induction chemotherapy could be used as justification for substitution of surgery by radiation. These trials represented the first attempt to move away from the old paradigm of surgery as the approach associated simultaneously with greatest cure rate and morbidity (organ removal) and radiation as the approach associated with lower cure rates but less morbidity (organ sparing).

The North Califonia Oncology Group used complete pathological response (pCR) at the primary site following 3 cycles of PF as a discriminator between subsequent radiation and surgery. [34] Those patients who achieved a pCR had 2 year relapse free and overall survivals of 60% and 70% respectively compared to 52% and 53% for the entire group entered on to the study. Demard and colleagues in Nice, France using clinical complete response rates (cCR) following 3 cycles of PF as their discriminant, found a 93% /69%(larynx/ hypopharynx) 2 year survival for the patients who achieved a cCR and subsequently received radiation versus 66%/40% for non cCR patients who were treated surgically. [35] The Radiation Therapy Oncology Group (RTOG) confirmed the high response rate and initial organ preservation rate associated with induction PF in a multi-institutional phase 2 trial in the US, further supporting the role of induction therapy as a discriminant. [36]

By the late 1980's the paradigm of radiation as a more palliative, less curative therapy than surgery was no longer universally accepted. The uncontrolled data cited above suggested that appropriately chosen patients could achieve similar if not superior results to surgery with radiation therapy in combination with chemotherapy. The role of chemotherapy was prognostic, if not therapeutic as well. Investigators set out to ask this question definitively in the phase 3 setting.

There have been at least three randomized phase 3 studies comparing induction chemotherapy followed by definitive loco regional therapy versus definitive loco regional (surgery + radiation) therapy alone. [37,38 39,40], with the endpoint of organ preservation. See Table 1. These studies differ with respect to chemotherapy used, sites and stages of SCCHN patients enrolled, and type of loco regional therapy in the control group. Despite these differences, these trials collectively established a standard framework into which induction chemotherapy based on a PF regimen became a standard of care.

Table 1. **Phase 3 studies of induction chemotherapy plus radiation versus surgery**

Study/ year/ # enrolled	Induction chemotherapy regimen	Locoregional treatment	Organ sites eligible	Study conclusion
VA/ 1991/332 37	P 100 mg/m2 iv, 5-FU 1000 mg/m2/d x5 ivci 2-3 cycles q 21 d	Radiation:1.8-2 Gy daily to 66-70 Gy total dose Or Laryngectomy= > XRT (50-64 Gy)	Larynx	Induction chemotherapy + XRT can be effective in preserving the larynx without overall survival compromise
EORTC/1996/2 02 40	P 100 mg/m2 iv, 5-FU 1000 mg/m2/d x5 ivci 3 cycles q 21 d	Radiation: 2 Gy daily to 70 Gy total dose Or Laryngectomy and partial pharyngectomy => XRT (50-64 Gy)	Hypopharynx (pyriform sinus)	Larynx preservation without jeopardizing survival appears feasible in hypopharynx cancer patients
GETTEC/1997/ 68 38	P 100 mg/m2 iv, 5-FU 1000 mg/m2/d x5 ivci 2-3 cycles q 21 d	Radiation: 2 Gy daily to 65-70 Gy total dose Or Laryngectomy	Larynx	Larynx preservation treatment cannot be considered a standard treatment

The Department of Veterans Affairs laryngeal cancer study group performed a prospective randomized study in patients with operable loco regionally advanced (AJCC stage III or IV) squamous cell carcinoma of the larynx (VA study). The primary question asked was whether induction chemotherapy with PF and definitive radiation and laryngectomy reserved for salvage was a better initial approach than total laryngectomy followed by adjuvant radiation. All patients in the experimental arm received induction PF chemotherapy. Any patient who experienced at least a clinical partial response (cPR) at the primary site after 2 cycles of PF received another cycle of PF followed by definitive radiation. Patients who failed to achieve a cPR underwent immediate surgical resection followed by adjuvant radiation. All patients in the control arm underwent laryngectomy followed by radiation therapy, and most had regional neck dissections at the time of laryngectomy. No significant differences in actuarial survival rates were seen between treatment groups. The overall survival rate at 3 years was 53%, with improved survival seen in patients achieving a cCR or pCR to chemotherapy.[41] Rates of distant metastases were diminished in the chemotherapy arm (11% versus 17%, p=0.001) and primary site recurrences were diminished in the surgical arm (2% versus 12%, p=0.001). Despite a shorter disease free interval in patients randomized to the experimental arm, the option for salvage surgery was successful in salvaging some of the patients initially treated with induction chemotherapy, which contributed to overall survival parity between the two groups. Two-thirds of all survivors in the chemotherapy arm retained a functioning larynx.

Conclusions drawn from this trial were that an initial strategy of organ preservation with sequential chemotherapy did not compromise overall survival and permitted the preservation of the larynx in two-thirds of survivors. Major issues not addressed in this trial included the quality of the function of the retained larynx and the therapeutic versus triage contribution of chemotherapy. Despite a significant reduction in metastases, induction chemotherapy did not lead to an increase in survival in the experimental group as a whole or any subgroup evaluated.

The EORTC head and neck cancer cooperative group extended the experience of the VA Study to patients with pyriform sinus cancer. [40] There is a higher risk of lymphatic involvement at presentation in patients with hypopharynx cancer when compared with patients with larynx cancer. Because hypopharynx cancer even in relatively early stages often causes organ dysfunction and debilitates patients, and because head and neck specialists felt that the risks involved with salvage surgery were higher than in patients with larynx cancer, investigators decided to evaluate an induction PF approach versus surgery in this specific group of patients in order to extend the question to another head and neck sub site. The design of this trial differed slightly form that of the VA trial in that patients must have achieved a clinical complete response (cCR) to induction PF chemotherapy in order to be eligible for radiation therapy. Patients who achieved a cCR after 2 cycles proceeded to radiation and patients who achieved a cPR after 2 cycles received an additional cycle and were re-assessed. All patients in the control arm and all patients who did not achieve a cCR to chemotherapy were supposed to proceed to definitive surgical resection, but 10 of the 60 patients who received radiation instead of surgery did so despite not fulfilling this criterion.

Overall survival for the chemotherapy and surgery arms of the EORTC trial were 57% and 43% at 3 years respectively and 30% and 35% at 5 years respectively. Based on the statistical power of the trial, overall survival was considered equivalent. While local and regional failures were similar between the two arms, the distant failure rate was significantly lower in the chemotherapy arm, 25%, versus 36% in the surgery arm. Forty-two percent of the surviving patients in the chemotherapy group had intact larynxes at 3 years. These investigators concluded that larynx preservation is possible without jeopardizing survival in patients with hypopharyngeal cancer, thus confirming the V.A. trial outcome at a different anatomical site.

The third and fourth trials suffer from sample size and trial design respectively. The Group d'Etude des Tumeurs da la Tete et du Cou (GETTEC) investigators in France focused on patients with laryngeal T3 cancers.[38] Patients were randomly assigned to induction PF or surgery, and any patient who did not experience tumor progression following two cycles of PF was to receive a third cycle of PF, then radiation. All other patients underwent laryngectomy. This trial was closed prematurely after accrual of only 68 patients because a majority of patients wished to receive chemotherapy. In this trial, overall 2 year survival was 69% in the chemotherapy group and 84% in the surgical group. There were more local, regional and metastatic relapses in the chemotherapy group.

With the exception of the small, prematurely closed GETTEC study, these data validated induction chemotherapy as part of an organ preserving strategy. While these studies and others clearly document a reduction in the risk of metastatic disease in association with the use of induction PF, this has not led to an improvement in overall survival. It is reasonable to suggest therefore that PF's contribution may be as a selector for radiation sensitivity.

In a recently published meta-analysis, French investigators take a different view of these data. [42] Their interpretation of the pooled data from the V.A., EORTC, and GETTEC studies is that the results do not exclude a negative impact of induction chemotherapy on survival and disease-free survival. It is worthwhile to note that these investigators have chosen to weigh the data from the GETTEC study equally with the other two studies despite the unusual premature closure of this study. It is also perplexing that patients on this study did not benefit in terms of a diminished rate of subsequent metastasis, a phenomenon observed virtually uniformly in all comparisons of chemotherapy and loco regional treatment versus loco regional treatment alone.

Meta-analyses of induction chemotherapy plus radiation and concurrent chemoradiation versus radiation alone

Three meta-analyses evaluating the randomized data concerning chemotherapy's role in addition to loco regional treatment have been performed in the last decade. [42-44] All three of these analyses grouped trials according to sequence of chemotherapy and radiation treatments. Table 2 summarizes the data for induction chemotherapy trials included in these meta-analyses. Note that many of the trials are represented in all 3 of these reviews, so the conclusions are not made on the basis of three independent datasets.

Table 2. **Recent meta-analyses of chemotherapy added to radiation in SCCHN**

Meta- analysis	# trials/patients/dates	Main conclusions
A.J.Munro [43]	54/ 7443/ 1963-93	absolute survival benefit to chemotherapy of 6.5% absolute concurrent therapy survival benefit 12% absolute neoadjuvant therapy survival benefit 3.7%
S. El- Sayed [44]	42/ 5583/ 1963-92	relative mortality rate reduction of 11% with chemotherapy 22% relative reduction with concurrent chemotherapy 5% relative reduction with induction chemotherapy (N.S.)
J.P. Pignon [42]	65 / 10850 / 1965-93	relative mortality rate reduction of 10% with chemotherapy 19% relative reduction with concurrent chemotherapy 5% relative reduction with induction chemotherapy (N.S.)

N.S.= non-significant

The Munro meta-analysis of 54 trials, 7443 patients concludes that in aggregate all forms of chemotherapy added to radiation in SCCHN might add modestly (6.5%)to absolute survival. [43] He goes on to make the point that when stratified by sequence of therapy, concurrent single agent chemotherapy seems to be the winner with an aggregate survival advantage of 12% over radiation therapy alone, while induction therapy yields only a 3.7% increase. However, what is not stressed in this analysis is the relative heterogeneity of the induction regimens in terms of drugs and schedules used in comparison to the concurrent regimens. Munro points out that PF therapy (without regard to sequence) in 8 trials was associated with a possible survival benefit of 10% versus radiation alone. What is not provided is a breakdown of patients receiving PF as induction versus PF as concurrent therapy. What is not addressed in this meta-analysis is the relative contributions of the specifics of the chemotherapy with respect to choice of agents versus sequence of agents relative to chemotherapy. It is possible that the benefit of PF as induction was diluted by all the ineffective other induction regimens aggregated together in the analysis.

Samy El- Sayed and colleagues performed a meta-analysis on 42 trials from the same era, with similar conclusions: a reduction in mortality of 11% (95% C.I. 1-19%) associated with chemotherapy. [44] Induction chemotherapy was associated with a 5% advantage, while concurrent yielded a 22% advantage. This meta- analysis made no attempt to evaluate the benefit of survival in relation to choice of chemotherapy agents, but noted a significant increase in toxicity was associated with the addition of chemotherapy to radiation.

J. P. Pignon and colleagues followed with a larger meta- analysis of published and unpublished data. [42] Their analysis yielded virtually identical results to those of Munro and El- Sayed, which is not surprising given the large overlap in data evaluated: a relative reduction in mortality of 10% associated with the addition of chemotherapy. Relative mortality reductions for concurrent and induction chemotherapy were 19% and 5% respectively. While PF was associated with a risk reduction of 16%, polychemotherapy regimens including platinum were associated with an increase in relative death risk by 5%, yet polychemotherapy without cisplatin and monochemotherapy were associated with risk reductions of 15 % and 11% respectively. There was no analysis of PF in the induction setting versus PF in the concurrent setting relative to radiation alone. There was, however, a 12% risk reduction with neoadjuvant PF, and a 16% risk reduction with PF overall, implying a favorable benefit with concomitant PF. It is difficult to rationally reconcile the observation that PF was associated with a risk reduction yet polychemotherpay with cisplatin was not unless one accepts that PF is fundamentally different from the other regimens in terms of its anti-tumor effects.

Randomized trials of concurrent versus induction chemoradiotherapy

The direct comparison between induction PF versus concurrent PF with radiation in patients with loco regionally advanced SCCHN has never been subjected to a large phase III randomized study. There are a series of randomized phase 2 or 3 trials which have asked sequence of therapy questions, but these studies are all hampered by lack of adequate statistical power, or use of different chemotherapy on different trial arms or nonstandard approach to surgical intervention. Therefore in 2001 there is still no definitive answer to the sequence of therapy question.

Salvajoli and colleagues conducted a 90 patient 3 arm trial of the following 3 regimens in patients with loco regionally confined stage IV SCCHN: Arm I: Radiation 2 Gy/ day to 70 Gy total dose.. Arm II: vinblastine(V), mitomycin(Mm), and cisplatin(P) q 21 days for two cycles followed by radiation 2 Gy/day to 70 Gy total dose. Arm III: Bleomycin(B) and cisplatin(low dose) every 21 days during radiation with 2 Gy/ day to 70 Gy total dose. [45]   Given the size of the trial (30 patients per arm) it is not surprising that response rates and overall survival were not significantly different.   Such a trial would almost certainly fail to detect a survival difference of 5-10% in a setting where the survival of the control arm could be expected to be about 50% at 2 years.   It is worth noting that not only were different drugs used in arms 2 and 3, the doses of cisplatin were different in the two arms (60 and 40 mg/m2/cycle), and substantially lower than the accepted 100 mg/m2/cycle standard dose for cisplatin in the PF regimen.

An Italian cooperative group compared sequential V, B and methotrexate (M), followed by radiation versus V, B, M alternating with radiation therapy in 116 patients. [46]   While this trial used identical chemotherapy in both arms, the choice of VBM would be regarded today as sub optimal therapy.   The radiation total dose and techniques were significantly different between the two arms, making assessment of drug sequence alone difficult.   Patients in the alternating therapy arm experienced a higher response rate (65% versus 52%) and an improved progression free survival, but there was no difference in overall survival.

SECOG investigators explored a comparison of VBMF or VBM given either sequentially or concurrently with conventional radiation in a two by two trial design. [47]   With 267 patients enrolled, this trial was more highly powered than the above trials, and the design included a comparison between what could be regarded as conventional sequential (S) versus concurrent (C) chemotherapy and radiation therapy. Results, published as rate ratios, were insignificantly different. The death rate ratio C:S was 0.96 and the event rate ratio was 1.23.

One can conclude, therefore, that in the pre-PF era of chemoradiotherapy, a series of small, mostly underpowered trials failed to demonstrate a significant, meaningful outcome difference between sequential and concomitant approaches. It is important to keep in mind that by today's standards for proof, these trials did not demonstrate that these approaches were not different. Rather, these trials were not designed to demonstrate what we would consider to be a meaningful difference in outcome, such as a survival advantage of 4%.

There have been four randomized studies of platinum- based chemotherapy addressing the sequential versus concurrent question. The first, published by Adelstein and colleagues, compared PF followed by radiation (SEQ) versus attenuated PF given concurrently with radiation (SIM). [48] This small trial of 48 patients included an interim analysis for resectability of patients with loco regional SCCHN. Approximately 40% of all patients entered into this trial underwent a surgical resection either after induction chemotherapy or halfway through concurrent chemoradiotherapy. Response rates to induction PF and the first half of concurrent therapy as assessed at surgery were high: 91% cR and 32 % cPR in the former and 100% cR and 67% cCR in the latter. The pCR rate for the patients in the SIM group who had resections was 100%, while no patients in the SEQ group who had resections achieved a pCR. It is important to note, however, that the time of evaluation could have a tremendous influence on responses reported. At the completion of all therapy, 79% of the SEQ patients and 88% of the SIM patients were alive and disease free. Overall survival at 24 months was 68% for the SIM arm and 43% for the SEQ arm. While these differences seem large, they were not statistically significant because of the small sample size.

Pinarro and colleagues compared sequential PF and radiation (SEQ) versus high dose cisplatin alone concurrent with radiation (SIM) in 97 patients with loco regionally advanced SCCHN. [49]. The vast majority of these patients had both stage IV disease with either T4 primaries or N3 regional nodal involvement. Despite the bulky disease, responses to therapy were high: complete responses were 47% and 40% respectively to SEQ and SIM. Overall response rates were 60% and 75% respectively. This study, set up to detect a standard error of 7% in cCR rate, was unable to show a significant difference in responses. Furthermore, the high response rates did not translate high survival or progression free survival rates, which were 16% and 20%, and 11% and 16% respectively for the SEQ and SIM arms.

Taylor and colleagues were the first to ask the question concerning SEQ versus SIM therapy using PF as induction and concurrent chemotherapy in a trial of sufficient magnitude to address clinically important differences between the arms. [50] Two hundred and fourteen patients were randomized to receive either standard dose PF for three cycles followed by radiation therapy

(SEQ) or seven cycles of attenuated PF administered with radiation every other week (SIM). While cCRs to SEQ and SIM were similar (50% and 52% respectively), the overall response rate to the SIM arm was 93% versus 78% in the SEQ arm. Virtually all patients in both arms who attained a cCR had negative confirmatory biopsies, but histologically positive biopsies were more common in patients who achieved a cPR with SEQ therapy(64%) than with SIM therapy(29%). While distant site failure rates were similar,   loco regional failure rates favored the SIM arm , 39% versus 55% in the SEQ arm. Uncorrected life table analysis failed to show a difference in progression-free or overall survival. The investigators performed a Cox regression analysis to assess significant prognostic variables. This corrected analysis favored SIM therapy with respect to progression free survival. The investigators found that the institution at which patients were treated was a significant variable, and they suggested that institutions with extensive prior experience with SIM therapy " may have been important in some, as yet, undetermined way". Noteably, however, acute toxicities were equivalent during the RT portions of both regimens. In almost all other studies of concomitant chemoradiation versus radiation alone, acute mucosal and skin toxicities are higher in the concomitant group. This may imply that the split course CRT given in this study utilized treatment breaks which were too long for effective cell kill.

The Radiation Therapy Oncology Group recently presented preliminary results of RTOG 91-11, a three arm study of patients with SCCHN of the larynx. [51] The primary endpoint of this 547 patient study was survival with preservation of laryngeal function. Patients were randomized to induction PF for 3 cycles followed by radiation (SEQ) versus concurrent high dose cisplatin and radiation (SIM), versus standard fractionation radiation alone (XRT). Patients all had potentially resected tumors, and any patient not responding to therapy was eligible for surgical salvage. The preliminary results presented demonstrate no difference in overall survival (see table3) but an advantage with respect to larynx preservation for the SIM arm. Additionally, this trial confirmed a decrease in distant disease in association with both chemotherapy arms, despite the fact that this did not translate into increased survival.

Table 3. Randomized trials, induction chemotherapy plus radiation versus concurrent (or alternating) chemoradiation.

Trial	# pts	Arms	Response rates (Complete response rates)	Outcomes
Buffolli [62]	49	A: B,M,H=> XRT 60 Gy B: XRT 20 Gy => B,M,H => XRT 40 Gy		No difference in response rates or overall survival
Salvajoli [45]	90	A ; XRT 70 Gy B : V, Mm,P => XRT C: P,B + XRT	A: 67% B: 60% C: 60%	No significant 2 year survival difference
Adelstein [48]	48	A : PF=> XRT B: PF + XRT	A: 91% (32%) (to PF) B: 100% (67%) (1st half of therapy)	Overall 24 month survival A: 43% B: 68% (N.S.)
SECOG I [47]	267	A: V,B,M,F or V.B.M => XRT B: V,B,M,F or V.B.M + RT	Death rate ratio A:B = 0.96 Event rate ratio A:B = 1.23 Both N.S.	
Merlano [46]	116	A: V,B,M => XRT B: V,B,M + XRT (alternating)	A: 52% (13%) B: 65% (31%)	Median survival, weeks. A: 41, B: 54. p=0.64
Taylor [50]	214	A: PF=> XRT B: PF + XRT (14 d cycle x 7)	A : 78% (50%) B : 93% (52%)	No survival difference
Pinnaro [49]	97	A: PF => XRT B: P + XRT	A: 60% (47%) B: 75% (41%) N.S.	5 yr. prog. free survival A: 16%, B: 20% p= N.S. 5 yr overall survival A: 11%, B: 16% p=N.S.
RTOG 91-11 [51]	547	A: PF => XRT B: P + XRT C: XRT	Overall survival, 5 yr: A: 59%, B: 54%, C: 53%. N.S. Larynx preservation, 5 year: A: 71%, B:85% (p=.0047 vs A), C: 64% Free of distant dz., 5 year: A: 87%, B: 86%, C: 76%	

Key: B= bleomycin. M= methotrexate. H=Hydroxyurea. "=>" = sequential. "+"= concurrent. V =vinblastine. Mm = mitomycin c. P = cisplatin. F = 5-fluorouracil.

The ideal trial to answer the question of the significance of the timing of PF with respect to radiation has not been performed. None of the above studies is an adequately powered trial of conventional once daily radiation given after or during PF. There are some observations one can make. The choice of chemotherapy is important. Full dose induction PF, high dose single agent cisplatin concurrent with radiation, and attenuated PF concurrent with radiation can deliver similar survival outcomes in this patient population. In potentially resectable patients, these therapies (performed for organ preservation) are equivalent to organ-removing surgical approaches, at least in patients with hypopharyngeal and laryngeal primary sites. Because recent preliminary data suggest concurrent therapy is associated with higher rates of larynx preservation and because concurrent therapy can be administered in half the time that sequential therapy can, it is reasonable to say that for most patients, a concurrent approach should be considered as the leading non-surgical approach.

Investigational induction chemotherapy regimens

Biochemical modulation of 5- FU with leucovorin to enhance thymidylate synthase inhibition and therefore increase 5-FU activity provided the basis for a number of trials which attempted to build on the activity of the induction PF regimen. [52] Aggressive combinations of cisplatin, 5-FU, and leucovorin (PFL) became the basis of several single arm trials of induction chemotherapy in patients with potentially curable loco regional SCCHN.(see Table 4)

Table 4. **Phase 2 trial of induction chemotherapy with cisplatin, 5-FU, and leucovorin, Response rates are to induction chemotherapy alone, assessed before radiation therapy**

STUDY	BOSTON[53]	CHICAGO[56]	Houston [54]	NY[55]
Cisplatin 5-FU leucovorin	25 mg/m2/CIx5 800 mg/m2/CIx5 500 mg/m2/CIx6	100 mg/m2/B 1000 mg/m2/CIx5 100mg/PO q4h	25 mg/m2/ CI x5 500 mg/m2/CIx5 500mgm2//CI x5	100 mg/m2/B 800 mg/m2/CIx5 100 mg/PO q4h
CYCLES	3	2	3	3
PATIENTS	102	29	47	22
CR%	54%	31%	30%	23%
CR + PR%	81%	90%	84%	45%
1º SITE CR	69%	NR	NR	32%
AGE (RANGE)	55 (13-70)	56 (29-74)	58 (32-73)	62 (42-82)
N2 (%)	48%	28%	34%	27%
N3 (%)	19%	38%	17%	5%
N2 + N3 (%)	67%	66%	51%	32%
Deaths on therapy	3%	7%	0%	14%

Key P-= cisplatin, F= 5-fluorouracil , l= leucovorin, CI= continuous infusion, B= bolus

The most extensive experience with PFL, at Dana-Farber Cancer Institute in Boston, suggests that the administration of PFL is feasible, associated with high overall complete and pathological response rates, but also is associated with severe side effects. [53] Clark and colleagues reported on 102 patients treated with an aggressive regimen consisting of a 5-day infusion of cisplatin at 125 mg/m2 with infusional 5-FU and leucovorin. CTC grade 2 or greater stomatitis was seen in virtually all patients. Twenty- seven percent of the patients experienced grade 3-4 stomatitis in the first cycle, and 19/102 patients required hospitalization to manage stomatitis and consequent dehydration. Approximately 40% of the patients had dose reductions in cycles 2 and 3 of therapy, and while these reductions did not decrease the overall incidence of stomatitis, episodes of grade 3-4 stomatitis were reduced to 5%. Response rates and survival data suggested the possibility of clinically relevant improvement over the PF regimen. (see table 4) Actuarial 5 year overall survival was 52% . Other institutions using identical versions of PFL produced lower complete response rates, and substantially diminished overall response rates with regimens using bolus cisplatin at lower doses and oral leucovorin.(See Table 4) [54-56] It is worth noting that the median age of the patients enrolled on the Boston, Houston, and Chicago trials was substantially below the typical age of head and neck cancer patients, and in the NY study, where the median age was higher, the incidence of PFL associated morbidity and mortality was substantially higher. PFL has never been tested against PF in a randomized clinical trial. Given the significant increase in toxicity and the failure in several phase 2 studies to reproduce the high response rates reported initially, it is unlikely that this regimen will be pursued further.

As a result of the promising single agent data reported with docetaxel, paclitaxel, and ifosfamide in patient with SCCHN, there have been a series of early phase clinical trials which have added these agents to cisplatin-based induction chemotherapy .

Colevas and colleagues built upon the PFL regimen in a series of phase one and two trials which combined docetaxel(T) with modified PFL. [57-59] These 3 sequential trials demonstrated that docetaxel could be added to modified PFL regimens (TPFL) as part of an induction regimen preceding hyper fractionated radiation therapy. As with the PFL series, gastrointestinal toxicity was formidable. More than 40% of all patients in these trials experienced grade 3 or greater mucositis and more than 50% experienced clinically relevant diarrhea. Despite this toxicity, virtually all patients completed both chemotherapy and radiation therapy without significant dose reductions or delays. This was in large part due to aggressive nursing and intravenous fluid administration during the episodes of TPFL induced mucositis and routine use of prophylactically placed gastrostomy feeding tubes during radiation therapy. These investigators were also able to show that TPFL could be administered on an outpatient basis in a comprehensive cancer center setting.

Response rates to the induction chemotherapy in the TPFL series were much higher than historically seen with PF or PFL regimens. Overall response rates exceeded 93% and cCRs averaged well above 50%, with primary site cCRs exceeding 67%. Virtually all patients achieved a cCR upon the completion of radiation therapy. The first two TPFL trials were associated with an actuarial survival at 24 months exceeding 83% in 53 patients. Data on the third trial are not yet available.

A multicenter phase 1-2 trial of docetaxel combined with modified PF (TPF) was subsequently conducted to see if such promising results would be reproducible without the use of leucovorin or continuous infusion cisplatin. Diarrhea and mucositis were much less prominent with this regimen, and response rates to TPF were high: 40% cCR, 93% cR, and 56% primary site cCR. Based on these promising preliminary data, a randomized phase 3 trial comparing TPF versus PF followed by concurrent platinum and radiation is underway.

Shin and colleagues have pursued a strategy of combining paclitaxel, ifosfamide, and either cisplatin or carboplatin in patients with metastatic or recurrent SCCHN . [60] [61] The phase 2 studies of this regimen in the palliative setting have demonstrated impressive cCR rates of 17% with cR rates exceeding 57%. Trials of this combination in the induction setting are presently being developed.

Several phase II studies have specifically examined organ preservation in resectable patients in sites outside the larynx using induction chemotherapy and definitive radiotherapy. In the first, 42 patients at the University of Michigan with resectable stage III or IV cancers of the oral cavity, oropharynx, hypopharynx, larynx, or sinuses were treated with three cycles of mitoguazone, 5-FU, and cisplatin[63] . Patients achieving a CR or who were downstaged to T1N1 or less were treated with definitive XRT. Sixty-nine percent of patients were initially spared surgery to the primary site and, at three-year median follow-up, 38 percent of all patients were disease-free and spared surgery at the primary site. Disease-free survival with organ preservation was significantly more common in the larynx and hypopharynx (11 of 18) versus the oral cavity or oropharynx (4 of 22). Thus, although possible, organ preservation outside of the larynx and hypopharynx using induction chemotherapy remains investigational.

The Dana Farber PFL series above examined 102 patients with stage III or IV previously untreated cancers of the head and neck [53]. Patients received up to three cycles of the PFL regimen. The overall response rate was 81 percent with a clinical CR in 69 percent of 97 patients who could be evaluated for organ preservation at the primary tumor site. Of the 78 patients with potentially resectable primary tumors, excluding three who died during induction and five with unknown primary lesions, the primary site was preserved in 78 percent. This included 30 of 32 cases of oropharyngeal cancer, 8 of 12 larynx cancer, and 23 of 31 others. Twenty-three patients total had a local recurrence without distant recurrence, 11 of whom had attempt at surgical salvage. With a median follow-up of five years, the overall survival rate was 52 percent.

CONCLUSION

Induction chemotherapy consisting of high dose cisplatin and infusional 5-FU (PF) followed by definitive radiation therapy for the past decade has been the organ-sparing alternative to surgery for patients with laryngeal and hypopharyngeal squamous cell carcinomas. Recent preliminary data from a large randomized trial, RTOG91-11, comparing this approach with concurrent cisplatin and radiation and radiation alone suggest that induction therapy achieves parity with concurrent therapy with respect to survival, but concurrent therapy seems to offer the possibility of greater rates of larynx preservation. If final results of RTOG 91-11 confirm the preliminary evaluation, it is probable that induction therapy will be displaced by concurrent platinum-based therapy as the standard of care.

In the case of loco regionally advanced disease not amenable to surgical resection and primary sites other than larynx or hypopharynx, the data supporting the routine use of induction chemotherapy prior to definitive radiation are far from definitive. Induction therapy is not part of the standard of care in these situations and should not be routinely used outside of a clinical trial.

The polemics of induction versus concurrent chemotherapy have persisted for more than a decade. However, many promising investigational approaches include incorporation of new agents into a combined approach of both induction chemotherapy and concurrent chemoradiotherapy. With the elucidation of more specific anti cancer targets, one can foresee the development of hybrid treatment plans of drug and radiation delivery that will optimize the anticancer effects of all modalities used.

REFERENCES

1.   Society AC. Five-Year Relative Survival Rates by Stage at Diagnosis, 1989-1995. In.; 2001.

2.   Greenlee RT, Murray T, Bolden S, Wingo P. Cancer Statistics. CA Cancer J Clin. 2000;50:13-30.

3.   McNeil BJ, Weichselbaum R, Pauker SG. Speech and survival: tradeoffs between quality and quantity of life in laryngeal cancer. N Engl J Med. 1981;305:982-7.

4.   Laccourreye O, Laccourreye L, Garcia D, Gutierrez-Fonseca R, Brasnu D, Weinstein G. Vertical partial laryngectomy versus supracricoid partial laryngectomy for selected carcinomas of the true vocal cord classified as T2N0. Ann Otol Rhinol Laryngol. 2000;109:965-71.

5.   Biacabe B, Crevier-Buchman L, Laccourreye O, Brasnu D. [Vertical partial laryngectomy with false vocal cord flap reconstruction: carcinologic and functional results]. Ann Otolaryngol Chir Cervicofac. 1998;115:189-95.

6.   Laccourreye O, Muscatello L, Laccourreye L, Naudo P, Brasnu D, Weinstein G. Supracricoid partial laryngectomy with cricohyoidoepiglottopexy for "early" glottic carcinoma classified as T1-T2N0 invading the anterior commissure. Am J Otolaryngol. 1997;18:385-90.

7.   Marcial V, Pajak T, Chang C, Tupchong L, Stetz J. Hyperfractionated photon radiation therapy in the treatment of advanced squamous cell carcinoma of the oral cavity, pharynx, larynx and sinuses, using radiation therapy as the only planned modality:(preliminary report) by the Radiation Therapy Oncology Group. International Journal of Radiation Oncology, Biology, Physics. 1987;13:41-47.

8.   Wang C, Nakfoor B, Spiro I, Martins P. Role of accelerated fractionated irradiation for supraglottic carcinoma: assessment of results. The Cancer Journal. 1997;3:88-91.

9.   Lusinchi A, Lartigau E, Luboinski B, Eschwege F. Acclerated radiation therapy in the treatment of very advanced and inoperable head and neck cancers. Int J Rad Oncol Biol Phys. 1994;29:149-152.

10.   Fu K, Pajak T, Trotti A, Jones C, Spencer S, Phillips T, Garden A, Ridge J, Cooper J, Ang K. A Radiation Therapy Oncology Group (RTOG) phase III randomized study to compare hyperfractionation and two variants of accelerated fractionation to standard fractionation radiotherapy for head and neck squamous cell carcinomas: First report of RTOG 9003. International Journal of Radiation Oncology, Biology, and Physics. 2000;48:7-16.

11.   Emami B, Purdy JA, Simpson JR, Harms W, Gerber R, Wippold JF. 3-D conformal radiotherapy in head and neck cancer. The Washington University experience. Front Radiat Ther Oncol. 1996;29:207-20.

12.   Willner J, Hadinger U, Neumann M, Schwab FJ, Bratengeier K, Flentje M. Three dimensional variability in patient positioning using bite block immobilization in 3D-conformal radiation treatment for ENT-tumors. Radiother Oncol. 1997;43:315-21.

13.   Bratengeier K, Pfreundner L, Flentje M. Radiation techniques for head and neck tumors. Radiother Oncol. 2000;56:209-20.

14.   Goodman LS, Wintrobe MM, Dameshek W, Goodman MJ, Gilman A, McLennan MT. Landmark article Sept. 21, 1946: Nitrogen mustard therapy. Use of methyl-bis(beta-chloroethyl)amine hydrochloride and tris(beta-chloroethyl)amine hydrochloride for Hodgkin's disease, lymphosarcoma, leukemia and certain allied and miscellaneous disorders. By Louis S. Goodman, Maxwell M. Wintrobe, William Dameshek, Morton J. Goodman, Alfred Gilman and Margaret T. McLennan. Jama. 1984;251:2255-61.

15.   Jesse RH, Goepfert H, Lindberg RD, Johnson RH. Combined intra-arterial infusion and radiotherapy for the treatment of advanced cancer of the head and neck. Am J Roentgenol Radium Ther Nucl Med. 1969;105:20-5.

16. Suzuki Y, Miyake H, Sakai M, Inuyama Y, Matsukawa J. Bleomycin in malignant tumors of head and neck. Keio J Med. 1969;18:153-62.

17. Friedman M, Daly JF. The treatment of squamous cell carcinoma of the head and neck with methotrexate and irradiation. Am J Roentgenol Radium Ther Nucl Med. 1967;99:289-301.

18. Kligerman MM, Hellman S, Bertino JR, Von Essen CF. Sequential chemotherapy and radiotherapy. Preliminary results of clinical trial with methotrexate in head and neck cancer. Radiology. 1966;86:247-50.

19. Higby DJ, Wallace HJ, Albert DJ, Holland JF. Diaminodichloroplatinum: a phase I study showing responses in testicular and other tumors. Cancer. 1974;33:1219-5.

20. Wittes RE, Brescia F, Young CW, Magill GB, Golbey RB, Krakoff IH. Combination chemothereapy with cis-diamminedichloroplatinum (II) and bleomycin in tumors of the head and neck. Oncology. 1975;32:202-7.

21. Elias EG, Chretien PB, Monnard E, Khan T, Bouchelle WH, Wiernik PH, Lipson SD, Hande KR, Zentai T. Chemotherapy prior to local therapy in advanced squamous cell carcinoma of the head and neck: Preliminary assessment of an intensive drug regimen. Cancer. 1979;43:1025-31.

22. Jacobs C, Bertino JR, Goffinet DR, Fee WE, Goode RL. Cis-platinum chemotherapy in head and neck cancers. Otolaryngology. 1978;86:ORL-780-3.

23. Petrovich Z, Block J, Kuisk H, Mackintosh R, Casciato D, Jose L, Barton R. A randomized comparison of radiotherapy with a radiotherapy--chemotherapy combination in stage IV carcinoma of the head and neck. Cancer. 1981;47:2259-64.

24. Davis RK, Perry DJ, Zajtchuk JT. Induction chemotherapy with vinblastine, bleomycin, and cis-diamminedichloroplatinum in squamous cell carcinoma of the head and neck. Otolaryngol Head Neck Surg. 1983;91:627-31.

25. Ervin TJ, Kirkwood J, Weichselbaum RR, Miller D, Pitman SW, Frei E, 3rd. Improved survival for patients with advanced carcinoma of the head and neck treated with methotrexate-leucovorin prior to definitive radiotherapy or surgery. Laryngoscope. 1981;91:1181-90.

26. Ensley JF, Jacobs JR, Weaver A, Kinzie J, Crissman J, Kish JA, Cummings G, Al-Sarraf M. Correlation between response to cisplatinum-combination chemotherapy and subsequent radiotherapy in previously untreated patients with advanced squamous cell cancers of the head and neck. Cancer. 1984;54:811-4.

27. Jacobs C, Lyman G, Velez-Garcia E, Sridhar K, Knight W, Hochster H, Goodnough L, Mortimer J, Einhorn L, Schacter L, Cherng N, Dalton T, Burroughs J, Rozencweig M. A Phase III randomized study comparing cisplatin and fluorouracil as single agents and in combination for advanced squamous cell carcinoma of the head and neck. Journal of Clinical Oncology. 1992; 10:257-263.

28. Clavel M, Vermorken J, Cognetti F, Cappelaere P, deMulder P, Schornagel J, Tueni E, Verweij J, J W, Clerico M, Dalesio O, Kirkpatrick A, Snow G. Randomized comparison of cisplatin. methotrexate, bleomycin, and vincristine (CABO) versus cisplatin and 5-fluorouracil (CF) versus csiplatin (C), in recurrent or metastatic squamous cell carcinoma of the head and neck. A Phase III stduy of the EORTC head and neck cancer cooperative group. Annals of Onocology. 1994;5:521-526.

29. Forastiere A, Metch B, Schuller D, Ensley J, Hutchins L, Triozzi P, Kish J, McLure S, VonFeldt E, Williamson S, Von Hoff D. Randomized comparison of cisplatin plus fluorouracil and carboplatin plus fluorouracil versus methotrexate in advanced squamous cell carcinoma of the head and neck: A southwest oncology group study. Journal of Clinical Oncology. 1992; 10:1245-1251.

30. Kish J, Ensley J, Jacobs J, Kinzie J, Weaver A, Crissman J, Al-Sarraf M. A randomized trial of cisplatin (CACP) + 5-fluorouracil (5-FU) infusion and CACP +

5-FU bolus for recurrent and advanced squamous cell carcinoma of the head and neck. Cancer. 1985; 56:2740-2744.

31.   De Andres L, Brunet J, Lopez-Pousa A, Burges J, Vega M, Tabernero J, Mesia R, Lopez J. Randomized trial of neoadjuvant cisplatin and flourouracil versus carboplatin and fluorouracil in patients with stage IV-M0 head and neck cancer. Journal of Clinical Oncology. 1995;13:1493-1500.

32.   Campbell JB, Dorman EB, McCormick M, Miles J, Morton RP, Rugman F, Stell PM, Stoney PJ, Vaughan ED, Wilson JA. A randomized phase III trial of cisplatinum, methotrexate, cisplatinum + methotrexate, and cisplatinum + 5-fluoro-uracil in end-stage head and neck cancer. Acta Otolaryngol. 1987;103:519-28.

33.   Group LHaNO. A phase III randomised trial of cisplatinum, methotrextate, cisplatinum + methotrexate and cisplatinum + 5-FU in end stage squamous carcinoma of the head and neck. Liverpool Head and Neck Oncology Group. Br J Cancer. 1990;61:311-5.

34.   Jacobs C, Goffinet D, Goffinet L, Kohler M, Fee W. Chemotherapy as a substitute for surgery in the treatment advanced resectable head and neck cancer. A report from the Northern California Oncology Group. Cancer. 1987;60:1178-1183.

35.   Demard F, Chauvel P, Santini J, Vallicioni J, Thyss A, Schneider M. Response to chemotherapy as justification for modification of the therapeutic strategy for pharyngolaryngeal carcinomas. Head Neck. 1990;12:225-31.

36.   Jacobs JR, Pajak TF, Kinzie J, Al-Sarraf M, Davis L, Hanks GA, Weigensberg I, Leibel S. Induction chemotherapy in advanced head and neck cancer. A Radiation Therapy Oncology Group Study. Arch Otolaryngol Head Neck Surg. 1987;113:193-7.

37.   Veterans Affairs Laryngeal Cancer Study Group. Induction chemotherapy plus radiation compared with surgery plus radiation in patients with advanced laryngeal cancer. New England Journal Medicine. 1991;324:1685-1689.

38.   Richard J, Sancho-Garnier H, Pessey J, Luboinski B, Lefebvre J, Dehesdin D, Stromboni-Luboinski M, Hill C. Randomized trial of induction chemotherapy in larynx cancer. Oral Oncology. 1998;34:224-228.

39.   Paccagnella A, Orlando A, Marchiori C, Zorat P, Cavaniglia G, Sileni V, Jirillo A, Tomio L, Fila G, Fede A, Endrizzi L, Bari M, Sampognaro E, Balli M, Gava A, Pappagallo G. Phase III trial of initial chemotherapy in stage III or IV head and neck cancers: A study by the Gruppo di Studio sui Tumori della Testa e del collo. Journal of the National Cancer Institute. 1994; 86:265-272.

40.   Lefebvre J, Chevalier D, Luboinski B, Kirkpatrick A, Collette L, Sahmoud T. Larynx preservation in pyriform sinus cancer: preliminary results of a European organization for research and treatment of cancer phase III trial. Journal of the National Cancer Institute. 1996;88:890-898.

41.   Spaulding M, Fischer S, Wolf G. Tumor response, toxicity, and survival after neoadjuvant organ-preserving chemotherapy for advanced laryngeal carcinoma. Journal of Clinical Oncology. 1994;12:1592-1599.

42.   Pignon J, Bourhis J, Domenge C, Designe L, Group M-NC. Chemotherapy added to locoregional treatment for head and neck squamous-cell cancer: three meta-analysis of updated individual data. The Lancet. 2000;355:949-955.

43.   Munro A. An overview of randomized controlled trials of adjuvant chemotherapy in head and neck cancer. British Journal of Cancer. 1995;71: 83-91.

44.   El-Sayed S, Nelson N. Adjuvant and adjunctive chemotherapy in the management of squamous cell carcinoma of the head and neck region: A meta-analysis of prospective and randomized trials. Journal of Clinical Oncology. 1996;14:838-847.

45.   Salvajoli J, Morioka H, Trippe N, Kowalski L. A randomized trial of neoadjuvant vs concomitant chemotherapy vs radiotherapy alone in the treatment of stage IV head and neck squamous carcinoma. European Archives of Oto-Rhino-Laryngology. 1992;249:211-215.

46. Merlano M, Rosso R, Sertoli R, Bonelli L, Margarino G, Grimaldi A, Benasso M, Gardin G, Corvo R, Scarpati D, Barbieri A, Pallestrini E, Castiglia G, Santelli A, Scasso F, Bottero G, Ciurlo E, Fracchia P, Moratti M, Santi L. Sequential versus alternating chemotherapy and radiotherapy in stage III-IV squamous cell carcinoma of the head and neck: a Phase III Study. Journal of Clinical Oncology. 1988;6:627-632.

47. SECOG. A randomized trial of combined multidrug chemotherapy and radiotherapy in advanced squamous cell carcinoma of the head and neck. An interim report from the SECOG participants. South-East Co-operative Oncology Group. Eur J Surg Oncol. 1986;12:289-95.

48. Adelstein D, Sharan V, Earle A, Shah A, Vlastou C, Haria C, Damm C, Carter S, Hines J. Simultaneous versus sequential combined technique therapy for squamous cell head and neck cancer. Cancer. 1990;65:1685-1691.

49. Pinnaro P, Cercato M, Giannarelli D, Carlini P, Del Vecchio M, Ambesi Impiombato F, Marzetti F, Milella M, Cognetii F. A randomized phase II study comparing sequential versus simultaneous chemo-radiotherapy in patients with unresectable locally advanced squamous cell cancer of the head and neck. Annals of Oncology. 1994;5:513-519.

50. Taylor S, Murthy A, Vannetzel J, Colin P, Dray M, Caldarelli D, Shott S, Vokes E, Showel J, Hutchinson J, Witt T, Griem K, Hartsell W, Kies M, Mittal B, Rebischung J-L, Coupez D, Desphieux J-L, Bobin S, LePajolec C. Randomized comparison of neoadjuvant cisplatin and fluorouracil infusion followed by radiation versus concomitant treatment in advanced head and neck cancer. Journal of Clinical Oncology. 1994;12:385-395.

51. Forastiere A, Berkey B, Maor M, Weber R, Goepfert H, Morrison WH, Glisson BS, Trotti A, Ridge JA, Chao C, Peters G, Lee D-J, Leaf A, Ensley J. Phase III Trial to Preserve the Larynx: Induction Chemotherapy and Radiotherapy Versus Concomitant Chemoradiotherapy Versus Radiotherapy Alone, Intergroup Trial R91-11. In: Annual meeting of the American Society of Clinical Oncology. San Francisco; 2001:2a Abst #4.

52. Rustum YM, Trave F, Zakrzewski SF, Petrelli N, Herrera L, Mittelman A, Arbuck SG, Creaven PJ. Biochemical and pharmacologic basis for potentiation of 5-fluorouracil action by leucovorin. NCI Monogr. 1987:165-70.

53. Clark J, Busse P, Norris C, Andersen J, Dreyfuss A, Rossi R, Poulin M, Colevas A, Tishler R, Costello R, Lucarini J, Lucarini D, Thornhill L, Lackey M, Peters E, Posner M. Induction chemotherapy with cisplatin, fluorouracil, and high-dose leucovorin for squamous cell carcinoma of the head and neck: Long-term results. Journal of Clinical Oncology. 1997;15:3100-3110.

54. Papadimitrakopoulou V, Dimery I, Lee J, Perez C, Hong W, Lippman S. Cisplatin, Fluorouracil, and L-Leucovorin induction chemotherapy for locally advanced head and neck cancer: the M.D. Anderson Cancer Center experience. The Cancer Journal. 1997;3:92-99

55. Pfister D, Bajorin D, Motzer R, Scher H, Louison C, Harrison L, Shah J, Strong E, Bosl G. Cisplatin, fluorouracil, and leucovorin. Increased toxicity without improved response in squamous cell head and neck cancer. Arch Otolaryngol Head and Neck Surg. 1994;120:89-95.

56. Vokes E, Schilsky R, Weichselbaum R, Kozloff M, Panje W. Induction chemotherapy with cisplatin, fluorouracil and high-dose leucovorin for locally advanced head and neck cancer: A clinical and pharmacologic analysis. Journal of Clinical Oncology. 1990;8:241-247.

57.   Colevas A, CM N, Tishler R, Lamb C, Fried M, Goguen L, Gopal H, Costello R, Read R, Adak S, Posner M. A Phase I/II trial of outpatient docetaxel, cisplatin, 5-fluorouracil, leucovorin (opTPFL) as induction for squamous cell carcinoma of the head and neck (SCCHN). American Journal of Clinical Oncology. 2001 accepted.

58.   Colevas AD, Norris CM, Tishler RB, Fried MP, Gomolin HI, Amrein P, Nixon A, Lamb C, Costello R, Barton J, Read R, Adak S, Posner MR. Phase II trial of docetaxel, cisplatin, fluorouracil, and leucovorin as induction for squamous cell carcinoma of the head and neck [see comments]. J Clin Oncol. 1999;17:3503-11.

59.   Colevas AD, Busse PM, Norris CM, Fried M, Tishler RB, Poulin M, Fabian RL, Fitzgerald TJ, Dreyfuss A, Peters ES, Adak S, Costello R, Barton JJ, Posner MR. Induction chemotherapy with docetaxel, cisplatin, fluorouracil, and leucovorin for squamous cell carcinoma of the head and neck: a phase I/II trial [see comments]. J Clin Oncol. 1998;16:1331-9.

60.   Shin DM, Glisson BS, Khuri FR, Ginsberg L, Papadimitrakopoulou V, Lee JJ, Lawhorn K, Gillenwater AM, Ang KK, Clayman GL, Callender DL, Hong WK, Lippman SM. Phase II trial of paclitaxel, ifosfamide, and cisplatin in patients with recurrent head and neck squamous cell carcinoma. J Clin Oncol. 1998;16:1325-30.

61.   Shin DM, Khuri FR, Glisson BS, Ginsberg L, Papadimitrakopoulou VM, Clayman G, Lee JJ, Ang KK, Lippman SM, Hong WK. Phase II study of paclitaxel, ifosfamide, and carboplatin in patients with recurrent or metastatic head and neck squamous cell carcinoma. Cancer. 2001;91:1316-23.

62.   Buffoli A, Morrica B, Frata P, La Face B. [Chemo-radiotherapy in advanced head and neck tumors. Personal experience]. Radiol Med (Torino). 1992;83:636-40.

63.   Urba SG, Forastiere AA, Wolf GT, Esclamado RM, McLaughlin PW, Thornton AF. Intensive induction chemotherapy and radiation for organ preservation in patietns with advanced resectable head and neck carcinoma. J Clin Oncol 1994;12:946-953.

Chapter 9

ORGAN PRESERVATION FOR ADVANCED HEAD AND NECK CANCER CONCOMITANT CHEMORADIATION

Bruce Brockstein, M.D.
Evanston Northwestern Healthcare, Evanston IL, Northwestern University, Chicago IL

INTRODUCTION

Despite advances in the understanding of the biology and pathogenesis of head and neck cancer (HNC), and despite improvements in imaging modalities, locoregionally advanced (stage III and stage IV) squamous cell carcinoma of the head and neck remains a difficult management problem. Traditionally, unresectable advanced head and neck cancer has been treated with RT alone, although more recently it has become evident that combined modality therapy with concomitant chemoradiation (CRT) provides a survival benefit over RT alone in this setting (1-3). The standard of care for resectable squamous cell carcinoma of the head and neck has traditionally been surgical excision followed by radiotherapy. Attempts at improving survival in the resectable setting with induction chemotherapy have generally failed to improve survival (1-3), although organ preservation for laryngeal cancer and hypopharyngeal cancer have been demonstrated to be possible using induction chemotherapy plus RT (4,5). Despite advances in surgical techniques, surgical excision followed by radiotherapy may lead to multiple problems with function and/or cosmesis. Attempts at using surgery as a radiation sparing modality are limited since most patients with stage III and stage IV head and neck cancer require radiotherapy postoperatively.

As a result, the last decade has seen a proliferation of studies which have strongly suggested that organ preservation using concomitant chemoradiotherapy, with surgery reserved for planned neck dissections or salvage, can provide survival as good or better than surgery plus radiation. With this strategy, organ preservation is possible in many patients, and in many of these patients organ function is preserved.

Much of the difficulty in assessing differences between outcome or function in studies of the various treatments for locoregionally advanced head and neck cancer arises from the lack of definition of resectablity, and the lack of distinction in studies between populations of patients who have unresectable head and neck cancer and those who have resectable head and neck cancer. Unresectable head and neck cancer generally implies biologically and anatomically more aggressive disease with a smaller chance for permanent eradication of the disease. It is difficult, however, to find a precise definition of resectability for these tumors. The limits of resectability vary between surgeons, institutions, and patients. Likewise, the acceptability of a near complete excision may alter the definition of resectability. Intimate involvement of the tumor with certain structures such as the base of the skull or prevertebral tissues may render a tumor unresectable. Involvement of carotid artery may render a tumor unresectable, although with proper planning even tumors involving the carotid artery may, in certain cases be considered resectable. Large tumors of the mid tongue or base of tongue may be "resectable", but require a total glossectomy. While this may be technically possible, this is unacceptable to many patients. Modern day reconstruction has allowed for vastly improved cosmetic outcomes and in some cases improved functional outcomes, and may extend the boundaries of resectability.

Nevertheless, a general definition of resectability implies that preoperatively, the tumor can be expected to be removed with negative margins with the possibility for reconstruction with acceptable cosmesis to patient and physician, and acceptable function, with or without reconstruction, to the patient and physician. Examples of resectable tumors include most oral cavity tumors, even though some require composite resection, and most laryngeal and hypopharyngeal tumors. Perhaps the greatest discrepancy in definition of resectability comes within the oropharynx, where some consider most tumors unresectable though these are sometimes considered resectable based on the technical ability to remove the tumor.

At least four studies have examined the role of induction chemotherapy followed by radiotherapy versus surgery plus radiotherapy with the goal of larynx preservation. In the Veterans Affairs Larynx Cancer Study (4), 325 patients with advanced laryngeal cancer were randomized to standard therapy with surgery and postoperative RT or two to three cycles of neoadjuvant cisplatin and 5-FU chemotherapy followed by definitive RT, with surgery reserved for tumor persistence or recurrence. Two goals were pursued in the study, improved survival and larynx preservation. The two-year actuarial overall survival rate was identical in the two groups at 68%. The most important finding was the high rate of larynx preservation: 64% of the patients in the chemotherapy arm had their larynx preserved at a median follow-up time of 33 months. Overall, 39% of patients remained disease free with an intact larynx. Similar findings were found in an EORTC conducted study in hypopharyngeal cancer (5). In this study, 194 patients were randomized to surgery plus RT or cisplatin and infusional 5-FU followed by radiotherapy, with surgery reserved for salvage. Again, there was no difference in overall survival between groups, but 28% of the chemotherapy patients were both alive and disease free with an intact larynx at three years (5). A recent US Intergroup trial, 91-11, was performed as a follow-up to VA larynx study. In this study, patients were randomized to receive induction chemotherapy followed by RT as on the VA larynx trial, RT alone, or RT plus concomitant cisplatin, 100 mg per m^2 delivered on weeks 1, 4 and 7 of a standard course of radiotherapy. There were no survival differences seen between groups. There was improved laryngectomy-free survival seen for both chemotherapy groups versus the radiotherapy alone group and improved time to laryngectomy in the concomitant group versus the sequential group (6).

The conclusions from the neoadjuvant chemotherapy strategy were that organ preservation was possible in laryngeal and hypopharyngeal cancer, but that no improvement in survival was seen despite the strategy. The Intergroup study further questioned the actual contribution of induction chemotherapy to radiation, and suggested that RT alone may even be an alternative to laryngectomy.

In addition to concomitant chemoradiation, other strategies have been employed to try to either improve the outcome with RT or to provide organ preservation. It should be noted that there have been no randomized trials directly comparing concomitant chemoradiation or altered fraction radiotherapy to surgery plus or minus radiation. A major study by the Radiation Therapy Oncology Group (RTOG), compared, in a phase III, randomized study, four regimens of RT administration in oropharyngeal cancer (7): 1) standard fraction radiation (2 Gy/day x 35 treatment days); 2) hyperfractionated radiation (1.2 Gy per fraction, twice daily, five days a week to 81.6 Gy); 3) accelerated fractionation with split (1.6 Gy twice daily to 67.2 Gy including a two-week rest after 38.4 Gy); 4) Accelerated fractionation with concomitant boost (1.8 Gy per fraction per day five days per week and 1.5 Gy per fraction per day to a boost field as a second daily treatment for last 12 treatment days to 72 Gy total). The patients treated with hyperfractionation and accelerated fractionation with concomitant boost had significantly better local regional control (P=0.045 and P=0.050 respectively) than those with standard fractionation. No survival difference has yet emerged. The patients treated with accelerated fractionation with a split had a similar outcome to those treated with standard fractionation. The outcome of this and other trials also have suggested that appropriate altered fractionation radiation may provide an alternative to surgery for resectable head and neck cancers.

An additional strategy, which has been explored, is alternating chemotherapy and radiation (8). Merlano and colleagues conducted a randomized study of RT alone or chemotherapy with cisplatin 20 mg/m^2/day times five days and 5-fluorouracil 200 mg/m^2/day for five consecutive days alternating with RT in three two-week courses (20 Gy per course). The median survival in the 80 combined therapy patients was 16.5 months versus 11.7 months in the radiotherapy alone group, and three-year survival was 41% versus 23%.

RADIATION RESISTANCE

Mechanisms of resistance to radiation

In general, mechanisms of radiation resistance can be divided into those based on characteristics of the tumor itself and those related to intrinsic cellular factors. An understanding of these theoretical mechanisms may allow for the development of strategies to overcome radiation resistance.

Tumor microenvironmental factors, which may contribute to radiation resistance include decreased tumor perfusion, increased interstitial pressure, and decreased oxygen tension. Blood flow, specifically oxygen flow, is necessary to initiate sustained free radical production, which is a cornerstone of radiation-induced tumor cell damage. Experimental and clinical tumors have been shown to have decreased perfusion and diffusion, compared with normal tissues (9). Adequate oxygen tension is required for radiation sensitivity and hypoxic cells are 2.5 to 3 times less likely to be radiosensitive than well-oxygenated cells. Large human tumors are likely to contain hypoxic areas. Additionally, several studies have demonstrated poor outcome for anemic patients compared to patients who are not anemic. (10)

Experimental models controlling for the above tumor factors still may demonstrate radioresistance. This represents inherent or intrinsic cellular radioresistance and may contribute to failure of radiation therapy. Conceptually, there are several reasons for this resistance.

1. Repair of sublethal x-ray damage - This term applies to the enhancement of cell survival seen, as a single dose of radiation is divided into smaller doses, so that cellular DNA is repaired before cell death is achieved

2. Potential lethal radiation damage repair (PLDR) - Radiation-induced damage, which may be lethal under specific conditions, may not be lethal under modified conditions (11).

3. Tumor cell repopulation - This is defined as the regrowth of tumor cells between fractions of radiation. At least one explanation is that tumors may recruit cells from the GO phase of cell cycle into an active phase, as there is tumor shrinkage. Long treatment interruptions allowing for recovery from toxicity may afford tumor cell repopulation to exceed cell kill and may limit the efficacy of the treatment of HNC.

4. Cell cycle specificity.- Cells in the S-phase of the cell cycle are radioresistant but may be sensitive to certain chemotherapy drugs (12).

The main principles of radiosensitization thus include the administration of chemotherapy or other drugs that may decrease tumor resistance or intrinsic cellular resistance.

Overcoming radioresistance

Strategies to overcome radioresistance should focus on the above mechanisms. Chemotherapy given with radiation or in alternating sequence may independently cause tumor cell kill and increase tumor blood flow, and decrease interstitial pressure, and decrease hypoxia in tumor cells. Numerous drugs have been used with marginal success with the aim of specifically acting as hypoxic cell sensitizers. These include Mitomycin C, nicotinamide, pentoxifylline, "perfluorocarbon chemicals" and hyperbaric oxygen.

Besides altering tumor characteristics, chemotherapy may overcome some of the specific intrinsic cellular resistance mechanisms. Cells in the S-phase of the cell cycle are radioresistant but may be sensitive to certain chemotherapy drugs (12).   Chemotherapy may lower the threshold for radiation induced cell kill, thus preventing sublethal x-ray damage repair. Several   chemotherapy   drugs   have   been   shown   to   inhibit   PLDR. Chemotherapy given with radiation or in an alternating fashion may decrease the tendency towards tumor cell repopulation between radiation fractions. Finally, chemotherapy has the potential to treat micro-metastases and subsequent distant metastases, which radiation cannot do.

Altered fraction radiation schema have been utilized in an attempt to decrease radiation resistance.   Hyperfractionated radiation may help to overcome problems related to tumor cell repopulation. Other schema such as high-dose fractions may overcome intrinsic cellular resistance or sublethal radiation damage repair.

SUPPORTING DATA FOR CHEMORADIATION

There are no known trials that have directly compared concomitant chemoradiation in a randomized fashion to surgery with or without radiation, in an attempt to assess for survival and organ or function preservation. Therefore, comparisons of these two modalities can only be made indirectly. Data such as that below should be carefully explained to patients who desire organ preservation so that they can account for factors such as potential differences in survival, likelihood of organ preservation, likelihood of function preservation, toxicity with treatment, duration of treatment and recovery, and cost and other factors related to the treatment.

Because of the lack of direct comparative trials, indirect comparisons must be made. Reported 5-year survival rates with surgery plus radiation for stage III and IV head and neck cancer range from 20% to 60% (4, 5,13-16). Of course there are differences in outcome between different head and neck sub-sites, making some of these indirect comparisons even be more difficult. Many studies of concomitant chemoradiation have failed to categorize patients as resectable or unresectable. It is likely that the outcome of these trials, which generally include some unresectable patients, represent a "worse case scenario" for chemoradiation since purely resectable patients would be expected to have an advantage with any treatment over unresectable patients.

It has been well demonstrated that concomitant chemoradiation improves survival over radiation alone for patient with unresectable disease, or when a surgical option is not possible (1-3). Three consecutive meta-analyses have demonstrated a relative overall survival advantage of about 20%. These meta-analyses generally included studies published from the early 1990s and earlier, and have omitted some of the modern studies that have demonstrated the largest percentage difference.

That data that most closely approach a direct comparison between chemoradiation and surgery plus radiation is the combination of the VA larynx study and the successor Intergroup 91-11. The first of these two studies demonstrated the equivalent survival between laryngectomy followed by radiation or induction chemotherapy followed by radiation. Two-thirds of patients receiving nonsurgical treatment retained a functional larynx. The successor, Intergroup 91-11, demonstrated that concomitant chemoradiation is at least as good as induction chemotherapy followed by radiation. The author believes that this demonstrates that CRT is probably the optimal choice for larynx preservation based on shorter treatment time and improved time to laryngectomy. It is possible that more intensive regimens than cisplatin alone, perhaps combining sequential and multiagent concomitant therapy, would improve survival over CRT or sequential therapy.

The remainder of the supporting data for organ preservation using concomitant chemoradiation comes from a series of phase III studies examining concomitant chemoradiation versus radiation alone and phase II studies of concomitant chemoradiation. The concomitant chemoradiation arms of the phase III studies as well as the phase II studies have consistently demonstrated 5-year overall survival rate of 30% to 60% with organ preservation in the majority of patients (17-27) (Table 1). Once again, some of these studies do not specify whether the patients were resectable or unresectable. Some specified a mix of resectable and unresectable patients were present while several of these studies were performed specifically on patients with resectable disease. Notably, these studies generally were performed in stage IV disease only, whereas most surgical series in advanced HNC have 60% stage IV and 40% stage III patients.

Table 1. **Randomized studies of concomitant chemoradiotherapy vs. radiotherapy alone.**

Author/ year	No. pts	Chemotherapy (+ RT in all)	O.S. (%)CRT/ RT	Comments
Phase III Studies				
Jeremic	130	Cisplatin, daily	5 yr 46/25 (p=0.008)	Hyperfractionated RT
Merlano	157	Cisplatin, 5FU	3 yr 41/23 (p< 0.05)	Chemo alternated with XRT
Brizel	116	Cisplatin, 5FU on wk 1, 6	3 yr 55/34 (p=0.07)	Hyperfractionated RT
Wendt	270	Cisplatin, 5FU weeks 1,4,7	3 yr 48/24 (p<0.0003)	Hyperfractionated RT
Adelstein	100	Cisplatin, 5FU weeks 1,4	5 yr 50/48	* Far less salvage surgery needed in chemo arm
Calais	226	Carboplatin, 5FU, weeks 1,4,7	3 yr 51/31 (p= 0.02)	
Phase II Studies				
Vokes	76	Cisplatin (cy 1,3,5), 5FU, hydroxyurea	3 yr 55%	Hyperfractionated, split course RT
Kies	64	Taxol (infusion), 5FU, hydroxyurea	3 yr 60%	Hyperfractionated , split course RT
Rosen	90	Taxol (1-hour), 5FU, hydroxyurea	2 yr 61%	Hyperfractionated, split course RT
Adelstein	42	Cisplatin, 5FU	2 yr 80%	Hyperfractionated RT
Leyvraz	91	Cisplatin, 5FU	4 yr 40%	Hyperfractionated, split course RT
Glicksman	74	Cisplatin/carboplatin	4 yr 51%	Hyperfactionated RT

Combined Chemoradiation Arms Of Phase III Studies

Numerous phase III studies of concomitant chemoradiation versus radiation alone have been performed over the past two-and-a-half decades. Five recent well-conducted large-scale studies are described here.

Adelstein et al randomized 100 (72% of whom were stage IV) resectable head and neck cancer patients to 66 to 72 Gy radiation with daily fractions without or with concomitant cisplatin and 5-FU, both given as continuous infusions on days, 1 to 4 and 22 to 25 (17). The patients not responding after 55 Gy and those with residual disease or recurrent disease underwent surgery. Overall survival between the two groups was not different (48% versus 50% for RT versus CRT at five years). Both relapse-free survival and overall survival with primary site preservation was improved in the CRT group. Fifty-four percent of patients receiving radiotherapy alone required surgical salvage, successful in 63%, versus 22% of those receiving

CRT, successful in 73%. Although no comparison was made in this study directly to surgery, these resectable mostly stage IV patients, had a five-year survival of 50% and 78% required no surgery. This compares very well with similarly staged surgical series.

Brizel et al randomized 122 patients with stage III or stage IV squamous cell head and neck cancer. Half received hyperfractionated radiation alone (125 cGy twice a day to 7500 cGy), and half received 125 cGy twice daily to 7000 cGy and five days of cisplatin plus 5-FU on days 1 through 5 of weeks 1 and 6 of radiotherapy. A seven day break was given midway through the CRT regimen. 47% of patients had resectable tumors. The three-year rate of overall survival was 55% in the combined therapy group versus 34% in the hyperfractionated group (p=0.07). Actuarial estimates of five-year overall survival were approximately 50% in the CRT group (20).

Wendt et al (19) randomized 278 assessable patients with locoregionally advanced head and neck cancer to radiotherapy administered in three courses, each of 13 fractions of 1.8 Gy twice daily or the same radiation with bolus cisplatin plus infusional 5-FU and leucovorin given on days 2 through 5 of each radiation course. The three-year overall survival rate was 48% in the combined therapy arm versus 24% with RT alone. There was no mention of specific assessment of resectability, however, slightly more than half the patients had tumors in the hypopharynx, larynx, or oral cavity so that about half the patients may have had "resectable" disease.

Jeremic et al randomized 130 patients to receive hyperfractionated radiation (1.1 Gy b.i.d. times 35 days) or the same hyperfractionated radiation plus low-dose bolus cisplatin given daily during radiation. No specific mention was made of resectability in these patients. Hyperfractionated CRT patients had a 68% 2-year survival (46% 5-yr survival versus 25% for radiation alone). Five-year local regional progression-free survival was 50% in the CRT arm.

Calais et al randomized 226 patients in a multicenter trial to radiotherapy alone (70 Gy in 35 fractions) or the same radiation plus four days of carboplatin plus infusional 5-FU for three cycles during radiation. The three-year overall actuarial survival rate was 51% (versus 31% for RT alone) and the three-year local regional control rate was 66% (versus 42%). Resectability was not assessed in the study.

Combined Chemoradiation Arms of Phase II Studies

A consortium of Chicago Hospitals led by the University of Chicago and Northwestern University has performed a series of five large phase two concomitant chemoradiation trials over the past decade. The last three of these trials have involved hyperfractionated radiation with chemotherapy, without any induction chemotherapy. The base chemotherapy of all three studies has included infusional 5-FU plus oral hydroxyurea. Radiation therapy was given in all three at 150 cGy b.i.d. 5 days a week, every other week to a total of 7500 cGy. In the first study, bolus cisplatin was given on treatment weeks 1, 3, and 5 (23). Three-year estimate of overall survival in this study was 55% and locoregional control was 92%. Ninety-seven percent of patients had stage IV disease. No specific attempt was made to determine resectability in these patients. Organ preservation was achieved in almost all patients, however, long-term studies of function showed a fairly high rate of chronic swallowing dysfunction in these patients, and this regimen was abandoned in favor of the subsequent two regimens. The subsequent two studies utilized the same 5-FU and hydroxyurea base, though at lower doses, and deleted cisplatin and substituted paclitaxel (24). In the first of these studies, paclitaxel was given by continuous infusion from days 1 through 5. In the second study,paclitaxel was given as a bolus on day 1 of each chemotherapy cycle. Overall survival at three years was 66%. 63 of 64 patients had stage IV disease. Only 3 of 64 patients required surgical salvage procedures, two laryngectomies, and one tongue base resection. (Neck dissections however were generally performed in patients with N2 or greater disease). In the second study, 90 patients, almost all with stage IV disease were treated with paclitaxel by bolus, infusional 5-FU and oral hydroxyurea, and hyperfractionated radiation as above. The overall survival rate at two years was 61%. Only seven locoregional recurrences occurred in 90 patients after two years (25).

Three phase II studies have examined chemoradiation specifically in patients with resectable disease. A multicentered phase-II study treated 20 stage III and 54 stage IV patients with 1.8 Gy daily for two weeks followed by 1.2 Gy twice daily to 46.8 Gy. Cisplatin was given by continuous infusion on days 1 through 4 and 22 through 25. The patients with a complete response continued with hyperfractionated radiation to 75.6 cGy plus simultaneous carboplatin, twice daily. Only 12 patients required surgical resection of the primary site. Actuarial overall survival at four years was 51% (26).

Adelstein et al treated 42 stage III and stage IV patients with hyperfractionated radiation (1.2 cGy b.i.d. to 72 Gy) and two courses of concurrent infusional cisplatin and 5-FU for four days during weeks 1 and 4 of radiation (18) Primary site resection was reserved for residual or recurrent primary disease in these resectable stage IV patients. The two-year projection of overall survival was 80%. At two years local control with salvage surgery was 97% and local control without the need for salvage surgery was 90%. The five-year projected disease-specific survival was 66%.

Leyvraz et al treated 91 patients with advanced head and neck cancer (69 of whom were resectable) with a regimen alternating split hyperfractionated irradiation 2 cGy t.i.d. over 30 to 40 days to a total of 48 to 60 Gy and chemotherapy with cisplatin bolus and infusional 5-FU plus or minus vindesine for two cycles. Amongst resectable patients, the organ preservation rate was 64%. The four-year overall survival was 40% (27).

Summary of phase II and phase III chemoradiotherapy data

1. There remain no good direct comparative studies of chemoradiation or radiation alone versus surgery for resectable disease. Therefore, the efficacy of chemoradiation, both in terms of cure and organ preservation must be extrapolated from studies such as those above.
2. The above studies generally contain a higher percentage of patients with stage IV disease than pure surgical series.
3. Overall survival on the above studies at five years is in the range of 40% to 55%. This compares favorably to historical reports of surgery plus RT.
4. Organ preservation with appropriate chemoradiation as in the above studies is possible in 50% to 90%. Surgical salvage is generally feasible in at least half of those patients who subsequently fail.
5. Functional evaluations are now an important endpoint in these studies and surgical series. Some of this is summarized in chapter 14 on Quality of Life and Late Toxicities in Head and Neck Cancer.
6. Aggressive concomitant chemoradiation, like surgery for advanced head and neck cancer should be performed at an institution experienced with these regimens and capable of shepherding patients throughacute toxicities and recovery, including functional rehabilitation, post-   treatment.
7. It is possible that the optimal treatment may include induction chemotherapy followed by CRT, or chemoradiation after surgery.

CONCLUSION

Treatment options for patients with locoregionally advanced head and neck cancer are now diverse. Surgery plus radiation or surgery plus chemoradiation remain options for patients with resectable disease. The same patients, however, appear to have an equally efficacious option of concomitant chemoradiation, with surgery reserved for salvage only. When performed in experienced settings, non-comparative data seem to indicate the outcome to be equivalent or perhaps even better. Direct comparisons between surgery and chemoradiation are unavailable. These would be extremely useful in terms of understanding optimal treatment, both in terms of cure, organ preservation, function preservation, and quality of life. All patients referred for resection of locoregionally advanced head and neck cancer should also have the option of concomitant chemoradiation discussed if an experienced treatment group is available to the patient.

REFERENCES

1. Pignon JP, Bourhis J, Domenge C, Designe L. Chemotherapy added to locoregional treatment for head and neck squamous cell carcinoma: three meta-analyses of updated individual patient data. Lancet 2000;355:949-955.
2. Munro, A. An overview of randomized controlled trials of adjuvant chemotherapy in head and neck cancer. Br J Cancer 1995; 71:83-91.
3. El-Sayed, S, Nelson, N. Adjuvant and adjunctive chemotherapy in the management of squamous cell carcinoma of the head and neck region: A meta-analysis of prospective and randomized trials. J Clin Oncol 1996; 14:838-847
4. Induction chemotherapy plus radiation compared with surgery plus radiation in patients with advanced laryngeal cancer. The Department of Veterans Affairs Cancer Study Group. N Engl J Med 1991; 324:1685-1690.
5. Lefebvre, JL, Chevalier, D, Luboinski, B, et al. Larynx preservation in pyriform sinus cancer: Preliminary results of a European Organization for research of cancer phase II trial. J Natl Cancer Inst 1996; 88:890-899.
6. Forastiere AA, Berkey B, Maor M, et al. Phase III trial to preserve the larynx: Induction chemotherapy and radiotherapy versus concomitant chemoradiotherapy versusu radiotherapy alone, Intergroup trial R91-11. Proc ASCO 2001;20:abstract 4.
7. Ku KK, Pajak TF, Trotti A, et al. A radiation therapy oncolgy group (RTOG) phase III randomized study to compare hyperfractionated and two variants of accelerated fractionation to standard fractionated radiotherapy for head and neck squamous cell carcinomas: First report of RTOG 9003. Int J Radiation Oncology Biol Phys 2000;48:7-16.
8. Merlano M, Benasso M, Corvo R, et al. Five-year update of a randomized trial of alternating radiotherapy and chemotherapy compared with radiotherapy alone in treatment of unresectable squamous cell carcinoma of the head and neck. J Natl Cancer Inst 1996;88:583-589.
9. Roh HD, Boucher Y, Kalnicki S, et al: Interstitial hypertension in carcinoma of uterine cervix in patients: Possible correlation with tumor oxygenation and radiation response. Cancer Res 1991; 51:6695

10. Bush RS, Jenkin RDT, Alh WEC et al: Definitive evidence for hypoxic cells influencing cure in cancer therapy. Br J Cancer 1978; 38(suppl 3):302

11. Weichselbaum RR, Little JB: Repair of potentially legal x-ray damage and possible applications to clinical radiotherapy. Int J Radiat Oncol Biol Phys 1993; 9:91

12. Kinsella TJ: Radiosensitization and cell kinetics: Clinical implications for s-phase-specific radiosensitizers. Semin Oncol 1992; 19(suppl 9):41

13. Laramore GB, Scott CB, Al-Sarraf M, et al. Adjuvant chemotherapy for resectable squamous cell carcinomas of the head and neck: report on Intergroup study 0034. Int J Radiat Oncol Biol Phys 1992;23:705-713.

14. Paccagnella A, Orlando A, Marchiori C, et al. Phase III trial of initial chemotherapy in stage III or IV head and neck cancers: a study by the Gruppodidi Studio SUI Tumori Della Testa E Del Collo. J Natl Cancer Inst 1994;86:265-272.

15. Schuller DE, Laramore G, Al-Sarraf M, Jacobs J, Pajak T. Combined therapy for resectable head and neck cancer. A phase III intergroup study. Arch Otolaryngol Head Neck Surg 1989;115:364-368.

16. Head and Neck Contracts Program. Adjuvant chemotherapy for advanced head and neck squamous carcinoma. Final report of the head and neck contracts program. Cancer 1987;60:301-311

17. Adelstein DJ, Lavertu P, Saxton JP et al. Mature results of a phase III randomized trial comparing concurrent chemoradiotherapy with radiation therapy alone in patients with stage III and IV squamous cell carcinoma of the head and neck. Cancer 2000;88:876-883.

18. Adelstein DJ, Saxton JP, Lavertu P, et al. Maximizing local control and organ preservation in advanced squamous cell head and neck cancer (SCHNC) with hyperfractionated radiation (HRT) and concurrent chemotherapy. Proc ASCO 2001;20:224a, abstract 893.

19. Wendt TG, Grabenbauer GG, Rodel CM. Simultaneous radiotherapy versus radiotherapy alone in advanced head and neck cancer: A randomized multicenter study. J Clin Oncol 16:1318-1324

20. Brizel DM, Albers ME, Fisher R, et al. Hyperfractionated irradiation with or without concurrent chemotherapy for locally advanced head and neck cancer. N Engl J Med 1998;338:1798-1804.

21. Jeremic B, Shibamoto Y, Milicic B, et al. Hyperfractionated radiation therapy with or without concurrent low dose cisplatin in locally advanced squamous cell carcinoma of the head and neck: A prospective randomized trial. J Clin Oncol 2000;18:1458-1464

22. Calais G, Alfonsi M, Bardet E et al. Randomized trial of radiation versus concomitant chemotherapy and radiation for advanced-stage oropharynx carcinoma, J Natl Cancer Inst 1999;15:2081-2086.

23. Vokes EE, Kies M, Haraf DJ, et al. Concomitant chemoradiotherapy as primary therapy for locoregionally advanced head and neck cancer. J Clin Oncol 2000;18:1652-1661.

24. Kies MS, Haraf DJ, Rosen F, et al. Concomitant infusional paclitaxel and fluorouracil, oral hydroxyurea, and hyperfractionated radiation for locally advanced squamous head and neck cancer. J Clin Oncol 2001;19:1961-1969.

25. Rosen FR, Haraf DJ, Brockstein B, et al. Multicenter randomized phase II study of 1-hour infusion paclitaxel, fluorouracil and hydroxyurea with concomitant hyperfractionated radiotherapy (2XRT) with or without erythropoietin for advanced head and neck cancer. Proc ASCO 2001;20:226a, abstract 902

26.   Glicksman AS, Wanebo HJ, Slotman G, et al. Concurrent platinum based chemotherapy and hyperfractionated radiotherapy with late intensification in advanced head and neck cancer. Int J Radiat Oncol Biol Phys 1997;39:721-729.

27.   Leyvraz, S, Pasche, P, Bauer, J, et al. Rapidly alternating chemotherapy and hyperfractionated radiotherapy in the management of locally advanced head and neck carcinoma; Four year results of a phase I/II study. J Clin Oncol 1994; 12:1876.

Chapter 10

UNRESECTABLE, LOCOREGIONALLY ADVANCED HEAD AND NECK CANCER

Fred Rosen.M.D.

University of Illinois at Chicago, Department of Medicine,Chicago, Illinois 60612

INTRODUCTION

Of the approximate 60,000 cases of squamous cell carcinoma of the head and neck diagnosed annually in the United States, approximately two thirds of patients present with locoregionally advanced disease (T3 or T4, N_{1-3}, M0). [1] The prognosis for patients with locoregionally advanced disease is poor. Historically, treatment consists of extensive surgery and post-operative radiation therapy, or if unresectable, extensive radiation therapy alone. Survival is poor with less than 30 percent of patients cured and treatment related sequelae including mucositits, xerostomia, loss of organ function (speech and swallowing), as well as, disfigurement from mutilative surgery. Chemotherapy, once used only for palliation in recurrent or metastatic disease, has become standard treatment when used concurrently with radiation therapy in advanced nasopharyngeal carcinoma, or arguably, as induction prior to definitive radiation therapy with the goal of organ preservation in advanced, resectable cancer of the larynx and hypopharynx.[2,3,4] Treatment strategies for metastatic disease, nasopharyngeal carcinoma, and organ preservation in resectable disease are discussed in other chapters.

Unresectable, locoregionally advanced head and neck cancer has been an area on intensive clinical research over the past two decades. Research has focused on the improvement of locoregional control, distant failure, and overall survival through the use of altered radiation fraction schedules and the integration of chemotherapy with the standard and altered radiation fraction schedules. Increased toxicity has also, unfortunately, accompanied the more intensified radiation and chemoradiation schedules, lowering the therapeutic index and prompting research on the use of cytoprotective agents to reduce toxicity.   Finally, newer chemotherapeutic agents, p53 gene therapy and epidermal growth factor receptor (EGFR)/tyrosine kinase inhibitor drugs are rapidly being integrated with standard therapy in phase II and III trials. Interpretations of the many trials to date is challenging because of the lack of a universally agreed upon definition of unresectability, and because most studies are not site specific (i.e. lumping all head and neck sites within the same eligible study population).   Because of a lack of formal definition, unresectability varies from one institution to another depending upon the experience of the surgeon and the availability of support staff, such as reconstructive surgeons and prosthodontists.[5]   An experienced surgeon considers a cancer unresectable if there is doubt that all gross tumor can be removed or that local control can be achieved after resection even with the addition of post-operative radiation therapy.   Such tumors typically involve the cervical vertebrae, brachial plexus, and deep muscles of the neck or carotid artery.[5,6]   Criteria used for unresectability in multiple randomized studies include 1) technical unresectability, 2) physician selection based on low surgical curability, and 3) medical contraindication to surgery.   Technical unresectability criteria included evidence for mediastinal spread, tumor fixation to the clavicle, base of the skull or the cervical vertebrae, and involvement of the nasopharynx. [6] Patients with medical contraindication to surgery, as well as patients who refuse surgery, regardless of resectability, may well be appropriate for non-surgical treatment, but inclusion of these patients in studies designed to address unresectable disease can bias the results.   Similarly, patients with definite evidence of distant metastases are considered unresectable and may be appropriate for localized and systemic treatment, but generally are ineligible for studies designed for locoregionally advanced head and neck cancer because of their overall poor prognosis and lack of curability.   There are a limited number of trials in locoregionally advanced head and neck cancers which are site specific because of the practical problem of accruing adequate numbers of patients, as well as an assumption that all patients with unresectable diseases have a similar prognosis.   Notable exceptions to this lack of site specific trials include larynx and hypopharynx where organ preservation is a primary endpoint and nasopharyngeal carcinoma where the biology of the disease differs from other head and neck sites.[2,3,4] These sites are addressed in other chapters.

Because of the complexity of the patient with advanced head and neck cancer, the multidisciplinary team approach is important in the management of advanced head and neck cancer.   Ideally, the multidisciplinary team consists of head and neck surgery, radiation oncology, medical oncology, plastic and reconstructive surgery, dentistry and prosthodontics, physical medicine and rehabilitation, speech and swallowing therapy, nutritional support, pathology, and diagnostic radiology.[7] Availability of neurosurgery and ophthalmology for specific circumstances is also essential for the multidisciplinary approach to advanced head and neck cancer.[5] In addition to specific treatment issues, the multidisciplinary team addresses multiple social issues which characterizes a large percentage of patients who present with advanced head and neck cancer in the United States. Malnutrition, speech, and swallowing difficulty are frequent presenting problems, as well as, sequelae of treatment. [8] Tobacco and alcohol addiction, lower social economic status, and associated decreased access to medical care contribute to patients' late presentation with advanced disease and present barriers to treatment once a diagnosis is made. [1]

Treatment of Locoregionally Advanced Head and Neck Cancer

Historically the primary treatment of unresectable head and neck cancer has been radiation therapy. However, after thirty years of clinical trials, there is a consensus that the integration of chemotherapy with radiation therapy improves survival in locoregionally advanced, unresectable head and neck cancer. [5,9] Early randomized studies by Ansfield, Lo, and Shanta demonstrated improved survival with the addition of single agent chemotherapy (5-FU or bleomycin) over radiation therapy alone. [10,11] Other studies (Fu et al.) demonstrated improved complete response rate, local regional control rate, and relapse free survival rate, but failed to demonstrate improved overall survival. [6]

As with many other solid tumor sites there are three strategies of integrating chemotherapy with definitive locoregional therapy (radiation therapy and/or surgery): neoadjuvant, adjuvant, and concomitant chemoradiotherapy. Each strategy has theoretical benefits and disadvantages. Neoadjuvant or induction chemotherapy, using standard doses of cisplatin and 5-FU prior to radiotherapy predictably results in a 60 to 90% response rate with 20-50% complete response rate in previously untreated locoregionally advanced head and neck cancer patients. [12,13] The incidence of distant metastases after induction chemotherapy is reduced presumably from the treatment of micrometastatic disease. There are also disadvantages to induction chemotherapy, such as the dependence on patient compliance to continue with definitive radiation and/or surgical therapy after a favorable response to induction chemotherapy, and most importantly, lack of a consistent survival benefit when compared to radiotherapy alone.[14] Concomitant chemoradiotherapy, using single or multiple chemotherapy agents ideally improves systemic, as well as, locoregional control by using chemotherapy agents with good systemic activity, and chemotherapy agents that are good radiopotentiators.[15,16] Concomitant chemoradiotherapy has been shown to improve survival in advanced head and neck cancer. The disadvantages of concomitant chemoradiotherapy include a significant increase in dermatitis, mucositits, and myelosuppression. [17,18,19,20] Adjuvant chemotherapy, following definitive radiation or surgery has the theoretical advantage of treating micrometastases, possibly growing at a faster rate following definitive locoregional treatment. Once again however, patients are often poorly compliant following extensive surgery and post-operative radiation therapy, and survival benefit in advanced disease has not been consistently shown in trials. [1]

Meta-Analysis

Of the three strategies, concomitant chemoradiotherapy appears to be the most promising in unresectable locoregionally advanced head and neck cancer according to three recent major meta-analyses. [18,19,20] The meta-analyses include randomized studies completed or published between 1963 through 1993 where the integration of chemotherapy with radiation is compared with radiation alone and survival or disease-free survival is a main endpoint. Munro's analysis included 54 trials including a total of 7828 patients. Significant findings included an absolute survival benefit of 6.5% in favor of patients who received chemotherapy in addition to radiotherapy, rather than radiotherapy alone. [18] The survival benefit was greatest, 12.1%, when chemotherapy was given concomitantly with radiotherapy. In this group the majority of the benefit was derived from single agent chemotherapy rather than cisplatin/5-FU regimens. Neoadjuvant chemotherapy was less effective than concomitant chemoradiotherapy with a survival rate difference of 3.9% over radiotherapy alone. The analysis of El-Sayed and Nelson also found a statistically significant benefit from chemotherapy when added to definitive local therapy. [19] The meta-analysis includes 42 trials and 5079 patients for assessment of toxicity from the addition of chemotherapy. There were 25 trials with 3708 patients with sufficient information for survival analysis. The addition of chemotherapy to definitive local therapy resulted in a 4% absolute survival benefit over local therapy alone. Once again the benefit was greatest in studies utilizing concomitant chemoradiotherapy with an 8% absolute survival benefit over radiotherapy alone. Within the meta-analysis there was a statistically significant benefit for concomitant chemoradiotherapy when compared to patients treated with neoadjuvant and adjuvant chemotherapy. Importantly, the analysis also demonstrated a statistically significant increase in toxicity when chemotherapy is added to local definitive treatment.

The Meta-Analysis of Chemotherapy in Head and Neck Cancer (MACH-NC) study, the largest and most recently published analysis, uses a different design from the prior two. Instead of relying on results published in the medical literature the MACH-NC analysis was based on individual patient data obtained from the principal investigators or the statistician of each trial. [20,21] The technique was felt to reduce bias inherent in published studies. The MACH-NC included 63 trials and 10,741 patients. Median follow-up of 6.8 years was longer than in the other meta-analyses and the authors were able to perform an intent-to-treat analysis. Despite the difference in design and number of patients, results from the MACH-NC were quite similar to those of El-Sayed and Nelson; absolute survival benefit at 2 and 5 years was statistically significant at 4%. Once again the majority of benefit, 8% at five years, was derived from concomitant chemoradiotherapy. Multiagent chemotherapy had a statistically significant increased effect over single agent chemotherapy when given concomitantly with radiotherapy. Neither the benefit from adjuvant nor neoadjuvant chemotherapy was statistically significant at 2 or 5 years. In summary, the major meta-analyses, although using different techniques and including different studies from the mid 1960's through 1993, demonstrate general agreement of a small but statistically significant survival benefit to the addition of chemotherapy to definitive local treatment with the majority if not all of the benefit from concomitant chemoradiotherapy rather than adjuvant or neoadjuvant chemotherapy. Although benefit from chemotherapy is small and toxicity is increased, if the MACH-NC is accepted as the most accurate and least biased analysis, 4% survival benefit in 10,000 patients included in the analysis would prevent 400 deaths at 5 years if all received chemotherapy. [21] Randomized studies conducted after 1993 further support the addition of chemotherapy to definitive radiotherapy.

Adjuvant Chemotherapy

Adjuvant chemotherapy following definitive local therapy has been least studied and is included for completeness. In the Head and Neck Contracts Program the addition of six cycles of monthly adjuvant cisplatin to standard surgical and post-operative radiotherapy resulted in a statistically significant reduction in the incidence of distant relapse compared to standard therapy or induction therapy followed by standard therapy. Overall survival and disease-free survival was not improved. [22]

More recently Intergroup 0034 compared patients with resectable, loco-regionally advanced disease randomized to standard therapy (surgery followed by post-operative radiotherapy) versus surgery followed by adjuvant chemotherapy, (cisplatin, and 5-FU for three cycles), preceding radiotherapy (sequential chemo-radiotherapy).[23,24] Although preliminary analysis appeared promising, in the final analysis there was no survival benefit to adjuvant chemotherapy , however, a high risk group with poor prognosis was identified. The high-risk group included patients with close surgical margins, multiple metastatic lymph nodes and/or extracapsular spread. Survival was decreased in patients in this high-risk group whether or not they received adjuvant chemotherapy.

A follow-up study, open only to patients with one or more high-risk features, has recently completed accrual. Patients found to be in the high-risk group after surgery were randomized to standard post-operative radiotherapy or concomitant, rather than sequential, cisplatin and radiotherapy. Results of this study are not yet available. It is hypothesized that the favorable interaction of concomitant chemotherapy and radiation therapy will result in a survival benefit for high-risk patients. Preliminary results of two similar smaller studies with post-operative weekly or every three week concomitant cisplatin and radiotherapy, resulted in improved disease-free survival and increased loco-regional control when compared to standard post-operative radiotherapy,[25,26] and one of the two studies showed a survival advantage (25). Adjuvant chemotherapy with three cycles of cisplatin and 5-FU is now considered part of the standard treatment for Stage III and IV nasopharyngeal carcinoma following loco-regional treatment with concomitant cisplatin and radiotherapy based on a strongly positive Intergroup study with statistically significant improvement in overall survival and disease free survival when compared to radiation therapy alone.[2] Because adjuvant chemotherapy independent of concomitant chemoradiotherapy was not included as a study arm it is unclear exactly what contribution the adjuvant chemotherapy adds to the treatment of nasopharyngeal carcinoma. Nasopharyngeal carcinoma is discussed in another chapter. Suffice it to say, that aside from nasopharyngeal carcinoma, there is no standard role for adjuvant chemotherapy in loco-regionally advanced head and neck cancer.

Neoadjuvant Chemotherapy

Neoadjuvant chemotherapy has been extensively reviewed as used in loc-regionally advanced resectable and unresectable disease elsewhere and in the appropriate chapters of this book.[14,15,27] The role of neoadjuvant chemotherapy in organ preservation has been established in carcinoma of the hypopharynx and larynx.[3,4] Its role in laryngeal carcinoma has recently been questioned in the follow-up study to the VA larynx preservation protocol, which resulted in a lack of statistically significant difference between induction chemotherapy compared to radiotherapy alone. Concomitant cisplatin and radiotherapy resulted in significantly prolonged recurrence free survival and preservation of the larynx.[28] As shown in the meta-analysis, neoadjuvant chemotherapy, with rare exception has not been shown to improve survival although several studies have demonstrated a significant reduction in distant metastases.[14,3,29] In a large study by Paccagnella, et al., which randomized operable and inoperable Stage III and IV to induction chemotherapy followed by definitive loco-regional therapy versus loco-regional therapy alone, there was no statistical advantage to induction chemotherapy.[29]   However, when operable and inoperable patients were analyzed separately, the lack of benefit remained for operable patients but there appeared to be a small, statistically significant benefit in inoperable patients. Decrease in loco-regional relapse, distant metastases and increase in overall survival were all statistically significant, although survival was poor, with or without induction chemotherapy, 24% versus 10% at 3 years respectively. Induction chemotherapy consisted of 4 rather than 3 cycles of cisplatin, $100mg/m^2$ day 1, and 5-FU, 1000 mg/m^2/day days 1-5. The complete response rate increased with each cycle. The authors hypothesize that the increased dose intensity of four cycles of induction chemotherapy rather than three contributed to the increased complete response rate and improved overall survival in the inoperable patients. Recent Phase II studies have focused on more dose intensive induction regimens [cisplatin, 5-FU, leucovorin (PFL), docetaxel, cisplatin, 5-FU with or without leucovorin (TPFL, TPF)] with complete response rates between 40-60%.[27,30] It remains to be seen whether or not these more dose intensive and toxic induction regimens will result in improved survival in randomized studies compared to or preceding concomitant chemo-radiotherapy. Until such evidence exists, induction chemotherapy is considered investigational in unresectable, loco-regionally advanced head and neck cancer.[5,31] Despite these recommendations Harari published results of a 1996 survey of practicing cancer specialists participating in the care of head and neck cancer patients (otolaryngologists, radiation oncologists, and medical oncologists) which revealed that induction chemotherapy, usually cisplatin and 5-FU, preceding radiation was the most common treatment approach reported for patients with loco-regionally advanced head and neck cancer (61% of participants).[32] A follow-up survey from 2000 however showed a shift in practice behavior with participants reporting concomitant chemoradiotherapy as the treatment of choice , more commonly used than induction chemotherapy (39% and 31% respectively).[33] This shift in practice is more consistent with accumulated results of recent studies in advanced head and neck cancer.

Concomitant Chemotherapy and Radiation Therapy

Concomitant chemoradiotherapy is now the standard treatment for unresectable, loco-regionally advanced head and neck cancer in those patients with adequate baseline performance status to tolerate the added toxicity of combined modality treatment.[5,9,17,18,19,20] This recommendation is based on the results of recent randomized studies, as well as, the small, but consistently statistically significant benefit of concomitant chemoradiotherapy in the meta-analyses. The optimal chemotherapy regimen (single agent or multi-agent), schedule or intensity is still the subject of Phase II and Phase III studies. The optimal radiation schedule is also under intense investigation with the growing evidence that altered radiation fractionation may prove superior to standard fractionation. In a large randomized study, RTOG 9003, accelerated fractionation with concomitant boost and hyperfractionation were superior to accelerated fractionation with split, or standard single fractionation.[34] Altered fractionation in advanced head and neck cancer is discussed in depth in chapter 8. Because the toxicity of concomitant chemoradiotherapy usually necessitates some type of break or split in treatment, the emergence of more affective radiation fractionation schemes re-opens the debate over sacrificing optimal, uninterrupted radiation therapy for the benefits of chemotherapy.[35] Single agent and combination chemotherapy combined with standard fractionated and hyperfractionated radiotherapy have been studied in advanced head and neck cancer.

Single Agent Chemotherapy

The use of single chemotherapy agents given concomitantly with standard fraction radiotherapy is supported by the meta-analyses and is more easily accomplished than multi-agent chemotherapy or altered fractionation. Single agents used in randomized studies loco-regionally advanced head and neck cancer can be divided between bioreductive alkylating agents which are selectively toxic to hypoxic cell and radiopotentiators. Both classes have single agent activity against head and neck cancer, but are more active when coupled with radiotherapy.[35,37] Mitomycin C is the most frequently studied bioreductive alkylating agent. Haffty et al. have studied the use of mitomycin C concomitantly with radiotherapy based on the rationale that the addition of a drug which is cytotoxic to hypoxic cells given concomitantly with radiotherapy, which is most effective against well oxygenated cells, would enhance the therapeutic index of both treatments.[38]

Chemoradiotherapy (mitomycin C 15 mg/m^2 week 1 and week 6 of radiotherapy) was given either post-operatively to patients with or without residual disease or high risk factors, as well as to patients treated primarily with radiotherapy for early or advanced disease, making it difficult to compare the results of this study to other chemoradiotherapy trials in advanced head and neck cancer. However, the results do favor concomitant mitomycin C and radiotherapy with significantly improved loco-regional control and disease free survival at five years when compared to radiotherapy alone. Overall, survival was not significantly improved on the chemotherapy arm. Aside from expected increase in hematologic toxicity, the addition of mitomycin C did not result in significant worsening of acute mucositis, dermatitis, chronic radiation fibrosis, or edema, when compared to radiotherapy alone. Since Mitomycin C is not a potent radiopotentiator, improved response was attributed to the cytotoxicity of mitomycin C on hypoxic cells. In contrast, other studies with 5-FU[39], methotrexate[40], bleomycin[6], and cisplatin[25] as single agents attributed improved disease control and sometimes improved survival to the radiopotentiation of these drugs. Browman chose infusional 5-FU, a potent radiopotentiator, to study in a randomized trial of single agent concomitant chemoradiotherapy versus radiotherapy alone in locally advanced head and neck cancer.[39] The study objectives were to improve response and survival without compromising delivery of radiation because of excessive toxicity. In the study 5-FU 1.2 grams/m^2/day as 72 hour continuous infusion was given on the first and third weeks of standard fraction radiation therapy. Despite significantly greater grade 3 or 4 mucositis, dermatitis, and weight loss, full dose radiotherapy could be delivered without significant delay. Complete response was significantly greater with chemoradiotherapy and progression free and overall survival approached statistical significance. Single agent 5-FU was chosen in this study as opposed to combination chemotherapy with cisplatin and 5-FU because of the belief that the latter would prove too toxic, necessitating a planned break in treatment (split course chemotherapy).

Combination Chemotherapy

A study by Taylor using a split course schedule of cisplatin, 5-FU, and concomitant radiotherapy resulted in improved disease control when compared to sequential (induction) chemotherapy and radiotherapy, but there was no overall survival benefit because of excess of deaths from other causes in the concomitant arm.[41] Patients treated with concomitant chemoradiotherapy required more supportive care and the experience of the treating institution was a significant variable for progression-free survival. In an attempt to avoid excessive toxicity while still taking advantage of the potentially favorable interaction of combination chemotherapy and radiotherapy, Merlano devised a schedule of alternating combination chemotherapy and radiotherapy, and compared it to standard fraction radiotherapy alone in a randomized study in unresectable head and neck cancer.[42] The chemotherapy consisted of 4 cycles of intravenous cisplatin (20 mg/m^2/day for 5 consecutive days) during weeks 1, 4, 7, and 10, which alternated with 3 courses of radiotherapy (20Gy per course) during weeks 2 and 3, 5 and 6, and 8 and 9. Complete response, progression-free survival, and overall survival were significantly improved with alternating chemotherapy and radiotherapy both at median follow-up at 3 years and in a follow-up report at 5 years.[42] Overall survival at 3 and 5 years was 41% and 24 % with alternating chemotherapy and radiotherapy compared 23% and 10% with radiotherapy alone. The low overall survival is consistent with a study population consisting of patients with unresectable disease. The incidence and severity of mucositis in the chemotherapy arm was similar to that observed with radiotherapy alone, 19% and 18% grade III-IV mucositis respectively, and chemotherapy did not necessitate significantly greater treatment delays. Alternating chemotherapy and radiotherapy appears superior to standard fractionated radiotherapy alone without an increase in toxicity, however, the relatively poor overall survival in both arms has prompted several investigators to continue to study more intensive concomitant chemoradiotherapy strategies.

Calais conducted a randomized trial of standard fraction radiation therapy versus concomitant chemoradiotherapy in advanced stage oropharyngeal carcinoma.[43] The study was unusual in that enough patients (N=226) could be accrued for a site specific study (oropharynx) rather than combining patients with multiple head and neck primary sites, with variable tumor natural histories, and prognoses. The chemotherapy in the experimental arm consisted of 3 cycles of 5-FU administered as a 24-hour continuous infusion at a dose of 600 mg/m^2/day for 4 days and carboplatin as a daily bolus of 70 mg/m^2/day for 4 days. Chemotherapy cycles were started on day 1, 22, and 43, given concomitantly with radiotherapy. The radiotherapy regimen was the same in both treatment arms with a total planned dose to the primary tumor and involved lymph nodes of 70Gy (2Gy per fraction, one fraction per day, and five fractions per week) without planned interruption. Similar to other studies, the chemoradiotherapy arm proved superior to radiotherapy alone. The median survival was nearly doubled, 15.4 months in the radiotherapy only group, and 29.2 months in the chemoradiotherapy group. Three years overall survival (51% versus 31%, p=0.02), three year disease-free survival (42% versus 20%, p=.04) and loco-regional control of the disease (66% versus 42%, p=.03) all favored chemoradiotherapy over radiotherapy alone. Acute toxicity was significantly increased with the addition of chemotherapy including hematologic toxicity, grade III and IV mucositis, dermatitis, and weight loss greater than 10% of body mass. Because of increased weight loss a higher percentage of patients receiving chemotherapy required placement of feeding gastrostomy tubes. There was also a trend toward greater late or chronic toxicity of severe cervical fibrosis. In summary, patients receiving chemoradiotherapy on this study had significantly improved survival but at the expense of greater toxicity and need for more supportive care. Improved survival was attributed to the increased loco-regional control rate as there was no statistically significant difference in the rate of distant metastases on either arm of the study.

Given the increased toxicity of concomitant chemoradiotherapy it is reasonable to ask whether or not it can be recommended in the community setting where adequate supportive care may not be readily available. It was found on one study that experience of the treating institution was a significant prognostic factor in overall survival.[41] The preliminary results of the much awaited Head and Neck Intergroup study may help answer the question of feasibility. The Head and Neck Intergroup conducted a large (N=295), but prematurely closed, three armed Phase III study comparing standard radiation versus standard radiation and concurrent single agent cisplatin versus split course radiation with concurrent cisplatin and 5-flourouracil in patients with unresectable, loco-regionally advanced head and neck cancer.[44] Chemotherapy in the single agent arm consisted of cisplatin 100 mg/m^2 IV on day 1, 22, and 43. Chemotherapy in the split course arm consisted of the 3 cycles of cisplatin 75 mg/m^2 on day 1 and 5-FU 1000 mg/m^2/day as a continuous infusion on days 1-4. Cycles were repeated every 4 weeks. Toxicity in both concomitant chemoradiotherapy arms was significantly greater that radiotherapy alone. Survival in the single agent cisplatin chemoradiotherapy arm, but not in the split course cisplatin/5-FU arm was significantly greater than radiotherapy alone, with a median follow-up of 25 months. The authors concluded that concomitant chemoradiotherapy could be safely administered with acceptable toxicity in the cooperative group setting, concurrent single agent cisplatin with standard radiotherapy is superior to radiotherapy alone and the use of multi-agent chemotherapy did not make up for the loss of efficacy resulting from split-course radiotherapy. Given the relative ease of administration, high dose single agent cisplatin given concurrently with standard fraction radiotherapy arguably could be considered the "standard" treatment for unresectable loco-regionally advanced head and neck cancer.

Chemotherapy and Hyperfractionated Radiotherapy

Weissler et al. compared hyperfractionated radiation therapy alone to hyperfractionated radiation with two cycles of concomitant cisplatin, 100 mg/m^2 day 1 and 5-FU 1000 mg/m^2/day continuous infusion for 96 hours days 1 through day 4 (repeated days 29-32).[45] For patients with unresectable disease chemotherapy significantly prolonged the mean time to death and the time to progression over hyperfractionated radiation alone. Although myelosuppression was increased in the chemotherapy arm, there was no increase in mucositis or dermatitis. Brizel et al also undertook a randomized study comparing chemoradiotherapy and radiotherapy alone.[46] Hyperfractionated radiotherapy was used in both arms but in the chemotherapy arm the radiation dose was decreased (7000cGy with chemotherapy, as opposed to 7500cGy) and a 7 day break after 4000cGy was planned in the chemotherapy arm to try to avoid excessive mucositis. Thus this trial compared "optimal" radiotherapy to concomitant chemotherapy and "sub-optimal" radiotherapy. The chemotherapy consisted of 2 cycles of cisplatin 12 mg/m^2/day for 5 days (60 mg/m^2 per cycle) and 5-FU, 600 mg/m^2/day for 5 days, administered during cycles 1 and 6. Two additional cycles of adjuvant chemotherapy with cisplatin and flourouracil were planned after completion of all local therapy in the chemoradiotherapy arm. More than half of the patients in both arms had unresectable disease. In general, treatment was well tolerated in both arms but confluent mucositis occurred in greater than 70% of patients in both arms. Only myelosupression was more common in the chemoradiotherapy arm. At three years follow-up loco-regional control of disease was superior with chemoradiotherapy (70% versus 44%, p=0.01) and there were trends towards improved relapse free survival and overall survival favoring chemoradiotherapy. Overall survival at 3 years was 55% with chemoradiotherapy. The primary site was the most common location of first recurrence in both arms with evidence of distant metastases similar in both arms. The authors concluded that despite the compromise in radiotherapy when combined with chemotherapy, concomitant chemotherapy and hyperfractionated radiotherapy was superior to hyperfractionated radiotherapy alone, without a significant increase in mucosal toxicity, which was severe in both arms.

Wendt also compared chemoradiotherapy with radiotherapy alone in loco-regionally advanced, unresectable head and neck cancer with both arms planned to receive the same dose (70.2Gy) and schedule of accelerated radiotherapy. Because of anticipated mucositis and dermatitis there were two planned treatment breaks on both arms.[47] Chemotherapy consisted of 3 cycles of cisplatin 60 mg/m^2 day 1, 5-FU 350 mg/m^2 by intravenous bolus, and leucovorin 100 mg/m^2/24 hrs. as a continuous infusion for day 2 to 5 of each cycle. Chemotherapy was repeated on days 22 and 44. Despite the planned treatment breaks in both arms, treatment was significantly prolonged in the chemoradiotherapy arm because of increased grade 3 and 4 mucositis (38% versus 16%, p<.001) and dermatitis (17% versus 7.3%, p<.05) in chemoradiotherapy and radiotherapy respectively, Despite prolongation of treatment time and increased mucosal toxicity, loco-regional tumor control and overall survival were significantly improved with concomitant chemoradiotherapy. At 3 years Kaplan-Meir estimates showed survival doubled (49% versus 24%, p<.0003) in favor of chemoradiotherapy. The improved survival was attributed to the improved loco-regional tumor control (35% versus 17%, p<.004) in favor of chemoradiotherapy rather than decreased distant failures which was the same in both arms, similar to Brizel's study.

Jeremic compared hyperfractionated radiotherapy (77GY in 70 fraction over 35 treatment days) with or without daily low dose cisplatin 6 mg/m^2/day. Once again, overall survival, progression-free survival, and loco-regional progression free-survival were significantly improved with the addition of chemotherapy without significant increase in mucosal toxicity. Unlike the other two studies, distant metastases were decreased significantly at 5 years on the chemotherapy arm.[48]

In summary, randomized studies comparing concomitant chemotherapy and hyperfractionated radiotherapy versus hyperfractionated radiotherapy alone favor the combined treatment approach. Although the addition of chemotherapy frequently caused an increase in toxicity and resulted in prolongation of treatment duration in some of the studies, survival consistently was superior with the addition of chemotherapy. Improved survival is surprisingly attributed more frequently to superior loco-regional control rather than decreased distant metastases with combined treatment.

Phase II Studies

Whereas recently completed and ongoing Phase III studies are still attempting to define the optimal integration of radiotherapy and chemotherapy, the integration of new active single chemotherapy agents and combination chemotherapy regimens with radiation therapy is being explored in Phase II studies. Of these agents, the taxanes, paclitaxel and docetaxel, are among the most important because of their single agent activity in head and neck cancer and their ability to act as potent radiopotentiators.[49] Paclitaxel causes cell-cycle arrest at the G_2/M phase, a particularly radiation-sensitive phase of the cell cycle, which is theorized to be the mechanism of radiopotentiation.[49]

Paclitaxel as a single agent has been given concomitantly with radiotherapy as a bolus and a prolonged infusion. [50,51,52] The combination of weekly paclitaxel and carboplatin in advanced head and neck cancer has been found to be feasible and active. Chougule studied the combination of weekly paclitaxel 60 mg/m^2/day, and carboplatin (AUC=1) with concomitant radiotherapy in operable and inoperable locally advanced head and neck cancer.[50] Operable patients were evaluated after 5 weeks (45Gy) for response. The complete response rate after 5 weeks in operable patients was 73%. Complete responders continued chemoradiotherapy for 3 additional weeks. Partial responders (23%) and non-responders at 5 weeks went on to have surgery. Inoperable patients were all to receive the entire 8 weeks of chemoradiotherapy. Response rate for the inoperable patients has not been reported. Toxicity was high with grade 3 and grade 4 mucositis occurring in 73% of patients. In a follow-up study with reduced dose paclitaxel (40 mg/m^2/week) response rate remained high but with reduced grade 3 and 4 toxicities.[53]

Over the past 15 years, Vokes et al have conducted multiple sequential Phase II studies, adding to or subtracting from an intensified chemoradiotherapy regimen consisting of 5-flourouracil, hydroxyurea, and radiotherapy given concomitantly on a week and week off schedule (FHX).[20,35] 5-FU and hydroxyurea have single agent activity in head and neck cancer, both agents are potent radiopotentiators, and hydroxyurea acts as a modulator of 5-FU activity.[54] In the initial Phase I-II study 5-FU was administered at 800 mg/m^2/day as a 5 day continuous infusion, hydroxyurea 1000 mg administered orally every 12 hours for 11 doses and concomitant radiotherapy 180 to 200 cGy single fraction per day was given for 5 consecutive days followed by a 9 day rest period (FHX). Patients with no prior radiation received 7 cycles of weekly chemoradiotherapy completed in a 14 week period.[55,56] This schedule, similar to that of Taylor[41],produced response rates greater than 90% in poor prognosis patients, some of which had received prior radiation. Loco-regional recurrence was uncommon, 1 out of 17, in patients who had not received prior local therapy.

Efforts have been made to improve loco-regional and systemic control with the addition of neo-adjuvant chemotherapy (cisplatin, 5-FU, leucovorin, and interferon), concurrent systemic agents, cisplatin (C-FHX) and paclitaxel (T-FHX) and hyperfractionated radiotherapy.[30,57,52] With the addition of intensive induction chemotherapy consisting of cisplatin, 5FU and leucovorin (PFL) followed by 6-8 cycles of FHX, overall survival at 5 years was 62% and progression-free survival was 68%. During induction, grade 3 and 4 mucositis was 57%, leucopenia 65%, and 5 deaths were secondary to toxicity. Grade 3 and 4 mucositis from FHX was 81%.[30] Despite the high response and overall survival rate, the induction regimen was felt too toxic and prolonged.

In the next Phase II study, induction chemotherapy was omitted and cisplatin 100 mg/m^2 was added to the first, third, and fifth cycles of FHX (C-FHX). [57] Radiation was given twice daily at 1.5 Gy/fraction on days 1 through 5 to reduce the number of cycles from 7 to 5 given over 10 weeks. 5-FU and hydroxyurea doses were the same as in the original FHX study. All patients received G-CSF during the off weeks. With 93% Stage IV disease and 75% N2 or N3, 3 year progression-free survival, loco-regional control, and systemic control were 72%, 92%, and 83% respectively. Overall survival was 55%. Toxicity was once again significant with 57% grade 3 and 4 mucositis, 39% grade 4 neutropenia, and 53% grade 4 thrombocytopenia.

In an attempt to maintain the high response rate and overall survival, but decrease toxicity, the next series of studies replaced cisplatin with paclitaxel. Paclitaxel, 100mg/m^2 ,was administered as a 120 hour continuous infusion with each cycle of FHX (5-FU 600 mg/m^2/day over 120 hours, HU 500 mg every 12 hours for 11 doses, radiation 1.5 Gy BID days 1-5 of each cycle for 5 cycles.[52] Because of anticipated myelosuppression from prolonged paclitaxel infusion, G-CSF was administered between cycles. Results were similar to C-FHX with 3 year progression-free survival, loco-regional control, systemic control, and overall survival of 63%, 86%, 79%, and 60% respectively. Grade 3 and 4 mucositis (84%) remained high and grade 3 and 4 leucopenia was 34% despite the use of G-CSF. A follow-up study replacing continuous infusion paclitaxel with a one hour infusion on day 1 of each cycle eased administration of the regimen with similar response rate, survival rate, and non-hematologic toxicity. Leucopenia was also similar but without the routine use of G-CSF reflecting the decreased myelosuppression of short infusion of paclitaxel when compared to prolonged infusion. [58]

Common to all of the intensified chemoradiotherapy studies, as well as a recently reported study by Adelstein using hyperfractionated radiotherapy and two cycles of concurrent chemotherapy (5-flourouracil, 1000 mg/m^{2}day and cisplatin 20 mg/m^2/day as 96 hour continuous infusions during weeks 1 and 4 of radiotherapy) have been high loco-regional complete response rates and control rates, but paradoxically, distant disease as the most common site of relapse.[59] This has once again prompted interest in the use of neoadjuvant chemotherapy prior to definitive chemoradiotherapy. To be effective, induction chemotherapy in advanced head and neck cancer should have a high complete response rate, but with tolerable toxicity so that patients can tolerate further definitive intensified chemoradiotherapy. Posner and Colevas, in a series of Phase II studies have combined docetaxel, cisplatin, 5-FU with and without leucovorin as induction chemotherapy with response rates between 93% and 100%, and complete response rates between 40% and 61%.[27] Both complete response and toxicity was greater with the addition of leucovorin. The authors believe that the addition of docetaxel improves the response rate of cisplatin and 5-FU alone without significantly adding to toxicity. A phase III trial comparing induction chemotherapy with three cycles of docetaxel, cisplatin, 5-FU versus cisplatin and 5-FU, followed by radiotherapy with concurrent weekly carboplatin is currently underway and open to patients with unresectable and resectable stage III and IV disease. Induction chemotherapy and its role in organ preservation is addressed in chapter 9.

The phase II studies have not yet defined a clear candidate to be studied in a randomized phase III study versus concurrent high dose cisplatin and radiotherapy as used in the Head and Neck Intergroup study. In a randomized phase II study, RTOG 9703, three multi-agent intensified chemoradiotherapy regimens were compared.[60,61] All arms included single daily fraction radiotherapy to a total dose of 70Gy. Patients in arm 1 received cisplatin 10 mg/m^2 and 5-FU 400 mg/m^2 daily for the last 10 days of therapy (XCF), patients in arm 2 were given chemoradiotherapy on alternate weeks with hydroxyurea 1 gram BID and 120 hour continuous infusion of 5-FU 800 mg/m^2/day (FHX), and in arm 3 patients received weekly cisplatin 20 mg/m^2 and paclitaxel 30 mg/m^2 during radiotherapy (XCT). Toxicities and 1 and 2 year survival rates were similar for all three regimens. What is interesting to note is that all three arms appear to have superior survival rates when compared to historical controls in the RTOG head and neck database who had received radiation alone or concomitant high dose cisplatin and radiotherapy.

Management of the Neck Following Chemoradiotherapy

Multiple studies of chemoradiotherapy in advance head and neck cancer have shown a higher complete response rate at the primary site as opposed to metastatic cervical lymph nodes. Response in the cervical lymph nodes is difficult to assess radiographically due to treatment related edema. When treatment includes planned neck dissection following definitive radiotherapy or chemoradiotherapy residual tumor has been found in approximately one third of the surgical specimens.[52,55,56,57,58,59,62] The risk of residual disease correlates to initial nodal stage N1-N3.[62,63] Current recommendations range from planned post-treatment neck dissection for all patients with pre-treatment N2 or N3 disease to neck dissection only in patients with radiographic or clinical evidence of residual disease. There is no question that post-treatment neck dissection adds morbidity to definitive chemoradiotherapy however this must be weighed against the potential long-term benefit in patients found to have occult residual disease. [64]

Management and Prevention of Toxicity

It is clear that the newer intensified chemoradiotherapy schedules are associated with increased toxicity. Grade 3 and 4 mucositis and dermatitis are common and dose limiting. As mentioned previously, building in breaks in treatment schedule such as split course, week on/week off, and rapidly alternating chemotherapy and radiotherapy have made toxicities manageable although still severe. Aggressive supportive care, including access to IV fluids, aggressive nutritional support, often via gastrostomy tube, and fastidious oral and skin care must be available to patients treated on intensive chemoradiotherapy protocols.

Cytoprotective agents have been studied to prevent mucosal toxicity during intensive chemoradiotherapy. An optimal cytoprotective agent is selectively taken up by normal tissue and not tumor so as to not interfere with cytotoxicity. Amifostine is a thiol-containing compound, which accumulates in many epithelial tissues with highest concentration in the salivary glands and kidneys, and acts as a scavenger of radiation and chemotherapy induced free-radicals.[65,66] Multiple small studies of amifostine administration prior to daily radiation have demonstrated a decrease in mucositis and xerostomia.[67,68] A large prospective randomized Phase III trial has now been reported comparing curative radiotherapy with or without daily amifostine (200 mg/m^2 IV) 15 minutes prior to daily radiation fraction.[69] There was a significant reduction in acute and chronic xerostomia without compromise of anti-tumor efficacy in the amifostine arm. Mucositis, however, was not significantly reduced. It is possible that higher and more toxic daily doses of amifostine may be necessary to reduce mucositis. Toxicity of high dose amifostine includes nausea, vomiting, and hypotension.

Pilocarpine, a stimulant of salivary glands via muscarinic receptors, has been approved for treatment of post-radiation induced xerostomia.[70,71] A Phase III study looking at concomitant oral pilocarpine and curative radiation therapy revealed a significant decrease in xerostomia in the concomitant arm, but once again, no difference in the reported incidence or severity of mucositits. Sweating was the most frequent toxicity reported with pilocarpine.[72] Given the relative lack of toxicity, it is reasonable to routinely offer pilocarpine to most patients undergoing radiation therapy for advanced head and neck cancer.

Future Considerations

Despite the progress made in the treatment of locally advanced unresectable head and neck cancer, the 5-year mortality rate remains high. Further reduction in mortality will hopefully be achieved with continued integration of newer agents with standard therapy. Newer conventional chemotherapy agents such a gemcitabine, a potent radiosensitizer with single agent activity in head and neck cancer has been used in Phase I studies combined with radiation, but hampered by excessive mucosal toxicity.[73] The use of high dose intra-arterial chemotherapy (cisplatin $150mg/m^2$) and concurrent hyperfractionated radiotherapy in phase I/II studies by Regine et al appears promising with high complete response rates and favorable toxicity profile. [74] These results will need to be verified in phase III studies comparing high-dose intra-arterial chemotherapy with similar regimens delivered by conventional systemic route.

The frequent observation of p53 gene deletion or mutation in head and neck cancer has prompted the development of gene therapy. Mutation of the p53 tumor suppressor gene has been associated with field cancerization, resistance to induction chemotherapy, increased risk for advanced disease, and poor prognosis. [75,76,77,78] Mutation of the p53 gene is higher among patients exposed to tobacco or alcohol than among patients without exposure.

Phase I and II studies of intratumoral injection of wild type p53 gene on a replication deficient adenoviral vector (AD5CMV-p53) have proved safe and demonstrated successful transduction of p53 gene into tumor cells, with tumor responses from p53 induced apoptosis or inhibition of angiogenesis.[79,80] Alternatively ONYX-015, an EIB 55kd gene deleted adenovirus that replicates in and destroys cancer cells lacking p53 function has induced responses in approximately one third of refractory head and neck cancer patients treated with 5 days of intratumoral injection in Phase I and Phase II studies.[81] Studies combining ONYX-015 with standard chemotherapy have been completed and are underway with AD5CMV-p53 and both agents are being considered for combination with potentially curative radiation therapy in advanced head and neck cancer.[82,83]

The epidermal growth factor receptor (EGFR), a transcellular membrane glycoprotein, and its ligand, transforming growth factor alpha is known to be over expressed in numerous epithelial malignancies including

85% of head and neck cancers and is felt to be responsible for increased cellular proliferation, decreased apoptosis, increased angiogenesis, and increased metastases. EGFR is currently being exploited as a therapeutic target for numerous newly developed agents.[84,85] Strategies for targeting EGFR include mono-clonal antibodies such as C225 (Cetuximab; Inclone Systems, Inc., New York, NY) which binds with high affinity to the extra-cellular membrane component of EGFR or small molecules such as ZD1839 (Iressa; Astra Zeneca, Wilmington, DE), which selectively inhibits intra-cellular EGFR–tyrosine kinase.[86] Both agents, in pre-clinical, and Phase I studies have shown activity against recurrent or refractory head and neck cancer. [87,88] In a Phase I study, Robert demonstrated the feasibility of combining C225 with radiation therapy in locally advanced unresectable head and neck cancer.[89] The treatment was well tolerated with the most common grade 3 toxicities, mucositis and odynophagia, similar to that seen in chemoradiotherapy or radiotherapy alone. Grade 3 skin toxicity, consisting of an acneiform rash, occurred in 6 of 15 patients and was most likely related to C225, possibly relating to the high concentration of EGFR residing normally in the skin. Surprisingly, 13 of 15 patients achieved a complete response. The actuarial 1 and 2 year disease-free survival rates were 73% and 75% respectively and median survival has not been reached. Although a small Phase I trial, the response and actuarial survival rates compare favorably to standard therapy and a multi-institutional Phase III study is currently underway comparing C225 combined with radiotherapy versus radiotherapy alone. Unfortunately, there is no chemoradiotherapy arm in the ongoing Phase III study. Ultimately, C225 will need to be shown to be superior to or less toxic than, chemoradiotherapy before being incorporated into standard therapy. Given the potential of the EGFR inhibitors in head and neck cancer, trials combining C225, ZD1839 or similar agents with standard chemotherapy and radiation therapy will undoubtedly be pursued in the near future.

CONCLUSION

There has been considerable progress in the treatment of locally advanced, unresectable head and neck cancer in the last 2 decades. Concurrent chemoradiotherapy has been proven superior to radiotherapy alone with 5 year survival rates of greater than 50% in some of the investigational intensified chemoradiotherapy programs. At this time the combination of high dose cisplatin and standard fractionated radiotherapy should be considered the community standard based on the results of the Head and Neck Intergroup Study which proved superior survival when compared to radiation therapy alone or split course multi-agent chemoradiotherapy and proved the feasibility of safely administering the regimen in the community setting. However, whenever possible, referral to institutions experienced in the treatment and care of patients receiving intensified chemoradiotherapy and enrollment in appropriate clinical trials should be encouraged.

REFERENCES

1.   Vokes E.E., Werchselbaum R.R., Lippman S.M., Hong W.K. Head and neck cancer. N Engl J Med 1993; 328: 184-194
2.   Al-Sarraf M., Le Blanc M., Giri P.G., et al. Chemoradiotherapy versus radiotherapy in patients with advanced nasopharyngeal cancer: phase III randomized Intergroup study 0099. J Clin Oncol 1998; 16: 1320-1317
3.   Department of Veterans Affairs Laryngeal Cancer Study Group: Induction chemotherapy plus radiation compared with surgery plus radiation in patients with advanced laryngeal cancer. N Engl J Med 1991; 324: 1685-1690
4.   Lefevre J.L., Chevalier D., Luboinski B., et al. Larynx preservation in pyriform sinus cancer: preliminary results of a European organization research and treatment of cancer phase III trial. J Natl Cancer Inst 1996; 88: 890-899
5.   Forastiere A., Goepfert H., Goffinet D., et al. NCCN practice guidelines for head and neck cancer. National Comprehensive Cancer Network. Oncology 1998; 12: 39-147
6.   Fu K.K., Phillips T.L., Silverberg I.J., et al. Combined radiotherapy and chemotherapy with bleomycin and methotrexate for advanced inoperable head and neck cancer: update of a northern California oncology group randomized trial. J Clin Oncol 1987; 5(9): 1410-1414
7.   Aisner J., Jacobs M., Sinabladi V., et al. Chemoradiotherapy for the treatment of regionally advanced head and neck cancers. Seminars in Oncology 1994; 21(5) Suppl 12: 35-44
8.   List M.A., Siston A., Haraf D., et al. Quality of life and performance in advanced head and neck cancer patients on concomtant chemoradiotherapy: a prospective examination. J Clin Oncol 1999; 17: 1020-1028
9.   Browman G.P., Hodson D.I., Mackenzie, R.G., et al. Concomitant chemotherapy and radiotherapy in squamous cell head and neck cancer (excluding nasopharynx). Head Neck 2001 (in press)
10.   Lo T.C., Wiley A.L. Jr., Ansfield F.J., et al. Combined radiation therapy and 5-flourouracil for advanced squamous cell carcinoma of the oral cavity and oropharynx: a randomized study. Am J Roentgenol 1976; 126: 229-235
11.   Shanta V., Krishnamurthi S. Combined bleomycin and radiotherapy in oral cancer. Clin Radio 1980; 31: 617-620
12.   Forastiere A.A. Overview of platinum chemotherapy in head and neck cancer. Seminars in Oncology 1994; 21(5) Supp 12: 20-27
13.   Al-Sarraf M. Cisplatin combinations in the treatment of head and neck cancer. Seminars in Oncology 1994; 21(5) Suppl 12: 28-34
14.   Adelstein D.J. Induction chemotherapy in head and neck cancer. Hematology/Oncology Clinics North America 1999; (13)4: 689-698
15.   Fu K.K. Combined-modality therapy for head and neck cancer. Oncology 1997; 11(12): 1781-1800
16.   Brockstein B.E., Vokes, E. E. Chemoradiotherapy for head and neck cancer. PPO Updates/Principles and Practice of Oncology. 1996; 10(9): 1-19
17.   Forastiere A. A., Trotti A. Radiotherapy and concurrent chemotherapy: a strategy that improves locoregional control and survival in oropharyngeal cancer. J Natl Cancer Inst 1999; 91(24): 2065-2066

18. Munro A.J. An overview of randomized trials of adjuvant chemotherapy in head and neck cancer. Br J Cancer 1995; 71: 83-91

19. El-Sayed S., Nelson N. Adjuvant and adjunctive chemotherapy in the management of squamous cell carcinoma of the head and neck region: a meta-analysis of prospective and randomized trials. J Clin Oncol 1996; 14(3): 838-847

20. Pignon J.P., Bourhis J., Domenge C., Designé L. Chemotherapy added to locoregional treatment for head and neck squamous cell carcinoma: three meta-analyses of updated individual data. Lancet 2000; 355: 949-955

21. Bourhis J., Pignon J.P. Meta-analyses in head and neck squamous cell carcinoma: what is the role of chemotherapy? Hematology/Oncology Clinics of North America 1999; 13(41): 769-775

22. Head and Neck Contracts Program. Adjuvant chemotherapy for advanced head and neck squamous carcinoma: final report of the head and neck contracts program. Cancer 1987; 60(3): 301-311

23. Laramore G.E., Scott C.B., Al-Sarraf M., et al. Adjuvant chemotherapy for resectable squamous cell carcinomas of the head and neck: report on Intergroup study 0034. Int Radiat Oncol Biol Phys 1992; 23: 705-713

24. Al-Sarraf M., Pajak T., Laramure G., et al. Radiotherapy versus chemotherapy followed by RT in resected and negative margins head and neck cancers. Intergroup study 0034: final analysis. Pro Am Soc Clin Oncol 1997; 16: 392a (abstr 1399)

25. Bachaud J.M., Cohen-Jonathan E., Alzieu C., et al. Combined post-operative radiotherapy and weekly cisplatin infusion for locally advanced head and neck carcinoma: final report of a randomized trial. Int J Radiat Oncol Biol Phys 1996; 36: 999-1004

26. Al-Sarraf M., Pajak T.F., Byhardt R.W., et al. Postoperative radiotherapy with concurrent cisplatin appears to improve locoregional control of advanced, respectable head and neck cancers: TROG 88-24. Int J Radiat Oncol Biol Phys 1997; 37(4): 777-782

27. Posner M.R., Colevas A.D., Tishler R.B. The role of induction chemotherapy in the curative treament of squamous cell caner of the head and neck. Seminars in Oncology 2000; 27(4) Suppl 8: 13-24

28. Forastiere A.A., Berlsey B., Maor M., et al. Phase III trial to preserve larynx: induction chemotherapy and radiotherapy versus concomitant chemoradiotherapy versus radiotherapy alone, intergroup trial R91-11. Proc Am Soc Clin Oncol 2001; 20: 2a (abstr 4)

29. Paccagnella A., Orlando A., Marchiori C., et al. Phase III trial of initial chemotherapy in stage III or IV head and neck cancers: a study by the Gruppo di Studio sui Tumori della Testa e del Collo. J Natl Cancer Inst 1994; 86(4): 265-272

30. Kies M.S., Haraf D.J., Athanasiadis I., et al. Induction chemotherapy followed by concurrent chemoradiation for advanced head and neck cancer: improved disease control and survival. J Clin Oncol 1998; 16: 2715-2721

31. Browman G.P. Evidence-based recommendation against neoadjuvant chemotherapy for routine management of patients with squamous cell head and neck cancer. Cancer Invest 1994; 12(6): 662-670

32. Harari P.M. Why had induction chemotherapy for advanced head and neck cancer become a United States community standard of practice? J Clin Oncol 1997; 15(5): 2050-2055

33. Harari P.M., Cleary J.F., Hartig G.K. Evolving patterns of practice regarding the use of chemoradiation for advanced head and neck cancer patients. Proc Am Soc Clin Oncol 2001; 20: 226a (abstr 903)

34.   Fu K.K., Pajak T.F., Trotti A., et al. A radiation therapy oncology group phase III randomized study to compare hyperfractionation and two variants of accelerated fractionation radiotherapy for head and neck squamous cell carcinomas: preliminary results of RTOG 9003. Int J Radiat Oncol Biol Phys 1999; 45 (Suppl): 145 (abstr 1)

35.   Vokes E.E., Haraf D.J., Kies M.S. The use of concurrent chemotherapy and radiotherapy for locoregionally advanced head and neck cancer. Seminars in Oncology 2000; 27(4) Suppl 8: 34-38

36.   Vokes E.E. Interactions of chemotherapy and radiation. Seminars in Oncology 1993; 20(1): 70-79

37.   Haffty B.G. Concurrent chemoradiation in the treatment of head and neck cancer. Hematology/Oncology Clinics of North America 1999; 13(4): 719-742

38.   Haffty B.G., Son Y.H., Rose P., et al. Chemotherapy as and adjunct to radiation in the treatment of squamous cell carcinoma of the head and neck: results of the Yale mitimycin randomized trials. J Clin Oncol 1997; 15(1): 268-276

39.   Browman G.P., Cripps C., Hodson D.J., et al. Placebo-controlled randomized trial of infusional flourouracil during standard radiotherapy in locally advanced head and neck cancer. J Clin Oncol 1994; 12(12): 2648-2653

40.   Gupta N.K., Pointon R.C.S., Wilkinson P.M. A randomized clinical trial to contrast radiotherapy with radiotherapy and methotrexate given synchronously in head and neck cancer. Clin Radiol 1987; 38: 575-581

41.   Taylor   S.G., Murthy A.K., Vannetzel J.M., et al. Randomized comparison of neoadjuvant cisplatin and fluorouracil infusion followed by radiation versus concomitant treatment in advanced head and neck cancer. J Clin Oncol 1994: 12(2):385-395

42.   Merlano M., Benasso M., Corvó R., et al. Five year update of a randomized trial of alternating radiotherapy and chemotherapy compared with radiotherapy alone in treatment of unresectable squamous cell carcinoma of the head and neck. J Natl Cancer Inst 1996; 88(19): 583-589

43.   Calais G., Alfonsi M., Bardet E., et al. Randomized trial of radiation therapy versus concomitant chemotherapy and radiation therapy for advanced-stage oropharynx carcinoma. J Natl Cancer Inst 1999; 91(24): 2081-2086

44.   Adelstein D.J., Adams G.L., Ly Y., et al. A phase III comparison of standard radiation therapy (RT) versus RT plus concurrent cisplatin (Ddp) versus split-course RT plus concurrent Ddp and 5-Flourouracil in patients with unresectable squamous cell head and neck cancer: an intergroup study. Proc Am Clin Oncol 2000; 19: (abstr 1624)

45.   Weissler M.L., Melin S., Sailer S.L., et al. Simultaneous chemoradiation in the treatment of advanced head and neck cancer. Arch Otolaryngol Head Neck Surg 1992; 118: 806-810

46.   Brizel D.M., Albers M.E., Fisher S.R., et al. Hyperfractionated irradiation with or without concurrent chemotherapy for locally advanced head and neck cancer. N Engl J Med 1998; 338(25): 1798-1804

47.   Wendt T. G., Grabenbauer G.G., Rödel C.M., et al. Simultaneous radiochemotherapy versus radiotherapy alone in advanced head and neck cancer: a randomized multicenter study. J Clin Oncol 1998; 16(4): 1318-1324

48.   Jeremic B., Shibamoto Y., Milici B., et al. Hyperfractionated radiation therapy with or without concurrent low-dose daily cisplatin in locally advanced squamous cell carcinoma of the head and neck: a prospective randomized trial. J Clin Oncol 2000; 18(7): 1458-1464

49.   Vokes E.E., Haraf D.J., Stenson K., et al. The role of paclitaxel in the treatment of head and neck cancer. Seminars in Oncology 1995; 22(5) Suppl 12: 8-12

50.   Chougule P., Wanebo M., Akerley W., et al. Concurrent paclitaxel, carboplatin, and radiotherapy in advanced head and neck cancers: a phase II study – preliminary results. Seminars Oncol 1997; 24(6) Suppl 19: 57-61

51. Conley B., Jacobs M., Suntharalingam M., et al. A pilot trial of paclitaxel, carboplatin, and concurrent radiotherapy for unresectable squamous cell carcinoma of the head and neck. Seminars Oncol 1997; 24(11) Suppl 2: 78-80

52. Kies M., Haraf D.J., Rosen F., et al. Concomitant infusional paclitaxel and flourouracil, oral hydroxyurea , and Hyperfractionated radiation for locally advanced squamous head and neck cancer. J Clin Oncol 2001; 19(7): 1961-1969

53. Wanebo H.J., Chougule P., Ready N., et al. Pre-operative therapy with reduced dose paclitaxel, and carboplatin and radiation achieves a similar complete response rate to a high dose regimen, but with reduced toxicity. Proc Am Soc Clin Oncol 2000; 19: (Abstr 1655)

54. Grem J.L. "Flourinated Pyrimidines." In Cancer Chemotherapy Principles and Practice, B.A. Chabner and J.M. Collins, eds. Philadelphia, PA: JB Lippincott, 1990

55. Haraf D.J., Vokes E.E., Panje W.R., Weichselbaum R.R. Survival and analysis of failure following hydroxyurea, 5-Flourouracil and concomitant radiation therapy in poor prognosis head and neck cancer. Am J Clin Oncol 1991; 14: 419-422

56. Vokes E.E., Panje W.R., Schilsky R.L., et al. Hydoxyurea, flourouracil, and concomitant radiotherapy in poor prognosis head and neck cancer: a phase I-II study. J Clin Oncol 1989; 7: 761-768

57. Vokes E.E., Kies M.S., Haraf D.J., et al. Concomitant chemoradiotherapy as primary therapy for locoregionally advanced head and neck cancer. J Clin Oncol 2000; 18(8): 1652-1661

58. Rosen F.R., Haraf D., Brackstein B., et al. Multicenter randomized phase III study of 1 hour infusion paclixel, flourouracil and hydroxyurea with concomitant Hyperfractionated radiotherapy with or without erythropoietin for advanced head and neck cancer. Proc Am Soc Clin Oncol 2001; 20: 226a (abstr 902)

59. Adelstein D.J., Saxton J.P., Lavertu P., et al. Maximizing local control and organ preservation in advanced squamous head and neck cancer with Hyperfractionated radiation and concurrent chemotherapy. Proc Am Soc Clin Oncol 2001; 20:224a (abstr 893)

60. Garden A.S., Pajak T.F., Vokes E., et al. Preliminary results of TROG 9703 – a phase II randomized trial of concurrent radiation and chemotherapy for advanced squamous cell carcinomas of the head and neck. Proc Am Soc Clin Oncol 2001; 20: 223a (abstr 891)

61. Garden A.S., Glisson B.S., Ang K.K., et al. Phase I/II trial of radiation with chemotherapy "boost" for advanced squamous cell carcinomas of the head and neck: toxicities and responses. J Clin Oncol 1999; 17(8): 2390-2395

62. Boyd T.S., Jarari P.M., Tannehill S.P., et al. Planned post radiotherapy neck dissection in patients with advanced head and neck cancer. Head Neck 1998; 20(2): 132-137

63. Sanguineti G., Corvo R., Benasso M., et al. Management of the neck after alternating chemoradiotherapy for advanced head and neck. Head Neck 1999; 21(3): 223-228

64. Naravan K., Crane C.H., Kleid S., Hughes P.G., Peters L.J. Planned neck dissection as an adjunct to the management of patients with advanced neck disease treated with definitive radiotherapy: for some or for all? Head Neck 1999; 21(7): 606-613

65. Yuhas J.M., Spellman J.M., Culo F. The role of WR-2721 in radiotherapy and/or chemotherapy. Cancer Clin Trials 1980; 3: 211-216

66. Utley J.F., Marlowe C., Waddell W.J. Distribution of 355 – labeled WR-2721 in normal and malignant tissues of the mouse. Radiat Res 1976; 68: 284-291

67. Buntzel J., Kuttner K., Frohlich D., et al. Selective cytoprotection with amifostine in concurrent radiochemotherapy for head and neck cancer. Ann Oncol 1998; 9: 505-509

68.   Rosen F.R., Chung T.D., Portugal L., et al. Amifostine, concomitant cisplatin, paclitaxel and re-irradiation in recurrent head and neck cancer. Proc Am Soc Clin Oncol 2000; 19: 427a (abstr 1686)

69.   Brizel D. M., Wasserman T.H., Henke M., et al. Phase III randomized trial of amifostine as a radioprotector in head and neck cancer. J Clin Oncol 2000; 18(19): 3339-3345

70.   Johnson J.T., Ferretti G.A., Nethery W.J., et al. Oral pilocarpine for post-irradiation xerostomia in patients with head and neck cancer. N Engl J Med 1993; 329(6): 390-395

71.   LeVeque F.G., Montgomery M., Potton D., et al. A multicenter, randomized, double-blind, placebo-controlled, dose-titration study of oral pilocarpine for treatment of radiation-induced xerostomia in head and neck cancer patients. J Clin Oncol 1993; 11(6): 1124-1131

72.   Scarantino C.W., Le Vegue F.G., Scott C.B., et al. A phase III study of concomitant oral pilocarpine to reduce hypo-salivation and mucositis associated with curative radiation therapy in head and neck cancer patients. RTOG 9709. Am Soc Clin Oncol 2001; 20:225a (abstr 897)

73.   Eisbruch A., Shewach D., Urba S., et al. Phase I trial of radiation concurrent with low dose gemcitabine for head and neck cancer: high mucosal and pharyngeal toxicity. Pro Am Soc Clin Oncol 1997; 16: 386a (abstr 1377)

74.   Regine W.F., Valentino J., Arnold S.M., et al. High-dose intra-arterial cisplatin boost with Hyperfractionated radiation therapy for advanced squamous cell carcinoma of the head and neck. J Clin Oncol 2001; 19(14): 3333-3339

75.   Bradford C. Predictive factors in head and neck cancer. Hematology Oncology Clinics of North America 1999; 13(4): 777-785

76   . Brennan J.A., Mao L., Hruban R.H., et al. Molecular assessment of histopathologic staging. N Engl J Med 1995

77.   Koch W. Biomarker predictors of response to chemoradiation therapy for head and neck squamous cell carcinoma. American Society of Clinical Oncology Educational Book: 36th Annual Meeting, Spring 2000, Michael C. Perry, ed.

78.   Teman S., Flahault A., Périé S., et al. p53 gene status as a predictor of tumor response to induction chemotherapy of patients with locoregionally advanced squamous cell carcinomas of the head and neck. J Clin Oncol 2000; 18(27): 385-399

79.   Clayman G.L., el-Naggar A.K., Lippman S.M., et al. Adenovirus-mediated p53 gene transfer in patients with advanced recurrent head and neck squamous cell carcinoma. J Clin Oncol 1998; 16: 2221-2232

80.   Goodwin W.J., Esser D., Clayman G., et al. Randomized phase II study of intratumoral injection of two dosing schedules using a replication-deficient adenovirus carrying the p53 gene (ADSCMV-p53) in patients with recurrent/refractory head and neck cancer. Proc Am Soc Clin Oncol 1999; 18: 445a (abstr 1717)

81.   Kirn D.H., Khuri F., Ganly I., et al. A phase II trial of ONYX-015, a selectively replicating adenovirus, in combination with cisplatin and 5-flourouracil in patients with recurrent head and neck cancer. Proc Am Soc Clin Oncol 1999; 18: 389a (abstr 1505)

82.   Khuri F.R., Nemunatis J., Ganly I., et al. A controlled trial of intratumoral ONYX-015, a selectively-replicating adenovirus, in combination with cisplatin and 5-fluorouracil in patients with recurrent head and neck cancer. Nature Medicine 2000; 6(8): 879-885

83.   Clayman G.L. The current status of gene therapy. Seminars in Oncology 2000; 27(4) Suppl 8: 39-43

84.   Grandis J.R., Melhern M.F., Gooding W.E., et al. Levels of TGF-alpha and EGFR protein in head and neck squamous cell carcinoma and patient survival. J Natl Cancer Inst 1998; 90: 824-832

85.   Mendelsohn J. Epidermal growth factor receptor inhibition by monoclonal antibody as anticancer therapy. Clin Cancer Res 1997; 3: 2703-2707

86.   Baselga J. New therapeutic agents targeting the epidermal growth factor receptor. J Clin Oncol 2000; 18(21s): 54s-59s

87.   Baselga J., Herbst R., La Russo P., et al. Continuous administration of ZD1839 (Iressa), a novel oral epidermal growth factor receptor tyrosine kinase inhibitor in patients with five selected tumor types: evidence of activity and good tolerability. Pro Am Soc Clin Oncol 2000; 19: 177a (abstr 686)

88.   Baselga J., Pfister D., Cooper M.R., et al. Phase I studies of anti-epidermal growth factor receptor chimeric antibody C225 alone and in combination with cisplatin. J Clin Oncol 2000; 18: 904-914

89.   Robert F., Ezekiel M., Spencer S., et al. Phase I study of anti-epidermal growth factor receptor antibody cetuximab in combination with radiation therapy in patients with advanced head and neck caner. J Clin Oncol 2001; 19(13): 3234-3243

Chapter 11

NASOPHARYNGEAL CANCER

Anthony TC Chan M.D., Peter ML Teo M.D.and Philip J Johnson M.D.
Chinese University of Hong Kong, HKSAR, China

Nasopharyngeal carcinoma is a major public health problem throughout southern China where it is the third commonest form of malignancy amongst men. Although much less common in the West, several features, including a consistent association with a virus (Epstein Barr Virus), a practical serological marker, and sensitivity to treatment such that cure is common even in patients with advanced disease, make this a model tumor of wide interest to workers in many fields of oncology.

EPIDEMIOLOGY

Nasopharyngeal carcinoma (NPC) occurs sporadically in the West where it is associated with the classical risk factors for other head and neck cancers, namely excessive alcohol consumption and tobacco smoking. In parts of Asia, in particular southern China, NPC is endemic with incidence rates of 15-50/100,000. There is an intermediate incidence in populations in the Mediterranean basin, and in Alaskan Eskimos. The median age at presentation is 40 - 50 years, a range that is significantly younger than that of other head and neck cancers. The incidence rises after the age of 20 and decreases after 60 years. The male-female ratio is around 3:1 [1].

ETIOLOGY

The striking geographical variation in incidence suggests a unique interaction of environmental and genetic factors. Consistent with other neoplasms it now appears that there is a recognizable stepwise progression of histological features that reflect underlying genetic events [Figure 1].

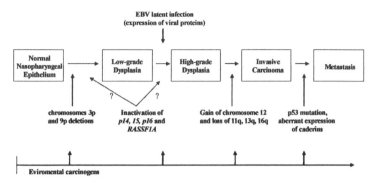

Figure 1. **Proposed tumorigenesis model for nasopharyngeal carcinoma (personal communication KW Lo ad DP Huong)**

Patches of dysplasia are the earliest recognizable lesions, presumably related to some environmental carcinogen. These are associated with allelic losses on the short arms of chromosomes 3 and 9 that result in inactivation of several tumor suppressor genes, particularly p14, p15 and p16 [2-5]. The relevant carcinogens have not been established but a link between the consumption of Chinese salted fish and other salted food items with the development of NPC has been suggested [1]. These dysplastic areas are the origin of the tumor but are probably insufficient in themselves to lead to further progression. At this stage latent EBV infection becomes critical and leads to the development of severe dysplasia. Gains of genes on chromosome 12 and allelic loss on 11q, 13q and 16q lead to invasive carcinoma; metastasis is associated with mutation of p53 and aberrant expression of cadherins. [6,7]

PATHOLOGY

Nasopharyngeal carcinomas are epithelia neoplasms. Three histopathological types are recognized in the WHO classifications [8].

Type I: squamous cell carcinoma (SCC) with varying degrees of differentiation
Type II: non keratinizing carcinoma
Type III: undifferentiated carcinoma

The latter is often referred to as a "lymphoepithelioma" although the term is probably inappropriate, as the lymphocytic infiltration is reactive and not neoplastic. There are similarities in the epidemiological, serological, clinical and natural history features of WHO types II and III and consequently it has been suggested that NPC should be divided into only two categories [9]: SCC and undifferentiated carcinoma of the nasopharyngeal type (UCNT). Most of non-keratinizing carcinomas (WHO type II) would be included under the heading of UCNT.

Prognostic significance of the histopathologic type

The histological types may be of prognostic significance. Some reports suggest that undifferentiated and poorly differentiated non-keratinizing carcinomas have a higher local control rate and a better prognosis than keratinizing squamous cell carcinomas. In line with this suggestion, Marks and others have shown that keratinizing squamous cell carcinomas are more radioresistant [10,11]. Furthermore, while keratinizing squamous NPC (WHO Type I) fails more locally than distantly, the undifferentiated of the poorly differentiated NPC (WHO Types II & III) fail more distantly than locally. The failures of keratinizing squamous NPC mostly occur within the first five years after treatment but the failures of the undifferentiated/poorly differentiated squamous histologies not infrequently occur later than 5 years.

PRESENTATION, IMAGING AND STAGING

The commonest presentation, occurring in half of cases, is with a neck mass that is found on examination to represent a non-tender, unilateral, subdigastric lymph node. Nasal complaints including blood-stained nasal discharge, nasal obstruction, posterior nasal discharge and epistaxis are encountered in almost one third of patients. Aural symptoms, particularly unilateral impairment of hearing of the conductive type, with or without tinnitus, is also a common presenting symptom that is caused by the obstruction of the Eustachian tube by the primary tumor. The obstruction may lead to serious otitis media. Consequently, if symptoms of otitis in an adult do not clear up within two to three weeks of conventional treatment, or if they relapse without an obvious cause, a thorough examination of the nasopharynx including biopsies should be carried out to exclude NPC.

Neurological complaints tend to occur at a later stage of the disease and comprise headache (in 20% of cases at presentation) and cranial nerve syndromes. Horner's syndrome occurs in 3 % of all patients, usually accompanied by paresis of one or more of the last four cranial nerves. The cranial nerves III-VI are affected within the cavernous sinus, the optic nerve by para-sellar involvement, and nerves IX-XII are primarily affected in the parapharyngeal region below the skull base.

Diagnostic work up

Once the diagnosis is suspected on the grounds of the above listed symptoms, histological confirmation of the diagnosis is mandatory. The technique of biopsy under local anesthesia has been found to have a diagnostic sensitivity comparable to that obtained by examination under general anesthesia. The biopsy is facilitated by direct visualization of the nasopharynx with a fiberoptic nasopharyngoscope. However, since the biopsy may cause soft tissue swelling and/or a hematoma, CT and MRI of the nasopharynx and the skull base should be undertaken before the biopsy.

The primary tumor extent should be evaluated by both computed tomography (CT) and magnetic resonance imaging (MRI). MRI is more sensitive than CT for the detection of the primary tumor, its direct soft tissue extent, regional nodal metastasis and perineural extension. Blood vessels are clearly shown by MRI even without the use of intravenous contrast. On the other hand, although MRI can also demonstrate erosion into the base of the skull by virtue of the change in signal of fatty bone marrow, CT is generally considered a better tool for defining bone erosion. The role of PET (positron emission tomography) scanning in NPC remains to be defined although preliminary reports indicate that PET can be useful in detecting both local failures after treatment and distant metastases.

Staging

Prior to 1997, several different stage-classifications were used but that described by Ho was found to be superior to the others in its ability to predict prognosis and treatment outcome [12]. However, the Ho's classification was not ideal as an international system because it comprised five overall stages (instead of the usual practice of four), included only three T-stages, and did not take into account CT-evidence of tumor infiltration of the parapharyngeal region, a factor of considerable prognostic significance [13].

In 1997, therefore, a new UICC/AJCC stage classification was formulated, which incorporated all the major prognostically significant tumor parameters (Table 1). It is noteworthy that tumors infiltrating the parapharyngeal region were associated with a higher rate of both local failure and distant metastasis; such cases were classified as T2b (Table 1). The presence of orbital, infratemporal fossal and hypopharyngeal disease was grouped together with the presence of cranial nerve(s) palsy and intracranial tumor extension as T4. The poor prognosis of supraclavicular nodal metastases was recognized and classified as N3, together with very large nodes (>6cm) (Table 1).

Table 1. **Staging criteria: UICC 1997 System**

Nasopharynx (T)	
T1	Nasopharynx
T2	Soft tissue of oropharynx and/or nasal fossa
T2a	Without parapharyngeal extension
T2b	With parapharyngeal extension
T3	Invades bony structure and/or paranasal sinuses
T4	Intracranial extension, involvement of cranial nerves, infratemporal fossa, hypopharynx, orbit

Regional lymph node (N)	
N1	Unilateral metastasis in lymph node(s), 6cm or less in greatest dimension,
N2	above supraclavicular fossa.
N3	Bilateral metastasis in lymph node(s), 6cm or less in greatest dimension, above supraclavicular fossa. Metastasis in lymph node(s) greater than 6cm in dimension in the supraclavicular fossa

Distant metastasis (M)	
M0	No distant metastasis
M1	Distant metastasis

Stage grouping				
Stage 0	T in situ N0	M0		
Stage I	T1	N0	M0	
Stage IIA	T2a	N0	M0	
Stage IIB	T2b	N0	M0	
	T1, T2a, T2b	N1	M0	
Stage III	T3	N0, N1	M0	
	T1, T2, T3	N2	M0	
Stage IVA	T4	N0, N1, N2	M0	
Stage IVB	Any T	N3	M0	
Stage IVC	Any T	Any N	M1	

Molecular monitoring

The demostration that tumor-derived DNA is detectable in the plasma and serum of cancer patients raised the possibility that non-invasive detection and monitoring of NPC may be feasible by EBV-DNA PCR analysis of plasma and serum samples. Using real-time quantitative PCR, cell-free EBV-DNA was found in the plasma of 96% NPC patients and 7% of controls. Advanced stage NPC patients had higher plasma EBV-DNA levels than tumors with early-stage disease [14]. Further studies have been undertaken demonstrating that EBV-DNA may be a valuable tool for monitoring of NPC patient response during radiotherapy, chemotherapy [15], as well as early detection of tumor recurrence [16]. In a cohort of 139 patients NPC patients treated with a uniform radiotherapy technique and followed up for a median period of 5.55 years, serum circulating EBV-DNA was found to be a significant prognosticator associated with NPC-related death in multiple Cox's regression analysis with a relative risk of 1.6 for each 10-fold increase in serum EBV-DNA concentration [17].

Thus the quantitation of EBV DNA appears to allow improved prognostication of NPC. The sensitivity and specificity also suggests the potential use as a screening test in endemic areas of NPC.

Prognosis

NPC is one of the very few common cancers in which cure can be anticipated even in patients with advanced disease. The prognosis is related to the disease extent as measured by the UICC staging system, the type of histology and, as emphasized by O'Sullivan et al [18] the extent to which patients have access to an experienced treatment team with access to modern oncological therapeutics. It seems likely that in the near future quantitation of EBV DNA, which appears independent of any of the above mentioned factors, will become routine and permit even more accurate prognostication.

RADIOTHERAPY

Up to early 90's, radical radiotherapy for NPC was delivered by 2-dimensional techniques such as the one described by Ho [1]. The conventional practice had been to deliver tumoricidal radiation dose (total 60-70Gy; 2.0-2.5Gy per fraction; 6-7 weeks course duration) to certain anatomical structures in the vicinity of the nasopharynx by 2 lateral opposing fields or multiple fields ($\geq$3) with appropriate shieldings positioned at predetermined distances from certain bony landmarks [1] to protect vital neural organs. The neck was usually separately irradiated by another portal with avoidance of midline structures such as the spinal cord and the larynx [1]. With 2-dimensional planning techniques, the local control rates for NPC were in the order of 80%, taking all T-stages together [13,19]. At the Prince of Wales Hospital, the overall survival figures after radiotherapy using Ho's technique were 85% for Ho's stages I and II and 55% for Ho's stages III and IV [Figure 2] [13].

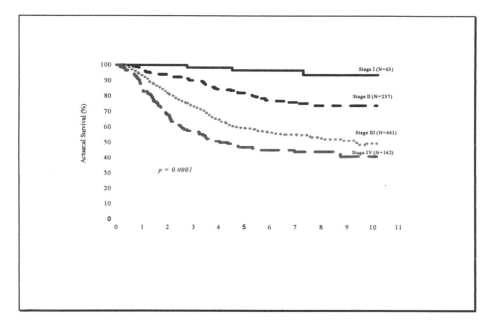

Figure 2. **Treatment results by Ho's Overall Stage [13]**

With advances in technology, the modern radiotherapy for NPC should be that of three-dimensional conformal (3DCRT) or intensity-modulated (IMRT) with inverse radiotherapy planning. Researchers at the University of California-San Francisco [20] have reported superior local control using such techniques when compared to standard 2D methods. Firstly, the success of 3DCRT or IMRT depends on better delineation of the tumor target (gross tumor volume – GTV) by CT and MRI, images of which can be co-registered, such that 'geographical misses' are largely avoided. Secondly, there is clear definition of the vital (mostly neural) organs in the vicinity of the NPC such that these organs are spared a heavy radiation dose, thus minimizing complications.

In general the clinical target volume (CTV) should include the whole GTV and the structures in the vicinity of the tumor, which are at substantial risk of subclinical infiltration. The sphenoid floor, the medial aspect of the greater wings of the sphenoid (and the foramin ovale, rotandum and lacerum), the vomer, the posterior choanae, the pterygoid plates, the pterygopalatine fossa, the posterior wall of the maxillary sinus, the parapharyngeal spaces bilaterally [21] and the prevertebral muscles and fascia are all at risk of tumor infiltration and should be included in the CTV. In T3 that infiltrates the clivus and T4 lesions, the entire clivus should be included in the CTV. However, in T1, T2, and less extensive T3 cases sparing the clivus, there has been no consensus on how much thickness of the clivus, if any at all, should be included in the CTV. Provided that the planning target volume (PTV) is not drawn too near to the brainstem (as described later), we recommend that the cortex of the clivus in juxtaposition to the tumor should be included in the CTV. In some T4 cases, the tumor has grossly infiltrated the inferior (or even the superior) orbital fissure and the whole bony orbit on that side should be included in the CTV. Intracranial extension via the foramen ovale when the tumor infiltrates laterally and superiorly through the pterygoid muscles is frequently associated with trigeminal nerve palsy. In such cases, the whole infratemporal fossal contents and the greater wing of sphenoid on the side of the lesion should be included in addition to the intracranial component of the cancer. Occasionally the tumor may infiltrate submucosally inferiorly to involve the oropharynx or even the hypopharynx. In these situations, the CTV has to be enlarged substantially in the inferior direction.

The PTV should, ideally, include the CTV with a safety margin that adequately caters for systemic and positional (set-up) errors (which can vary from center to center). Usually a 5mm safety margin should be adequate. However, the addition of safety margins in the posterosuperior direction on the CTV is hindered by the proximity of critical neural organs such as the brainstem, the spinal cord, and the optic chiasma. To facilitate maximal dose sparing, we recommend that the PTV be drawn not closer to 5mm of the critical neural organs. In the very advanced cases where the CTV is already within 5mm for the critical neural organs, a phasic reduction in the PTV is required during the course of radiotherapy to avoid severe neurological sequelae.

Although the overall local control rate of NPC (all T-stages together) has been improved from 80% to 90% after using 3DCRT or IMRT, the major benefit is likely to be in the advanced T-stages (T3 and T4). The early T-stages were usually adequately irradiated with 2D-planning methods with little chance of geographical misses [1,19], even though conventional 2D-planning methods such as the Ho's technique [1] has been shown to adequately circumscribe in high radiation dose only the GTV but not the CTV or the PTV (as described above)[20]. Indeed when 2-dimensional external radiotherapy was supplemented by intracavitary brachytherapy, long-term local tumor control as high as 94% was reported for T1 and T2a [22]. For the more advanced T-stages, local failures occurred in one-third to two-thirds of cases after conventional 2-dimensional planning methods [13,19]. These should benefit most from 3DCRT or IMRT in terms of improvement in long-term local control by avoidance of geographical misses. On the other hand, the major benefit of 3DCRT/IMRT in the early T-stages should be reduction of severe late radiation complications such as chronic xerostomia which subtracts significantly from the quality of life of the long-term survivors of the disease.

Altered fractionation

In addition to improved radiotherapy techniques, use of altered fractionation and radiation dose escalation have been reported to improve the local control. Although an RTOG Trial [23] has proved the superiority of both concomitant boost (accelerated hyperfractionated radiotherapy) and hyperfractionation over the conventional daily fractionation (2Gy per fraction, 5 fractions per week) for head and neck cancers in general, the benefit for NPC has not been addressed specifically. Subgroup analysis for NPC was not possible in the RTOG trial due to the small numbers of NPC cases.

Recently, we have reported a significant increase in neurological complications, especially temporal lobe encephalopathy and cranial nerve(s) palsy, after a late-course 'bid' hyper-/accelerated fractionated radiotherapy in a randomized comparison with conventional daily fractionation [24]. The temporal lobe and some other neurological complications arose despite keeping the interfraction time interval to 6 hours or more. These observations have led us to conclude that the sublethal damage repair half-life of the central nervous tissue is likely to be longer than previously thought [24]. Clearly, the routine practice of a 'bid' radiotherapy regimen together with a 2-dimensional planning method should be avoided unless specific measures to avoid irradiation to neural organs are implemented [24]. This precaution is especially relevant to the advanced T-stage NPC, the tumor target of which is often in very close proximity to major neural organs such as the optic chiasma and the brainstem. On the other hand, improved local control by treating 6 fractions per week rather than 5 fractions per week has been recently reported [25]. By keeping most interfraction intervals to 24 hours, the problem of inadequate sublethal damage repair of neurons of the 'bid' technique appears to be avoided.

Meanwhile, a definite relationship between total radiation dose and the local tumor control has been established in early T-stage NPC when the effect of dose escalation by intracavity brachytherapy after 66-70Gy of external beam radiation was studied [22]. However, brachytherapy is unable to deliver a significant dose to bulky parapharyngeal infiltration significant skull base involvement, or intracranial extension, due to the geometrical dose fall-off with distance from the radioactive sources. Thus, the bulky T2b and the T3 and the T4 in general cannot benefit much from this approach.

COMBINED MODALITY TREATMENT FOR LOCOREGIONALLY ADVANCED DISEASE

About 60% of patients present with locoregionally advanced, UICC stages III and IV disease. These cases have significant rates of both local and distant failures after conventional radiotherapy. Since NPC appears to be highly sensitive to chemotherapy as well as radiotherapy, it was logical to incorporate some form of chemotherapy into the primary treatment with a view to improving the outlook of those with locoregionally-advanced disease.

Following encouraging response rates to platinum containing regimens in phase II studies in patients with metastatic disease, the use of neoadjuvant and adjuvant chemotherapy, combined with radiotherapy was investigated in patients with locoregionally advanced disease in four prospective randomized trials (Table 2) [26-29]. None of these trials demonstrated an improvement in overall survival. Although the International NPC study group trial showed a significant improvement in progression free survival (PFS) [28], this was only achieved at the expense of an 8% treatment related mortality. Hence, outside the context of a clinical study, the use of adjuvant chemotherapy cannot be recommended as a standard therapeutic approach.

Table 2. **Randomized trials of neoadjuvant chemotherapy in advanced NPC**

Institution	No.	Chemotherapy	Median Followu p	Results
Prince of Wales Hospital	82	Cisplatin + 5FU x2 cycles neoadjuvant x4 cycles adjuvant	28.5 months	DFS no difference OS no difference
Institute Nationale Tumori	229	Vincristine, cyclophosphamide, Adriamycin x6 cycles adjuvant	48 months	DFS no difference OS no difference
International NPC Study Group	339	Bleomycin + epirubicin + cisplatin x3 cycles neoadjuvant	49 months (74 months)	DFS improved OS no difference
Asian Oceanian Clinical Oncology Association	334	Cisplatin + epirubicin x2-3 cycles neoadjuvant	30 months	DFS no difference OS no difference

DFS = disease free survival OS = overall survival

Concurrent chemoradiotherapy

Early results using concurrent cisplatin-radiotherapy in head and neck cancers, including NPC, were encouraging. Cisplatin acts both as a cytotoxic agent and as a radiation sensitizer. The optimal scheduling of cisplatin and radiation has not yet been firmly established, but daily low dose, weekly intermediate dose, or 3-weekly high dose regimens, have all been used.

The head and neck Intergroup conducted a study comparing concurrent cisplatin and adjuvant cisplatin-5fluorouracil (5FU) with radiotherapy against radiotherapy alone in patients with stages III and IV NPC using the UICC 1987 classification [30]. The study was closed early after demonstrating significant overall and progression free survival advantage for the chemotherapy-radiotherapy group. Since the publication of this trial in 1998, the standard practice in North America has been concurrent chemotherapy-radiotherapy using cisplatin 100 mg/m^2 every 3 weeks x 3, followed by adjuvant cisplatin 80 mg/m^2 D1 and 5-FU 1 g/m^2 D1-4 every 3 weeks x 3. However, it is noteworthy that in this trial WHO III histology (undifferentiated carcinoma) was present in only 44% of the patients. In endemic areas such as southern China, the proportion of WHO III histology will be more than 90%. Whether the results of a clinical trial derived from a heterogenous histological mix of patients can be directly applied to WHO III undifferentiated NPC is not certain. Another factor that may have influenced the results of the trial was that the radiotherapy technique was not uniform among the participating Intergroup centers.

Furthermore, the benefit of concurrent chemotherapy during radiotherapy and adjuvant chemotherapy after radiotherapy cannot be separated in the Intergroup study. A randomized trial of 229 patients treated in the Institute Nazionale Tumori in Milan failed to demonstrate any survival benefit for patients receiving 4 cycles of vincristine, cyclophosphamide and doxorubicin compared with the patients receiving no adjuvant therapy [27]. In addition, the MACH-NC meta-analysis results of head and neck cancer in general have indicated no survival benefit of adjuvant chemotherapy [31]. These data suggest that most of the benefit of the Intergroup 0099 regimen may have been derived from concurrent chemotherapy-radiotherapy.

Based on the success of concurrent chemoradiation in head and neck cancers and the encouraging phase II data in NPC, we embarked on a study in locoregionally advanced NPC comparing radiotherapy with concurrent cisplatin-radiotherapy. Patients with Ho's N2 or N3 stage or N1 stage with nodal size ≥ 4 cm were eligible. Patients were randomized to receive cisplatin 40 mg/m^2 on a weekly basis concurrently with external radiotherapy or radiotherapy alone. Three hundred and fifty eligible patients were entered between April 1994 and November 1999. A preliminary PFS analysis demonstrated a trend towards benefit for the concurrent chemotherapy-radiotherapy arm. [32] Moreover, there was a very clear PFS benefit favoring chemotherapy-radiotherapy in the subgroup of Ho's T3 (UICC T3/T4) patients with a hazards ratio of 2.49 (95% C.I. 1.28-4.8) [Figure 3]. The benefit in the subgroup of advanced T stage patients was mainly attributable to a reduction in the rate of distant metastases. Based on the evidence of this latter study and Intergroup 0099 study, the use of concurrent-cisplatin-radiotherapy should become standard therapy for endemic locoregionally advanced T and N stage NPC patients.

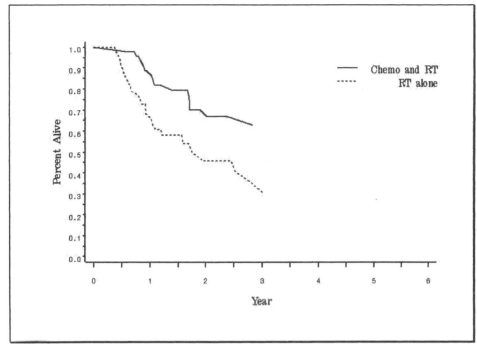

Figure 3. **Progression-free survival subgroup analysis of Ho's Stage T3**

SALVAGE OF LOCAL FAILURE AFTER RADIOTHERAPY

Locoregional failures without distant metastases are potentially curable and should be treated aggressively. In the 1970's when the primary radiotherapy was often suboptimal in dose and tumor target coverage, the salvage rates of locally recurrent NPC by re-irradiation, mainly using external beams, were reported to be between 20-30% [33,34]. However, as the primary radiotherapy improved, resulting in more adequate dose to the major part of the tumor, the rate of 'geographical misses' lessened. The tumors that fail such treatment should, at least theoretically, be more radioresistant. Indeed, we reported little success of re-irradiation to a high dose using 2-dimensionally planned external beams for the salvage of local relapse [35]. Moreover, the complications of re-irradiation were many and severe. These included severe trismus that disrupted the patient's speech and ability to eat and also radiation-induced temporal lobe encephalopathy and cranial nerve damage causing diplopia (VI) and dysphonia (VIII-XII) and even aspiration (VIII-XII). In view of limited success but significant morbidity, we do not recommend 2-dimensionally planned external radiotherapy as a salvage for NPC local relapses [35].

In small (<5cm in largest dimension) and suitably located recurrences that spare the nasal septum and the Eustachian cushions, over 60% long-term control was reported using Au-198 implantation [36]. This interstitial brachytherapy delivered a very high dose to the local tumor but spared the important organs in the vicinity because of the inverse square law. However, it was associated with a not insignificant rate of troublesome headache and nasopharyngeal radiative necrosis that causes a foul-smell and occasional epistaxis. In addition, palatal wound problems and even chronic non-healing palatal fistulas were also reported after Au-198 implantation. The greatest drawback of this method is that it could be applied to only a minority of cases. Even though the procedure can be performed under endoscopic guidance, a split-palatal approach had been advocated [36] for improved visualization and hemostasis. Tumor infiltration of the parapharyngeal region is also a contraindication to Au-198 implantation.

For tumors not amenable to Au-198 implantation, in the absence of significant skull base erosion and intracranial extension or cranial nerve(s) palsy, surgical resection of the recurrent or persistent local tumor becomes the mainstay salvage treatment [37,38]. There are various approaches to the nasopharyngectomy: transcervical, transoral and transpalatal, postero-lateral, transmaxillary (maxillary swing) [38], and, midface deglove [39]. There is no 'ideal' surgical approach that suits all cases of local relapses and there are advantages and disadvantages associated with each approach. The surgical procedure should therefore be tailored to the individual patients depending on the disease extent.

TREATMENT FOR DISTANT METASTASES

The median survival for patients with distant metastases is around 9 months. Wide ranges of chemotherapeutic agents have been used in the treatment of patients with locally recurrent and metastatic NPC. Older agents including methotrexate, bleomycin, 5-fluorouracil (5-FU), cisplatin, and carboplatin are the most active agents, with response rates varying from 15% to 31% [40]. Newer active agents include paclitaxel and gemcitibine. Cisplatin-containing regimens have been used in phase II trials with encouraging response rates of 50 - 90% (Table 3) [40]. The response rates were clearly improved with more intensive chemotherapy. However, the question of whether the gain is sufficient to justify the added toxicities remains to be answered. Hence the current standard first-line therapy for metastatic NPC remains one containing platinum.

Table 3. **Combination chemotherapy in metastatic NPC**

Institution	Pat-ients	Chemo-therapy	OR	CR	Toxicities	Median Survival
Prince of Wales Hospital	42	Carboplatin + 5FU	38%	17%	Mild	12 mos
Prince of Wales Hospital	27	Paclitaxel + carboplatin	59%	11%	Mild	14 mos
Singapore General Hospital	31	Paclitaxel + carboplatin	71%	3%	Moderate	15 mos
Institute Gustav Roussy	41	Cisplatin + bleomycin + 5FU	79%	19%	Moderate	25mos for patients with CR
Princess Margaret Hospital, Toronto	44	CAPABLE	80%	7%	Severe	14 mos

Investigational strategies

Overexpression of the epidermal growth factor receptor (EGFR) is a significant predictor of adverse disease-free survival and correlates with overall survival in head and neck cancers. Zheng et al reported that a strong expression of EGFR in Chinese patients with NPC [41], and we have recently demonstrated that EGFR staining correlated with poor survival in advanced stage NPC patients [42]. C225 (cetuximab), a chimeric counterpart of the murine M225 antibody, is directed against the ligand-binding site of EGFR. Encouraging preliminary data in the use of C225 in combination with cisplatin in head and neck cancers have been reported. We have recently initiated a multicenter, open-label study to evaluate the efficacy of C225 in combination with carboplatin in patients with recurrent or metastatic NPC who have failed one line of platinum-based chemotherapy.

Immunotherapy

There is evidence that HLA class I-restricted cytotoxic-T-lymphocytes (CTL) play a major role in controlling EBV infections, and if CTL-mediated control is reduced e.g. in transplant patients receiving immunosuppressive treatment or in HIV-infected individuals, the cell growth-transforming ability of EBV is apparent, and life-treating EBV-driven lymphoproliferative diseases may occur. Furthermore, these often regress following relaxation of immunosuppressive treatment with recovery of the cellular immune response. Hence there is considerable interest in the possibility of targeting this virus-specific immune response to treat human tumors that carry EBV. We have shown that functional CTLs are present in NPC tumor biopsies, and LMP 2-specific CTL response can be detected in untreated NPC patients [43]. Studies in NPC cell lines indicate that the tumor is capable of processing endogenously expressed EBV antigens for recognition by HLA class I-restricted CTL and this results in lysis of the malignant cell. There is hence a sound basis for treating NPC by boosting LMP2-specific CTL response. We are currently investigating several strategies that involve immunization with LMP 2 peptide epitopes presented on autologous dendritic cells in metastatic NPC.

REFERENCES

1.   Ho JHC. An epidemiologic and clinical study of nasopharyngeal carcinoma. Int J Radiat Oncol Biol Phys 1978;4:183-205.
2.   Lo KW, Cheung ST, Leung SF, et al. Hypermethylation of the p16 gene in nasopharyngeal carcinoma. Cancer Res 1996;56:2721-5.
3.   Chan AS, To KF, Lo KW, et al. High frequency of chromosome 3p deletion in histologically normal nasopharyngeal epithelia from southern Chinese. Cancer Res 2000;60:5365-70.
4.   Lo KW, Teo PM, Hui AB, et al. High resolution allelotype of microdissected primary nasopharyngeal carcinoma. Cancer Res 2000;60:3348-53.
5.   Lo KW, Kwong J, Hui AB, et al. High frequency of promoter hypermethylation of RASSF1A in nasopharyngeal carcinoma. Cancer Res 2001;61:3877-81.
6.   Huang DP, Lo KW, van Hasselt CA, et al. A region of homozygous deletion on chromosome 9p21-22 in primary nasopharyngeal carcinoma. Cancer Res 1994;54:4003-6.
7.   Hui AB, Lo KW, Leung SF, et al. Detection of recurrent chromosomal and losses in primary nasopharyngeal carcinoma by comparative genomic hybridization. Int J Cancer 1999;82:498-503.
8.   Shanmugaratnam K, Sobin LH. The World Health Organization histological classification of tumours of the upper respiratory tract and ear. A commentary on the second edition. Cancer1993;71:2689-97.

9.   Krueger GR, Wustrow J. Current histological classification of nasopharyngeal carcinoma at Cologne University, in Grundman (ed): Cancer Campaign; Nasopharyngeal Carcinoma Vol 5, Stuttgart, Germany, Gustay Fisher verlag, pp. 11-15; 1981.
10.   Reddy SP, Raslan WF, Gooneratne S, Kathuria S, Marks JE. Prognostic significance of keratinization in nasopharyngeal carcinoma. Am J Otolaryngol 1995;16(2):1038.
11.   Marks JE, Phillips JL, Menck HR. The National Cancer Data Base report on the relationship of race and national origin to the histology of nasopharyngeal carcinoma. Cancer 1998;83(3):582-8.
12.   Teo PML, Leung SF, Yu P, Tsao SY, Foo W, Shiu W. A comparison of Ho's, International Union Against Cancer, and American Joint Committee Stage Classifications for Nasopharyngeal Carcinoma. Cancer 1991;67:434-439.
13.   Teo PML, Yu P, Lee WY, et al. Significant prognosticators after primary radiotherapy in 903 nondisseminated nasopharyngeal carcinoma evaluated by computer tomography. Int J Radiat Oncol Biol Phys 1996;36:291-304.
14.   Lo Y.M.D., Chan L.Y.S., Lo K.W., et al. Quantitative analysis of cell-free Epstein-Barr virus DNA in plasma of patients with nasopharyngeal carcinoma. Cancer Res 1999;59:1188-91.
15.   Chan A.T.C., Lo Y.M.D., Chan L.Y.S., et al. EBV DNA monitoring during chemotherapy for patients with undifferentiated nasopharyngeal carcinoma : A strong predictor of tumor response. (Abst.) Proc ASCO 2001;20:928.
16.   Lo Y.M.D., Chan L.Y.S., Chan A.T.C., et al. Quantitative and temporal correlation between circulating cell-free Epstein-Barr virus DNA and tumor recurrence in nasopharyngeal carcinoma. Cancer Res 1999;59:5452-5.
17.   Lo Y.M.D., Chan A.T.C., Chan L.Y.S., et al. Molecular prognostication of nasopharyngeal carcinoma by quantitative analysis of circulating Epstein-Barr virus DNA. Cancer Res 2000;60:6878-81.
18.   O'Sullivan B, Chong V, Gospodarowicz MK et al. Nasopharyngeal carcinoma. Prognostic factors in Cancer 2nd edition. UICC TNM Project and Prognostic Factors Committee, 2001.
19.   Lee AWM, Poon YF, Foo W, et al. Retrospective analysis of 5037 patients with nasopharyngeal carcinoma treated during 1976-1985: Overall survival and patterns of failure. Int J Radiat Oncol Biol Phys 1992;23:261-270.
20.   Xia P, Fu KK, Wong GW, Akazawa C, Verhey LJ. Comparison of treatment plans involving intensity-modulated radiotherapy for nasopharyngeal carcinoma. Int J Radiat Oncol Biol Phys 2000;48:329-337.
21.   Chau RMC, Teo PML, Choi PHK, Cheung KY, Lee WY. Three-dimensional dosimetric evaluation of a conventional radiotherapy technique for treatment of nasopharyngeal carcinoma. Radioth Oncol 2001;58:143-153.
22.   Teo PML, Leung SF, Lee WY, Zee B. Intracavitary brachytherapy significantly enhances local control of early T-stage nasopharyngeal carcinoma: The existence of a dose-tumour-control relationship above conventional tumoricidal dose. Int J Radiat Oncol Biol Phys 2000;46:445-458.
23.   Fu KK, Pajak TF, Trotti A, et al. A radiation therapy oncology group (RTOG) phase III randomized study to compare hyperfractionation and two variants of accelerated fractionation to standard fractionation radiotherapy for head and neck squamous cell carcinomas: first report of RTOG 9003. Int J Radiat Oncol Biol Phys 2000;48:7-16.
24.   Teo P.M.L., Leung S.F., Chan A.T.C., et al. Final report of a randomized trial on altered-fractionated radiotherapy in nasopharyngeal carcinoma prematurely terminated by significant increase in neurologic complications. Int J Radiat Oncol Biol Phys 2000;48:1311-22.

25.   Lee AWM, Sze WM, Yau TK, Yeung RM, Chappell R, Fowler JF. Retrospective analysis on treating nasopharyngeal carcinoma accelerated fractionation (6 fractions per week) in comparison conventional fractionation (5 fractions per week): report on control and normal tissue toxicity. Radiother Oncol 2001;58:121-130.

26.   Chan ATC, Teo PML, Leung TWT, et al. A prospective randomized study of chemotherapy adjunctive to definitive radiotherapy in advanced nasopharyngeal carcinoma. Int J Radiat Oncol Biol Phys 1995;33:569-577.

27.   Rossi A, Molinari R, Boracchi P, et al. Adjuvant chemotherapy with vincristine, cyclophosphamide, and doxorubicin after radiotherapy in local-regional nasopharyngeal cancer : Results of a 4-year multicenter randomized study. J Clin Oncol 1988;6:1401-1410.

28.   International Nasopharynx Cancer Study Group. Preliminary results of a randomized trial comparing neoadjuvant chemotherapy (cisplatin, epirubicin, bleomycin) plus radiotherapy vs. radiotherapy alone in stage IV ($\geq$ N2, M0) undifferentiated nasopharyngeal carcinoma : A positive effect on progression-free survival. Int J Radiat Oncol Biol Phys 1996;35:463-469.

29.   Chua DTT, Sham JST, Choy D, et al. Preliminary report of the Asian-Oceanian clinical oncology association randomized trial comparing cisplatin and epirubicin followed by radiotherapy versus radiotherapy alone in the treatment of patients with locoregionally advanced nasopharyngeal carcinoma. Cancer 1998;83:2270-2283.

30.   Al-Sarraf M, LeBlanc M, Giri PGS, et al. Chemoradiotherapy versus radiotherapy in patients with advanced nasopharyngeal cancer : Phase III randomized intergroup study 0099. J Clin Oncol 1998;16:1310-1317.

31.   Pignon JP, Bourhis J, Domenge C, Designe L. Chemotherapy added to locoregional treatment for head and neck squamous-cell carcinoma : Three meta-analyses of updated individual data. Lancet 2000:355.

32.   Chan AT, Teo PM, Ngan RK, et al. A phase III randomized trial comparing concurrent chemotherapy-radiotherapy with radiotherapy alone in locoregionally advanced nasopharyngeal carcinoma. (Abst.) Proc ASCO 2000;19:1637.

33.   Lee AWM, Law SCK, Foo W, et al. Retrospective analysis of patients with nasopharyngeal carcinoma treated during 1976-1985 : Survival after local recurrence. Int Radiat Oncol Biol Phys 1993;26:773-782.

34.   Wang CC. Re-irradiation of recurrent nasopharyngeal carcinoma : Treatment techniques and results. Int J Radiat Oncol Biol Phys 1987;13:953-956.

35.   Teo PML, Kwan WH, Chan ATC, et al. How successful is high-dose ($\geq$ 60Gy) reirradiation using mainly external beams in salvaging local failures of nasopharyngeal carcinoma? Int J Radiat Oncol Biol Phys 1998;40:897-913.

36.   Choy D, Sham JST, Wei WI, Ho CM, Wu PM. Transpalatal insertion of radioactive gold grain for the treatment of persistent and recurrent nasopharyngeal carcinoma. Int J Radiat Oncol Biol Phys 1993;25:505-512.

37.   King WWK, Ku PKM, Mok CO, Teo PML. Nasopharyngectomy in the treatment of recurrent nasopharyngeal carcinoma : a twelve-year experience. Head and Neck 2000;22:215-222.

38.   Wei WI, Lam KH, Sham JST. New approach to nasopharynx : The maxillary swing approach. Head and Neck 1991;13:200-207.

39.   To EWH, Teo PML, Ku PKM, Pang PCW. Nasopharyngectomy for recurrent nasopharyngeal carcinoma : an innovative transnasal approach through a mid-face deglove incision with stereotactic navigation guidance. Brit J Oral Maxillofacial Surgery 2001;39:55-62.

40.   Chan A.T.C., Teo P.M.L., Leung W.T., Johnson P.J. Role of chemotherapy in the management of nasopharyngeal carcinoma. Cancer 1998;82:1003-12.

41.   Zheng X, Hu L, Chen F, Christensson B. Expression of Ki67 antigen, epidermal growth factor receptor and Epstein-Barr virus-encoded latent membrane protein (LMP1) in nasopharyngeal carcinoma. Eur J Cancer Oral Oncol 1994;30B5:290-295.

40.   Chan A.T.C., Teo P.M.L., Leung W.T., Johnson P.J. Role of chemotherapy in the management of nasopharyngeal carcinoma. Cancer 1998;82:1003-12.
41.   Zheng X, Hu L, Chen F, Christensson B. Expression of Ki67 antigen, epidermal growth factor receptor and Epstein-Barr virus-encoded latent membrane protein (LMP1) in nasopharyngeal carcinoma. Eur J Cancer Oral Oncol 1994;30B5:290-295.
42.   Poon TCW, Chan ATC, To KF, et al. Expression and prognostic significance of epidermal growth factor receptor and HER2 protein in nasopharyngeal carcinoma. Proc ASCO 2001;20:913.
43.   Lee SP, Chan ATC, Cheung ST, et al. Cytotoxic T lymphocyte control of Epstein-Barr virus in nasopharyngeal carcinoma (NPC) : EBV-specific CTL response in the blood and tumour of NPC patients and the antigen processing function of the tumour cells. J Immunology 00;165:573-82.

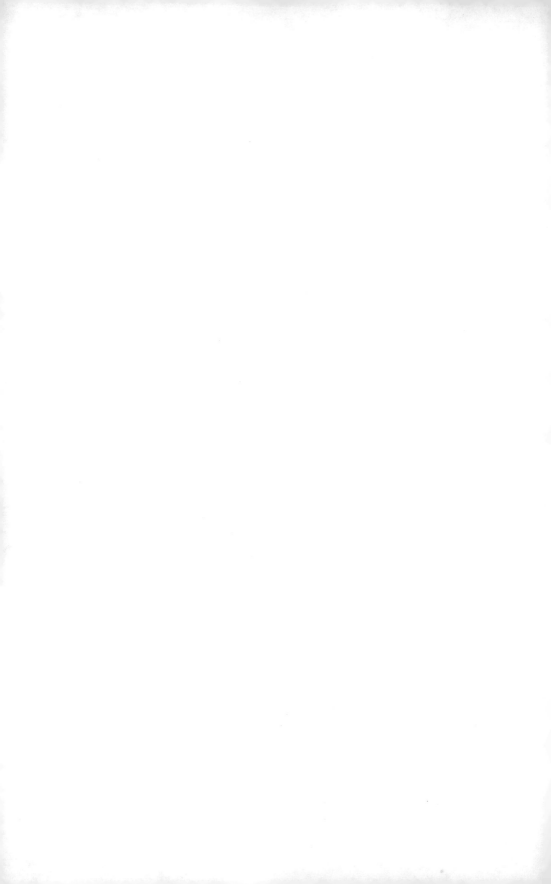

Chapter 12

TREATMENT OF METASTATIC HEAD AND NECK CANCER: CHEMOTHERAPY AND NOVEL AGENTS

Edward S. Kim and Bonnie S. Glisson.
University of Texas M. D. Anderson Cancer Center, Houston, TX 77030

For more than a decade, the de facto "standard of care" for palliative management of recurrent head/neck squamous carcinoma (HNSCC) has been the combination of cisplatin/5-fluorouracil. With the advent of new cytotoxins, such as the taxanes, and of the molecularly targeted agents, eg., the EGFR inhibitors, the number of options for treatment in this setting has increased. However, none of these new approaches has yet been proven to be more effective than cisplatin/5-fluorouracil. Further, despite the palliative intent of therapy in this setting, the palliative effects have been only infrequently assessed, with many studies relying on response as a surrogate for palliation.

This chapter will focus on clinical and translational research efforts in the past decade focusing on the patient with incurable locoregionally recurrent or metastatic HNSCC. Ongoing and planned future trials will also be discussed.

INTRODUCTION

Head and neck squamous cell carcinoma (HNSCC) is a complex challenging disease resulting in more than 500,000 cases worldwide in 2001. In the United States, 37,800 cases with over 11,000 deaths are estimated in 2002, making it the 7th leading cause of cancer and the 12th leading cause of cancer-related death (1). The vast majority of head and neck cancer in the United States is squamous cell carcinoma, with the major risk factors being tobacco, and frequently alcohol, exposure.

Early stage disease (stages I and II) is successfully treated with a single local modality, either radiation or surgery. Two-thirds of patients are initially diagnosed with local or regionally advanced disease (stage III or IV) and cure rates in this setting are approximately 30-40% (2). The treatment of locally advanced disease typically requires multi-modality therapy including surgery and radiation or radiation and chemotherapy. All three modalities may be required to increase the chance of cure in some patients.

Once patients experience locoregionally recurrent or metastatic HNSCC, chemotherapy is only palliative in nature with a median survival of approximately 6-9 months and a 20-30% one-year survival rate. This chapter will review the data extant regarding the use of conventional cytotoxins as well as several classes of novel biologic compounds in the setting of recurrent HNSCC.

CHEMOTHERAPY

Single-Agent Treatment

Active single agents and response rate ranges in the treatment of recurrent HNSCC are listed in table 1. Cisplatin, methotrexate, 5-fluorouracil and the taxanes (paclitaxel and docetaxel) have been the best studied.

Table 1. **Active Single Agents in HNSCC***

Drug	N	RR% (Range)[+]
Cisplatin	376	19 (16-29)
Carboplatin	60	25 (24-26)
Methotrexate	540	22 (10-35)
5-Fluorouracil	201	14 (13-15)
Docetaxel	106	35 (24-25
Paclitaxel	95	37 (35-54)
Ifosfamide	135	24 (4-43)
Gemcitabine	54	13
Navelbine	96	12 (8-16)

*This topic is reviewed in references 9-11.
[+] RR = Response Rate

Methotrexate was more commonly used prior to the "platinum era". Doses ranged from 40-60 mg/m2 weekly with relatively low toxicity, primarily from stomatitis. Phase II studies have shown improved response rates (30% or greater) with high dose methotrexate requiring leucovorin rescue; however, no survival benefit has been demonstrated in several randomized trials (3-8). Further, response rates in a modern randomized trial, in which CT scanning was used to assess response, demonstrated only a 10% response rate with a 40 mg/m^2 weekly dose (*vide infra*).

Cisplatin is a widely used drug in the treatment of HNSCC with a dose range of 60-100 mg/m^2 every 3-4 weeks (10, 11). A dose response relationship has been studied as higher doses have produced higher response rates in some trials (12,13); however, randomized trials comparing lower and higher doses have found no difference in response or survival (14). Carboplatin is a cisplatin analogue which offers a better side effect profile with less renal, otologic, and neurologic toxicity and lessened risk for nausea and vomiting. In combination with 5-fluorouracil, it is associated with somewhat lower response rates than cisplatin. However, in the palliative setting, its use seems reasonable given the improved tolerance and ease of administration (15).

5-Fluorouracil (5-FU) was initially tested as a salvage chemotherapy option; thus response rates ranged from 0-33%. Continuous infusion of 5-FU at 1 gm/m2/d for 4-5 days was associated with increased activity in HNSCC relative to bolus administration when given in combination with cisplatin in one randomized trial (16).

The taxanes, docetaxel and paclitaxel, are quite similar in single agent activity in recurrent HNSCC with mean rates of approximately 35% (16-20). The doses of docetaxel studied range from 60-100 mg/m^2 given every 3 weeks. The largest study of paclitaxel as a single agent was conducted using 50 mg/m^2 as a 24 hour infusion given every 3 weeks (17). As discussed below, this schedule has proven excessively toxic in combination with cisplatin and in a randomized trial was not associated with response benefit relative to a better-tolerated 3 hour infusion (21).

COMBINATION THERAPY

In order to improve efficacy and survival, combination chemotherapy regimens have been developed for treating patients with locoregional recurrent or metastatic HNSCC. Numerous single-arm trials have been published using the combination of cisplatin and 5-FU and have suggested increased response rates over either agent alone (10,11).   Several large multicenter trials have reported results using cisplatin-based regimens. Jacobs et al. (22) (Table 2a) reported that the cisplatin and infusional 5-FU combination had a higher response rate than either cisplatin or 5-FU alone, (32% vs. 17% vs. 15%, p = 0.035), but no survival advantage. Another randomized trial by Forastiere et al. (23) (Table 2b) showed that the combination of cisplatin and 5-FU was superior to both methotrexate alone (32% vs. 10%, p < 0.001) as well as the carboplatin/5-FU combination (response rate =21%, p=0.05). Again the response advantage did not translate into improved survival. Other trials including one by Clavel et al. (24) observed similar findings with the cisplatin/5-FU combination as compared to monotherapy.   A review analysis of these and other randomized trials in recurrent HNSCC confirmed the findings from the trials discussed above without evidence of significant impact on survival with combination vs monotherapy approaches (25).

Table 2a. **Combinations vs. Monotherapy in HNSCC**

Jacobs et al [22]	N	RR (%)	Med. Surv. (mos)
Cisplatin/FU	79	32	5.5
Cisplatin	83	17	5
FU	83	13	6.1

FU=5-fluorouracil; RR= response rate; mos = months

Table 2b. **Combinations vs. Monotherapy in HNSCC**

Forastiere et al [23]	N	RR (%)	Med. Surv. (mos)
Cisplatin/FU	87	32	6.6
Carboplatin/FU	86	21	5
Methotrexate	88	10	5.6

FU= 5-fluorouracil; RR = response rate; mos. = months

Despite lack of survival impact with combination therapy, combinations are generally preferred in practice given a belief that higher response rates are associated with greater palliative effect. However, this belief is not supported by firm evidence and the issue of response as a surrogate for palliation deserves rigorous evaluation in future randomized trials.

The demonstrated single agent activity of the taxanes led to several studies evaluating efficacy in combination regimens.   Phase II studies with taxane-based therapy in the setting of recurrent HNSCC have included doublets with cisplatin or 5-FU. Data are also available with 5-FU or ifosfamide added to a taxane/cisplatin or carboplatin doublet. With a few notable exceptions, these studies have not yielded response rates significantly different from monotherapy with the taxanes, although to date there are no randomized trials which specifically address this issue (26-30).

The Eastern Cooperative Oncology Group (ECOG) has completed and reported two randomized trials with taxane-based therapy in recurrent HNSCC. The first investigated the impact of two different doses of paclitaxel (135 vs. 250 mg/m^2 in 24 hrs) in combination with cisplatin (31) (Table 3a).

Table 3a. **Cisplatin/Paclitaxel in HNSCC**

Forastiere et al [31]	N	RR (%)	Med. Surv. (mos.)	1-year Surv. (%)	Tx-Related Death (%)
Paclitaxel 250 mg/m^2 (24 h) Cisplatin 75 mg/m^2 G-CSF	101	35	7.6	29	8
Paclitaxel 135 mg/m^2 (24 h) Cisplatin 75 mg/m^2	98	36	6.8	29	5

N= number of patients; tx = treatment; G-CSF = granulocyte colony stimulating factor

No benefit in response or survival was observed with the higher dose. In fact, the rates for response and survival in both arms were quite similar to those previously reported by ECOG with the cisplatin/5-FU combination. Both arms of this trial were viewed as excessively toxic by the investigators and neither arm was taken to further study. Another randomized trial that investigated a 24-hour schedule of paclitaxel (vs. 3-hour paclitaxel vs. methotrexate) also led to a conclusion that the 24-hour infusion was excessively toxic without benefit in response (21).

The second ECOG trial, reported only in abstract form, tested a less toxic regimen of paclitaxel given in 3-hours with cisplatin compared to cisplatin/5-FU (32) (Table 3b). Preliminary data suggest the two arms were equally effective as regards response and survival outcome. Somewhat surprising, the median and one year survival rates on both arms were improved relative to previous ECOG trials with the cisplatin/5-FU combination. The paclitaxel arm, with a lower dose of cisplatin and devoid of 5-FU's mucosal toxicity, was, perhaps predictably, better tolerated, although not associated with improved quality of life as assessed by the FACT-HN. A similarly designed industry-sponsored trial of docetaxel/cisplatin compared to cisplatin/5-FU is accruing and these data are awaited with interest. One arm of this trial, docetaxel/5-FU has been closed due to inferior response rates in the first stages of the trial.

Table 3b. **Cisplatin/Paclitaxel in HNSCC**

Murphy et al [32]	N	RR (%)	Med. Surv. (mos.)	1-Year Surv. (%)
Paclitaxel 175 mg/m^2 (3 h) Cisplatin 75 mg/m^2	101	25	9	34
5-FU 4 gm/m^2 (96 h) Cisplatin 100 mg/m^2	98	27	9	41

N= number of patients; tx = treatment; FU = 5-fluorouracil

SUMMARY OF CHEMOTHERAPY

For the patient with recurrent HNSCC, outside of a study setting, there are many options for palliative chemotherapy. Based on improved tolerance and equal effectiveness, some hold that the paclitaxel/cisplatin combination is preferred over the old "standard" of cisplatin/5-FU. Others extrapolate from this that paclitaxel/carboplatin should be chosen, although the evidence to support that specific regimen in this setting are not strong (33, 34). Because of familiarity, some will choose cisplatin/5-FU. One could even argue that given its low cost, low toxicity, and ease of administration, methotrexate is still a viable option. Choosing the patient with recurrent HNSCC for whom chemotherapy is appropriate is likely far more important than the particular drugs selected. Patients with poor performance and those with rapid recurrence after initial chemotherapy in the concomitant or neoadjuvant setting have a low likelihood of benefit from additional therapy with conventional cytotoxins.

Despite significant improvements in diagnosis, local management, and chemotherapy of head and neck cancer, there has been no significant increase in long-term survival over the past 30 years. This is especially true for management of the patient with recurrent disease. As little progress has been made, new treatment approaches are needed. In the following section experience with investigational agents which target cancer-specific receptors or mutations and appear promising in the treatment of recurrent HNSCC is described.

EPIDERMAL GROWTH FACTOR RECEPTOR

Epidermal growth factor receptor (EGFR/erb-B1) is a member of the erb-B family of receptor tyrosine kinases, which also include erb-B2/Her2-neu, erb-B3/Her3 and erb-B4/Her4 (35, 36). It plays a critical role in cellular proliferation of epithelium. EGFR is a 170 kiloDalton transmembrane protein composed of three domains: an extracellular ligand-binding domain, a transmembrane lipophilic region, and an intracellular protein tyrosine kinase domain. EGF, tgf-alpha, heparin-binding EGF (HB-EGF), amphiregulin (AR) and betacellulin (BTC) are some of the endogenous ligands (35). Erb-B family members can form homodimers or heterodimers upon ligand binding to the cytoplasmic domain of the receptors, which leads to phosphorylation of tyrosine residues on EGFR and further activation of the downstream signal transduction pathways, including *ras*/MAP kinase, phosphatidylinositol-3 kinase and STAT-3. This signal transduction cascade can result in cell proliferation, resistance to apoptosis, enhanced angiogenesis, and increased capacity for invasion and metastasis (36-38).

Overexpression of EGFR is commonly observed in human epithelial malignancies (36-45). In HNSCC, EGFR expression is reported in over 90% of tumors and increasing levels of expression are correlated with poor prognosis (44, 45). Therefore, a number of strategies to inhibit EGFR have been developed in order to improve overall clinical outcome (46). These include tyrosine kinase inhibition, use of monoclonal antibodies to the epidermal growth factor receptor, ligand-linked toxins, and antisense approaches (47).

Because of EGFR's interrelated role in proliferation and resistance to apoptosis, combinations of anti-EGFR therapy with chemotherapy and/or radiation have been studied pre-clinically and frequently result in evidence of additive or synergistic antitumor effect (36, 48,49).

Anti-EGFR monoclonal antibodies target the extracellular domain and thus are able to effectively block the EGFR pathways in a highly specific manner, but may require a threshold level of EGFR expression for activity. The small molecule tyrosine kinase inhibitors (TKIs), which target the intracellular tyrosine kinase domain, also inhibit EGFR activation, and may be less dependent on EGFR expression for effect. The TKIs, are less specific than antibody, however, given a degree of promiscuity in inhibiting other tyrosine kinases.

Monoclonal Antibodies

IMC-C225 (ImClone), a chimeric monoclonal antibody targeting EGFR, has been studied in a variety of tumors types. Early phase I studies of IMC-225 alone and in combination with cisplatin were performed in patients with advanced epithelial tumors expressing EGFR (50). The doses for single-agent IMC-C225 ranged from 5 mg/m^2 up to 100 mg/m^2 given as a single, one-time dose, or given weekly. With the combination of IMC-C225 and cisplatin, the dose of IMC-C225 was increased to 400 mg/m^2 weekly. The cisplatin dose, initially fixed at 100 mg/m^2, was later readjusted to 60 mg/m^2 every 4 weeks due to toxicity. IMC-C225 at doses of 200-400 mg/m^2 was associated with complete saturation of systemic clearance, and clearance did not appear to be affected by repeated administration or by co-administration of cisplatin. Furthermore, only 1 of 19 patients developed a humoral response to IMC-C225. Toxicities included fever, chills, aesthenia, transaminitis, nausea, and skin toxicities (flushing, seborrheic dermatitis and acneiform rashes). Rashes were observed at doses higher than 100 mg/m^2 and were mostly grade 1 in severity. Four patients experienced more serious allergic reactions including anaphylactoid reactions and/or urticara. In the combination therapy with cisplatin, nine (69%) of 13 patients treated with antibody doses ≥ 50 mg/m^2 completed 12 weeks of therapy, and two partial responses were observed (50).

To determine the tumor EGFR saturation dose of IMC-C225, a phase I trial in combination with cisplatin was initiated (51). Twelve patients with recurrent or metastatic HNSCC who had high levels of EGFR expression (2-3+ by immunohistochemistry) were enrolled, and 3 different doses of IMC-C225 up to 500 mg/m^2 were administered intravenously as loading doses with cisplatin at 100 mg/m^2 every three weeks. The weekly maintenance dose of IMC-C225 given was 250 mg/m^2 during each 6-week cycle. Tumor EGFR saturation increased up to 95% at the higher dose level as assessed by immunohistochemistry. In 4 cases analyzed for EGFR tyrosine kinase activity, the assay showed a significant reduction in activity after the first IMC-C225 infusion, suggesting functional blockade of EGFR with antibody. Major responses were observed in 6/ 9 (67%) evaluable patients including 2 (22%) complete responses. Toxicity was mild and essentially related to allergic reactions (1 with grade 2 and 1 with grade 3) and folliculitis-like rashes (2 patients with grade 3). Thus, the loading dose of 400 mg/mg^2 with a maintenance dose of 250 mg/m^2 weekly was recommended for further study (51).

Further evaluation of IMC-C225 and cisplatin in patients with recurrent head and neck squamous cell cancers includes two phase II trials in cisplatin-refractory patients and one phase III trial of the combination vs. cisplatin as initial therapy for patients with recurrent disease. These studies are summarized in Table 4. The trials of Kies et al (52) and Baselga et al (53) both entered patients who were progressing on platin –based therapy. They were then treated with the agent (Baselga- cisplatin or carboplatin; Kies-cisplatin) on which they were progressing, and IMC-225. Both trials are reported only in abstract form. Preliminarily response rates are in the 10-15 % range, suggesting either that IMC-225 overcomes cisplatin resistance in a subset of patients or alternatively that IMC-225 has single agent activity in this setting. Burtness et al used a time to progression endpoint in their small randomized trial of cisplatin/placebo vs. cisplatin/IMC-225 (54) . There were some trends to improved response and time to progression in the IMC-225 arm, but no statistically significant differences.

Table 4. **Phase II/III Trials of IMC-225 in HNSCC**

Author	Experimental Regimen	Trial Design	Eligibility	RR (%)
Kies et al (52) (N=56)	CDDP/ IMC-225	Phase II	recurrent/refractory	11
Baselga et al[53] (N=96)	CDDP/ IMC-225	Phase II	recurrent/refractory	14
Burtness et al [54] (N=121)	CDDP/ IMC-225 (vs. CDDP)	Phase III	recurrent	21 vs. 9 (NS)

RR = response rate; CDDP = cisplatin

IMC-225 is worthy of further evaluation in HNSCC; however, the likelihood that it will have a major impact on the outcome of treatment in the patient with recurrent disease seems low given the data now at hand. Study of its integration into curative-intent therapy with radiation, chemoradiation, or with neoadjuvant chemotherapy is either underway or planned.

Tyrosine Kinase Inhibitors

ZD1839 (Iressa, AstraZeneca Pharmaceuticals) is a selective EGFR TKI. Phase I trials have now confirmed mild toxicities and antitumor activity when used as monotherapy in patients with refractory carcinomas. Preclinically, ZD1839 also appears to potentiate the antitumor effects of a number of cytotoxic agents, including the platins and taxanes, against a number of human tumor xenografts including non-small cell lung cancer, vulvar, and prostate carcinomas (54, 55). A small study reported enhanced cisplatin-induced apoptosis in oral squamous cell carcinoma (SCC) cell lines by pre-exposure of cells to ZD1839 (56). When combined with radiation, ZD1839 demonstrated dose-dependent inhibition of cellular proliferation in human SCC cell lines grown in culture. Additionally, this study found that ZD1839 inhibited tumor angiogenesis in tumor xenograft models in vivo (57).

In the phase I trials, consistent dose-related, mechanism-based toxicities have been commonly confined to the skin (rash or erythema) and gastrointestinal system (diarrhea, nausea and vomiting); transient hepatic enzyme elevation has also occurred. These studies have identified dose-limiting toxicity of diarrhea at ZD1839 doses of 800 to 1000 mg/d given continuously orally (58-61).

In four phase I monotherapy trials, 252 patients were treated with dosages ranging from 50 mg to 1000 mg. In the largest trials, 5 select tumor types were eligible, including non-small cell lung, hormone refractory prostate, colorectal, ovarian and head and neck cancer. None of these trials included an eligibility criterion for tumor to express or over-express EGFR. Patients in these trials were typical phase I patients who had been heavily pre-treated. Responses were primarily seen in patients with non-small cell lung cancer. Stabilization was observed for patients with recurrent HNSCC (58-61).

Use of ZD 1839 has been reported to be associated with tumor response/stabilization and quality of life improvement in the second and third line settings for patients with non-small cell lung cancer (62,63). A phase II trial of ZD1839 has been reported in refractory HNSCC by Cohen et al (64). These data and those from a similar trial with OSI-774 (65), another EGFR tyrosine kinase inhibitor, are summarized in Table 5. The results of these two trials, which are reported in abstract only, suggest a modicum of effect for these agents in the chemotherapy-refractory patient and are reminiscent of the activity seen in the IMC-225 trials. Both of these drugs will be further developed in HNSCC in combination with chemotherapy and radiation. Their advantage, relative to IMC-225, may be lack of dependence on overexpression of EGFR, convenient oral dosing, and lack of hypersensitivity reaction.

Table 5. **EGFR-TKIs in HNSCC**

Regimen	N	RR (%)	Stable Dis. (%)	Toxicity
ZD 1839 500 mg/d Cohen et al (64)	47	11	45	Rash Diarrhea
OSI-774 150 mg/d Senzer et al (65)	124	6	29	Rash Diarrhea

RR = response rate; N= number of patients

Other small molecules targeting EGFR and its family of receptors have also been developed and are ongoing in phase 1. CI-1033 (Pfizer) is an orally active 4-anilinoquinazoline that acts as a pan-erbB tyrosine kinase inhibitor. PKI166 is a selective inhibitor of the tyrosine kinase of EGFR and the erbB2 (her2/neu) receptor. It is likely that these drugs will be further evaluated in HNSCC.

RAS AND FARNESYL TRANSFERASE INHIBITORS

One report indicates that 27% of oral cavity cancers have mutations in the h-ras gene (66). Farnesyl transferease inhibitors (FTIs) are a class of compounds that inhibit a critical enzymatic step in the constitutive expression of mutated ras genes (67). These agents include SCH66336, a novel tricyclic peptidomemetic compound designed by Schering Plough, R115777 (Janssen Pharmaceuticals), and BMS-214662 (Bristol-Meyers Squibb). FTIs appears to have activity in pre-clinical studies utilizing head and neck squamous cell carcinoma and non-small cell lung cancer cell lines (68).

A phase I B randomized trial of patients with newly diagnosed HNSCC scheduled for surgery were enrolled to a 4-arm trial testing the effects of SCH66336 in tumor. The intent of this trial was to show "proof of principle" by demonstrating the inhibition of farnesylation in two proteins known to require farnesylation in the differentiated state, relative to pre-treatment biopsies. Both DNA-J, a heat shock protein, and prelamin-A, typically found in tissue as lamin-A, were assayed following an 8-14 day schedule of oral SCH66336 at 3 doses; 100 mg BID, 200 mg BID, and 300 mg BID. Patients were randomized to one of 3 dosing arms or placebo. Preliminary data indicates potent inhibition of protein farnesylation, in both target proteins. Somewhat surprisingly, four patients experienced tumor reduction, despite the short course of therapy (8-14 days). In fact, one patient who had a large bulky oral cavity tumor had only microscopic disease after 3 days of therapy at 300 mg BID of SCH66336 (69).

Pre-clinical data indicates that the addition of farnesyl transfererase inhibitors to either paclitaxel or epothilones, resulted in reversal of acquired resistance to these tubulin toxins in a variety of different cancer cell lines (68). Based on these observations, a phase I/II trial of SCH66336 in combination with paclitaxel was performed in patients with solid tumors. Through the phase I portion of the study, a phase II dose of SCH66336 100 mg po BID and paclitaxel 175 mg/m^2 was established (70). Additionally, responses and disease stabilization were observed in HNSCC and NSCLC. Extension of the phase I for patients with taxane-refractory NSCLC showed promising response rates. (71). Trials in NSCLC (phase III) and HNSCC (phase II) with SCH66336 are planned in combination with chemotherapy.

TARGETING p53

p53 mutations occur in 45% - 70% of HNSCC cases; alcohol and tobacco use are associated with these mutations (72,73). In tumors with a normal p53 gene sequence, loss of p53 function can occur through p53 protein inhibition and/or degradation (74,75). p53 is a multi-functional protein which can be induced by DNA damage and plays a significant role in the detection and repair of damaged DNA. p53 can also induce apoptosis or programmed cell death in severely damaged cells and has been associated with both carcinogesis and overall prognosis in HNSCC (76). Thus, strategies targeting the p53 gene and protein may halt or reverse the process of tumorogenesis and metastasis.

ONYX-015 is an E1B-55 kD gene-deleted replication selective adenovirus which replicates and causes cytopathic changes in cells that are deficient in p53 function (77,78). Although pre-clinical *in vitro* results have varied, initial clinical data with regards to safety and antitumor activity following intratumoral injection of ONYX-015 have been promising. Selective intratumoral replication and tumor-selective tissue destruction of ONYX-015 have been documented in phase I and II clinical trials of intratumoral administration in patients with recurrent/refractory HNSCC (77-81). However, durable responses and clinical benefit were seen in less than 15% of these end-stage patients. As predicted, p53 mutant tumors underwent necrosis at a higher rate than did tumors with a wild-type gene sequence (58% and 0% respectively) (80).

Both *in vitro* and nude mouse-human tumors xenograft model studies have shown additive or potentially synergistic efficacy of ONYX-015 in combination with cisplatin-based chemotherapy compared with that of either ONYX-015 or chemotherapy alone (75). ONYX-015 was able to enhance the efficacy of cisplatin both in p53 deficient and p53-functional tumor cells. Recent data indicate that viral replication of ONYX-015 virus is largely influenced by, and can be dependent on the status p14 arf (82). Sensitization of p53-functional tumor cells may involve expression of the adenovirus E1A gene product, which is a potent chemosensitizer, induction of high levels of p53 protein, or both (81-87).

A phase II multi-center trial of intratumoral ONYX-015 in combination with cisplatin and 5-FU in patients with recurrent HNSCC was recently reported (88). This study demonstrated enhanced response in injected lesions versus those exposed to systemic chemotherapy alone. Other studies include a phase II trial of ONYX-015 administered to patients with HNSCC at 2 different dose schedules (89). Forty patients received injections, 30 for 5 consecutive days (standard) and 10 for twice daily for 2 weeks (hyperfractionated). Responses and disease stabilization were observed in both groups. Systemic toxicity was similar although there was a higher reported injection site pain with the hyperfractionated regimen (80% vs 47%). Because of this side effect, a dose escalation study of intravenous ONYX-015 has been tested (90). Doses ranged from 2 x 10(10) to 2 X 10(13) particles via weekly infusion in 10 patients with advanced NSCLC. This dose was well tolerated but was associated with rapid development of anti-ONYX-015 antibody in high titers.

Ongoing trials of ONYX-015 in patients with recurrent HNSCC include a randomized trial of the virus with chemotherapy versus chemotherapy alone in patients therapy-naïve for recurrent disease. A second trial is targeted to the second-line setting and randomizes to the virus alone versus methotrexate. Feasibility of these trials has been low so far with slow accrual in large part likely attributable to the requirement for injectable disease.

Another approach targeting p53 mutations has been gene replacement strategies using an adenovirus containing the wild-type p53 gene (Ad-p53 or RPR-INGN-201). Ad-p53 is a vector system in which the wild-type p53 gene is inserted into a first-generation adenoviral vector. In pre-clinical studies, Ad-p53 gene treatment induced apoptosis of cancer cells without affecting normal cells. It was not only active against p53 mutant cancer cells, but also against cancer cells with a wild-type p53 genomic sequence. Ad-p53 also reduced tumor growth in mouse xenograft models of HNSCC and other cancers (91,92).

Clayman et al. conducted a phase I trial of Ad-p53 gene transfer in patients with advanced recurrent HNSCC (93). Thirty-three patients received intratumoral injections of Ad-p53 at a dose of 1×10^{11} plaque-forming units (PFU) 3 times a week, which consisted of one course. Patients with resectable tumor received one full course of treatment followed by two additional administrations, one during surgery, and one 72 hours after surgery in the surgically resectable group. Patients with unresectable disease received a treatment every 4 weeks. The treatment regimen was well tolerated, the most common adverse effect being injection site pain, which did not seem to be related to the dose or the anatomic site of injection. Other common side effects included transient fever, headache, pain, and edema with these symptoms mainly occurring at doses of 1×10^{10} PFU or greater. No allergic reactions or evidence of systemic hypersensitivity was observed. Two (11.8%) of 17 evaluable patients with unresectable disease at a dose of 1×10^{10} and 1×10^{11} PFU had brief major responses. The duration of the responses were 7 weeks and 18 days respectively. Among resectable tumor patients, 1 had a pathologic complete response at the time of surgery and remained free of disease 26 months. Another patient also had no evidence of disease at 24 months. Ad-p53 was detected in blood, urine, and the sputum of patients, but no patients reported viremic symptoms. Similar to the design of the ongoing ONYX-15 trials, Ad-p53 is being further studied in randomized studies for patients with recurrent HNSCC. One tests the combination of Ad-p53 with cisplatin/5-FU versus cisplatin/5-FU alone in the front-line setting. A second-line trial compares Ad-p53 injection versus methotrexate.

CONCLUSIONS

Recurrent HNSCC remains a complex and frustrating disease. Given the experience of the past decade, expectations that improvements in outcome with traditional cytotoxins will ensue have been dampened. Molecularly targeted agents are under active investigation and hold more promise for improving the plight of our patients. These agents will likely have the greatest impact when used in combination with chemotherapy. It seems unlikely, however, that we will begin to cure these patients who currently have a life expectancy of 6-9 months. Palliation will remain the intent of therapy in the recurrent setting and for this reason it is paramount that we focus on these effects in our research.

REFERENCES

1. Jemal A, Thomas A, Murray T, Thun M. Cancer Statistics, 2002. CA Cancer J Clin 2002; 52:23-47.
2. Vokes EE, Weichselbaum RR, Lippman SM, Hong WK: Medical progress: head and neck cancer. N. Engl J Med 328: 184-194, 1993.
3. Mitchell MS, Wawro NW, DeConti RC, et al: Effectiveness of high-dose infusion of methotrexate followed by leucovorin in carcinoma of the head and neck. Cancer Res 1968;28:108.
4. Kirkwood JM, Millder D, Pitman S, et al: Initial high dose methotrexate-leucovorin in advanced squamous carcinoma of the head and neck. Proc Am Assoc Cancer Res 1978;19:398.
5. Levitt M, Mosher MB, DeConti RC, et al: Improved therapeutics of methotrexate with leucovorin rescue. Cancer Res 1973;33:1729.
6. Woods RL, Fox RM, Tattersall MHN. Methotrexate treatment of advanced head and neck cancers: a dose-response evaluation. Cancer Treat Rep 1981;65:155.
7. DeConti RC, Schoenfeld D. A randomized prospective comparison of intermittent methotrexate, methotrexate with leucovorin, and a methotrexate combination in head and neck cancer. Cancer 1981;48:1061.
8. Taylor SG, McGuire WP, Hauck WW, et al: A randomized comparison of high-dose infusion methotrexate versus standard-dose weekly therapy in head and neck squamous cancer. J Clin Oncol 1984;2:1006.
9. Urba SG. Palliative chemotherapy for recurrent or metastatic head and neck cancer. ASCO Educational Book, Spring 2002,573-77.
10. Pinto HA, Jacobs CJ: Chemotherapy for recurrent and metastatic head and neck cancer. Hematol/Oncol Clin North Am 1991;5:667.
11. Al-Sarraf M. Chemotherapeutic management of head and neck cancer. Cancer Metastasis Rev 1987;6:191.
12. Forastiere AA, Takasugi BJ, Baker SR, et al: High dose cisplatin in head and neck cancer. Cancer Chemother Pharmacol 1987;19:155.
13. Havlin KA, Kuhn JG, Myers JW, et al: High-dose cisplatin for locally advanced or metastatic head and neck cancer. Cancer 1989;63:423.

14.   Veronesi A, Zagonel V, Rirelli U, et al: High dose versus low dose cisplatin in advanced head and neck squamous carcinoma. A randomized study. J Clin Oncol 1985;3:1105.

15.   Al-Sarraf M.   Management strategies in head and neck cancer: the role of carboplatin. In: Bunn PA, Canetta R, Ozols RF, Rozencqeig M, eds. Current perspectives and future directions. Philadelphia: WB Saunders, 1990.

16.   Kish JA, Ensley JF, Jacobs J, et al: A randomized trial of cisplatin (CACP) + 5-fluorouracil (5-FU) infusion and CACP + 5-FU bolus for recurrent and advanced squamous cell carcinoma of the head and neck. Cancer 56:2740-2744, 1985.

17.   Forastiere AA, Shank D, Neuberg D, Taylor SG 4th, DeConi RC, Adams G. Final report of a phase II evaluation of paclitaxel in patients with advanced squamous cell carcinoma of the head and neck: an Eastern Cooperative Oncology Group Trial (PA390). Cancer 1998, 82:2270-2274.

18.   McWilliams JE, Cohen II, Everts EC, Andersen PE, Henner WD. A phase II trial of lower dose paclitaxel in recurrent and metastatic and neck squamous cell carcinoma (HNSCC) (abstract). Proc Am Soc Clin Oncol 1998, 17:407a.

19.   Dreyfuss AI, Clark JR, Norris CM, et al: Docetaxel: an active drug for squamous cell carcinoma of the head and neck. J Clin Oncol 1996; 14:1672-8.

20.   Catimel G, Verweij J, Mattijssen V, et al: Docetaxel: an active drug for the treatment of patients with advanced squamous cell carcinoma of the head and neck. Ann Oncol 1994;5:533.

21.   Vermorken JB, Catimel G, De Mulder P, Hoekman K, Hupperts P, Ruggeri E, et al. randomized phase II trial of weekly methotrexate versus two schedules of triweekly paclitaxel (Taxol) in patients with metastic or recurrent squamous cell carcinoma of the head and neck (abstract) Proc ASCO 1999, 18:295a.

22.   Jacobs C; Lyman G; Velez-Garcia E, et al: A phase III randomized study comparing cisplatin and fluorouracil as single agents and in combination for advanced squamous cell carcinoma of the head and neck. J Clin Oncol 10(2):257-63, 1992

23.   Forastiere AA; Metch B; Schuller DE, et al: Randomized comparison of cisplatin plus fluorouracil and carboplatin plus fluorouracil versus methotrexate in advanced squamous-cell carcinoma of the head and neck: a Southwest Oncology Group study. J Clin Oncol 10(8):1245-51, 1992

24.   Clavel M, Vermorken JB, Cognetti F, et al: Randomized comparison of cisplatin, methotrexate, bleomycin and vincristine (CABO) versus cisplatin and 5-fluorouracil (CF) versus cisplatin (C) in recurrent or metastatic squamous cell carcinoma of the head and neck. Ann Oncol 1994;5:521.

25.   Browman GP, Cronin L. Standard chemotherapy in squamous cell head and neck cancer: what we have learned from randomized trials. Semin Oncol 1994;21:311.

26.   Hussain M; Gadgeel S; Kucuk O, et al: Paclitaxel, cisplatin, and 5-fluorouracil for patients with advanced or recurrent squamous cell carcinoma of the head and neck. Cancer 1999;86(11):2364-9.

27.   Shin DM; Glisson BS; Khuri FR, et al: Phase II trial of paclitaxel, ifosfamide, and cisplatin in patients with recurrent head and neck squamous cell carcinoma. J Clin Oncol 1998;16(4):1325-30.

28.   Thodtmann F, Theisis F, Kemmerich M, Heinrich B. Laubenbacher C. Quasthoff S, et al. Clinical phase II evaluation of paclitaxel in combination with cisplatin in metastic or recurrent squamous cell carcinoma of the head and neck. Ann Oncol 1998, 9:335-337.

29.   Janinis J, Papadakou M, Xidakis E, et al. Combination chemotherapy with docetaxel, cisplatin, and 5-fluorouracil in previously treated patients with advanced/recurrent head and neck cancer: a phase II feasibility study. Am J Clin Oncol. 2000;23(2):128-31.

30. Glisson BS, Murphy BA, Frenette G, Khuri FR, Forastiere AA. Phase II trial of docetaxel and cisplatin combination chemotherapy in patients with squamous cell carcinoma of the head and neck. J Clin Oncol 2002;20:1593-1599.

31. Forastiere AA, Leong T, Rowinsky E, Murphy BA, Vlock DR, DeConti RC, Adams GL. Phase III comparison of high-dose paclitaxel + cisplatin + granulocyte colony-stimulating factor versus low-dose paclitaxel + cisplatin in advanced head and neck cancer: Eastern Cooperative Oncology Group Study E1393. J Clin Oncol 2001;19:1088-1095.

32. Murphy B, Li Y, Cella D, Karnad A, Hussain M, Forastiere A. Phase III study comparing cisplatin (C) & 5-flurouracil (F) versus cisplatin & paclitaxel (T) in Metastatic/Recurrent Head & Neck Cancer (MHNC). (abstract 894) Proc ASCO 2001, 20:224a.

33. Fountzilas G, Athanassiades A, Kalogera-Fountzila A, Samantas E, Bacoyiannis C, et al. Paclitaxel in combination with carboplatin or gemcitabine for the treatment of advanced head and neck cancer. Semin Oncol 1997;24(suppl 19):S19-28-S19-32.

34. Stathopoulos GP, Rigatos S, Papakostas P, Fountzilas G. Effectiveness of paclitaxel and carboplatin combination in heavily pretreated patients with head and neck cancers. Eur J Cancer 1997; 33:1780-1783.

35. Salomen DS, Brandt R, Ciardiello F, et al: Epidermal growth factor-related peptides and their receptors in human malignancies. Crit Rev Oncol/Hematol 1995;19:183-232.

36. Harari PM, Huang SM: Modulation of molecular targets to enhance radiation. Clin Cancer Res 2000, 6: 323-325

37. Thompson DM, Gill GN: The EGF receptor: structure, regulation and potential role in malignancy. Cancer Surv 1985, 4: 767-788

38. Shin DM, Ro JY, Hong WK, et al: Dysregulation of epidermal growth factor receptor expression in multistep process of head and neck tumorigenesis. Cancer Res 1994; 54: 3153-3159.

39. Gullick WJ. Prevalence of aberrant expression of the epidermal growth factor receptor in human cancers. Br Med Bull 1991;47:87-98.

40. Lofts FJ, Gullick WJ. C-erbB2 amplification and overexpression in human tumors, in Dickson RB, Lippman ME (eds.): Genes, Oncogenes, and Hormones: Advances in Cellular and Molecular Biology of Breast Cancer. Boston: Kluwer Academic Publishers, 1991, pp 161-179

41. Bruns CJ, Harbison MT, Davis DW, et al: Epidermal growth factor receptor blockade with C225 plus gemcitabine results in regression of human pancreatic carcinoma growing orthotopically in nude mice by antiangiogenic mechanisms. Clin Cancer Res 2000;1936-1948.

42. Fischer-Colbrie J, Witt A, Heinzl H, et al: EGFR and steroid receptors in ovarian carcinoma: Comparison with prognostic parameters and outcome of patients. Anticancer Res 1997;17:613-620.

43. Chow N-H, Liu H-S, Lee EI, et al: Significance of urinary epidermal growth factor and its receptor expression in human bladder cancer. Anticancer Res 1997;17:1293-1296.

44. Ke LD, Adler-Storthz K, Clayman GL, et al: Differential expression of epidermal growth factor receptor in human head and neck cancers. Head Neck 1998;20:320-327.

45. Grandis JR, Melhem MF, Barnes EL, et al: Quantitative immunohistochemical analysis of transforming growth factor-α and epidermal growth factor receptor in patients with squamous cell carcinoma of the head and neck. Cancer 1996;78:1284-1292.

46.　　　Modjahedi H, Affleck K, Stubberfield C, et al: EGFR blockade by tyrosine kinase inhibitor or monoclonal antibody inhibits growth, directs terminal differentiation and induces apoptosis in human squamous cell carcinoma HN5. Int J Oncol 1998;13:335-342.

47.　　　He Y, Zeng Q, Drenning SD, et al: Inhibition of human squamous cell carcinoma growth in vivo by epidermal growth factor receptor antisense RNA transcribed from the U6 promoter. J Natl Cancer Inst 1998;90:1080-1087.

48.　　　Huang S-M, Bock JM, Harari PM. Epidermal growth factor receptor blockade with C225 modulates proliferation, apoptosis, and radiosensitivity in squamous cell carcinomas of the head and neck. Cancer Res 1999;35-1940.

49.　　　Baselga J, Norton L, Masui H, et al: Antitumor effects of doxorubicin in combination with anti-epidermal growth factor receptor monoclonal antibodies. J Natl Cancer Inst 1993;27-1333.

50.　　　Baselga J; Pfister D; Cooper MR, et al: Phase I studies of anti-epidermal growth factor receptor chimeric antibody C225 alone and in combination with cisplatin. J Clin Oncol 2000;904-14.

51.　　　Shin DM, Donato NJ, Cooper M, et al: Epidermal growth factor receptor targeted therapy with humanized chimeric monoclonal antibody, C225 in combination with cisplatin in patients with head and neck cancer. Clin Cancer Res 2001:1204-13.

52.　　　Kies MS, Arquette MA, Nabell L, Quinn D, Shin D, Needle MN, Waksal H, Hong WK, Herbst RS. Final report of the efficacy and safety of the anti-epidermal growth factor antibody Erbitux (IMC-C225), in combination with cisplatin in patients with recurrent squamous cell carcinoma of the head and neck (SCCHN) refractory to cisplatin containing chemotherapy. Proc Am Soc Clin Oncol 21:232a, 2002 (abstr 925)

53.　　　Baselga J, Trigo JM, Bourhis J, Tortochaux J, Cortes-Funes H, Hitt R, Gascon P, Muesser M, Harstrick A, Eckardt A. Cetuximab (C225) plus cisplatin/carboplatin is active in patients (pts) with recurrent/metastatic squamous cell carcinoma of the head and neck (SCCHN) progressing on a same dose and schedule platinum-based regimen. Proc Am Soc Clin Oncol 21:226a, 2002 (abstr 900)

54.　　　Burtness BA, Li Y, Flood W, Mattar BI, Forastiere AA. Phase III trial comparing cisplatin (C) + placebo (P) to C + anti-epidermal growth factor antibody (EGF-R) C225 in patients (pts) with metastic/recurrent head & neck cancer (HNC). Proc Am Soc Clin Oncol 21:226a, 2002 (abstr 901)

55.　　　Baselga J, Averbuch SD. ZD1839 ('Iressa') as an anticancer agent. Drugs. 60 Suppl 1:33-40; discussion 41-2, 2000

56.　　　Al-Hazzaa AA, Bowen ID, Birchall MA, et al: p53-independent apoptosis induced by cisplatin and enhanced by the combination of cisplatin with ZD1839 (Iressa) an EGFR-TK inhibitor in an oral squamous cell carcinoma cell line. Proceedings AACR-NCI-EORTC International Conference, 2001 348(abstract).

57.　　　Huang S, Harari PM: Modulation of radiation response and tumor-induced angiogenesis following EGFR blockade by ZD1839 (Iressa) in human squamous cell carcinomas. Proceedings AACR-NCI-EORTC International Conference, 2001 259(abstract).

58.　　　Kris M, Ranson M, Ferry D, et al.: Phase I study of oral ZD1839 (Iressa), a novel inhibitor of epidermal growth factor tyrosine kinase (EGFR-tK): evidence of good tolerability and activity. Clin Cancer Res 5:3749S.

59.　　　Negoro S, Nakagawa K, Fukuoka M, et al.: Final results of a phase I intermittent dose-escalation trial of ZD1839 (Iressa) in Japanese patients with various solid tumors. Proc Am Soc Clin Oncol 20:324a, 2001.

60.　　　Baselga J, Herbst R, LoRusso P, et al. Continuous administration of ZD1839 (Iressa), a novel oral epidermal growth factor receptor tyrosine kinase inhibitor (EGFRj-TKI), in patients with five selected tumor types: evidence of activity and good tolerability. Proc Am Soc Clin Oncol 19:1771 (686), 2000.

61. Ferry D, Hammond L, Ranson M, et al. Intermittent oral ZD1839 (Iressa), a novel epidermal growth factor receptor tyrosine kinase inhibitor (Egfr-tki), shows evidence of good tolerability and activity: final results from a phase I study. Proc Am Soc Clin Oncol 19:3a, 2000. (Abstract 5E)

62. Baselga J, Yano S, Giaccone G, et al: Initial results from a phase II trial of ZD1839 (Iressa) as second- and third-line monotherapy for patients with advanced non-small cell lung cancer (IDEAL-1). Proceedings AACR-NCI-EORTC International Conference, 2001 630A(abstract).

63. Kris MG, Natale RB, Herbst RS, Lynch TJ, Prager D, et al. A phase II trial of ZD1839 ('IRESSA') in advanced non-small cell lung cancer (NSCLC) patients who had failed platinum- and docetaxel-based regimens (IDEAL 2). Proc Am Soc Clin Oncol 21:292a(1166), 2002.

64. Cohen EE, Rosen F, Dekker A, Bajda C, Stenson K, Shulman KL, Lamont E, Kozoloff M, Vokes EE. Phase II study of ZD1839 (Iressa) in recurrent or metastatic squamous cell carcinoma of the head and neck (SCCHN). Proc Am Soc Clin Oncol 21:225a, 2002. (abstract 899)

65. Senzer NN, Soulieres D, Siu L, et al: Phase II evaluation of OSI-774, a potent oral antagonist of the EGFR-TK in patients with advanced squamous cell carcinoma of the head and neck. Proc Amer Soc Clinic Onc 2001, 6 (abstract).

66. Glisson S, Huber J, Gaugler M, et al: Smokeless Tobacco Induced Oral Cavity Tumors in Kentucky Have a High Incidence of H-ras Mutations. ASCO Volume 17, 1998

67. Sepp-Lorenzino L, Ma Z, Rands E, et al: A peptidomimetic inhibitor of farnesylprotein transferase blocks the anchorage-dependent and -independent growth of human tumor cell lines. Cancer Res 55(22):5302-9, 1995

68. Moasser MM, Sepp-Lorenzino L, Kohl NE, et al: Farnesyl transferase inhibitors cause enhanced mitotic sensitivity to taxol and epothilones. Proc Natl Acad Sci U S A. 1998;95;1369-74, 1998

69. Kies MS, Clayman GL, El-Naggar AK, et al: Induction therapy with SCH 66336, a farnesyltransferase inhibitor,in squamous cell carcinoma (SCC) of the head and neck. Proc Am Soc Clin Oncol 2001 896 (abstract)

70. Kim ES, Glisson BS, Meyers ML, et al: A phase I/II study of the farnesyl transferase inhibitor (FTI) SCH66336 with paclitaxel in patients with solid tumors. Proc Amer Assoc Cancer Res 2001, 2629 (abstract)

71. Kim ES, Kies MS, Fossella FV, et al: A phase I/II study of farnesyl transferase inhibitor (FTI) SCH66336 (lonafarnib) with paclitaxel in taxane-refractory/resistant patients with non-small cell lung cancer: final report. Proc Amer Assoc Cancer Res 2002, (abstract) submitted and accepted.

72. Boyle JO, Hakim J, Koch W, et al: The incidence of p53 mutations increases with progression of head and neck cancer. Cancer Res 1993;53:4477-4480.

73. Brennan JA, Boyle JO, Koch WM, et al: Association between cigarette smoking and mutation of the p53 gene in squamous cell carcinoma of the head and neck. N Engl J Med 1995;332:712-717.

74. Werness BA, Levine AJ, Howley PM: Association of human papillomavirus type 16 and 18 E6 proteins with p53. Science 1990;248:76-79.

75. Gillison ML, Koch WM, Capone RB, et al: Evidence for a causal association between human papillomavirus and a subset of head and neck cancers. J Natl Cancer Inst 2000;92:709-720.

76. Cabelguenne A, Blons H, de Waziers I, et al: p53 alterations predict tumor response to neoadjuvant chemotherapy in head and neck squamous cell carcinoma: a prospective series. J Clin Oncol 2000;18:1465-73.

77.   Bischoff JR, Kirn DH, Williams A, et al: An adenovirus mutant that replicates selectively in p53-deficient human tumor cells. Science 1996;274:373-376.

78.   Heise C, Sampson-Johannes A, Williams A, et al: ONYX-015, an E1B gene-attenuated adenovirus, causes tumor-specific cytolysis and antitumoral efficacy that can be augmented by standard chemotherapeutic agents. Nat Med 1997; 3:639-45.

79.   Kirn D, Hermiston T, McCormick F. ONYX-015: clinical data are encouraging. Nat Med 1998; 4:1341-2.

80.   Kirn D, et al: A phase II trial of intratumoral injection with an E1B-deleted adenovirus, ONYX-015, inpatients with recurrent, refractory head and neck cancer. Proc am Soc Clin Oncol 1998;17:391a

81.   Ganly I, Eckhardt SG, Rodriguez GI, et al: A phase I study of Onyx-015, an E1B attenuated adenovirus, administered intratumorally to patients with recurrent head and neck cancer. Clin Cancer Res 2000;6:798-806.

82.   Ries SJ; Brandts CH; Chung AS, et al: Loss of p14ARF in tumor cells facilitates replication of the adenovirus mutant dl1520 (ONYX-015). Nat Med 2000;6:1128-33, 2000.

83.   Lowe SW, Ruley HE, Jacks T, et al: p53-dependent apoptosis modulates the cytotoxicity of anticancer agents. Cell 1993;24:957-67.

84.   Lowe SW, Bodis S, McClatchey A, et al: p53 status and the efficacy of cancer therapy in vivo. Science 1994;266:807-10.

85.   Sanchez-Prieto R, Quintanilla M, Cano A, et al: Carcinoma cell lines become sensitive to DNA-damaging agents by the expression of the adenovirus E1A gene. Oncogene 1996;5;13(5):1083-92.

86.   Lowe SW, Ruley HE: Stabilization of the p53 tumor suppressor is induced by adenovirus 5 E1A and accompanies apoptosis. Genes Dev 1993;7:535-45.

87.   Barker DD, Berk AJ: Adenovirus proteins from both E1B reading frames are required for transformation of rodent cells by viral infection and DNA transfection. Virology 1987;156:107-21.

88.   Khuri FR, Nemunaitis J, Ganly I, et al: A controlled trial of intratumoral ONYX-015, a selectively-replicating adenovirus, in combination with cisplatin and 5-fluorouracil in patients with recurrent head and neck cancer. Nat Med 2000;6:879-85.

89.   Nemunaitis J, Khuri F, Ganly I, et al: Phase II trial of intratumoral administration of ONYX-015, a replication-selective adenovirus, in patients with refractory head and neck cancer. J Clin Oncol 2001;19:289-98.

90.   Nemunaitis J, Cunningham C, Buchanan A, et al: Intravenous infusion of a replication-selective adenovirus (ONYX-015) in cancer patients: safety, feasibility and biological activity. Gene Ther 2001;8:746-59.

91.   Horio Y, Hasegawa Y, Sekido Y, et al: Synergistic effects of adenovirus expressing wild-type p53 on chemosensitivity of non-small cell lung cancer cells. Cancer Gene Ther 2000;7:537-44.

92.   Ishida S, Yamashita T, Nakaya U, et al: Adenovirus-mediated transfer of p53-related genes induces apoptosis of human cancer cells. Jpn J Cancer Res 2000; 91:174-80.

93.   Clayman GL, El-Naggar AK, Lippman SM, et al: Adenovirus-mediated p53 gene transfer in patients with advanced recurrent head and neck squamous cell carcinoma. J Clin Oncol 1998;16:2221-32.

Chapter 13

NEW THERAPIES FOR LOCOREGIONALLY ADVANCED AND LOCOREGIONALLY RECURRENT HEAD AND NECK CANCER

Barry L. Wenig, M.D., M.P.H.
Feinberg School of Medicine, Northwestern University
Division of Otolaryngology - Head and Neck Surgery
Evanston Northwestern Healthcare

INTRODUCTION

The majority of head and neck cancers are squamous cell malignancies that arise on the mucosal surfaces of the upper aerodigestive tract. Histopathological classification of these tumors ranges from poorly differentiated to well-differentiated lesions. Approximately 42,000 new cases are documented in the United States annually resulting in more than 12,500 deaths each year. Surgery and radiotherapy are highly effective in the treatment of stage I and II head and neck cancers, but more than 70% of patients present with loco-regionally advanced (stage III and IV) disease (1). Loco-regional disease recurs often and metastatic disease develops in as many as 30% of patients (2,3).

THE BIOLOGY OF THE METASTATIC PROCESS

The biology of the metastatic process relates to the spread of cancer from the primary tumor to distant sites. Metastasis is a characteristic of malignancy. It results from the process of angiogenesis or neovascularization whereby new blood vessels are produced. In tumorigenesis, neovascularization is most commonly the rate-limiting step. Malignant cells are incapable of growing beyond the limits of oxygenation permitted by diffusion without the induction of new blood vessels. Early work by Tomlinson and Gray (4) showed that tumor necrosis develops in tumor cords with a central vessel and a radius exceeding 160 μm.

The hypothesis that tumor growth is dependent on the induction of neovascularization was originally proposed by Folkman (5). Tumor growth beyond the immediate borders of the tumor requires recruitment of new blood vessels. This new blood vessel formation involves interactions between endothelial cells and the extracellular matrix. Without this interaction the process cannot take place as tumors are angiogenesis-dependent diseases. This process is necessary for primary tumor growth, progression, and metastasis and is triggered by the release of polypeptide growth factors and cytokines by the tumor cells and cells of the host response to the tumor.

Metastasis, or the spread of tumor from the primary site to distant sites within the body, is one of the characteristics that determines a cancer's lethality. In head and neck malignancies, distant spread beyond the loco-regional area is equivalent to incurable disease. Hart and Saini (6) described the properties necessary for a cancer cell to acquire prior to being able to metastasize. As a general rule the first organ of metastasis tends to be the first capillary bed that detached cells from a clinically manifest tumor encounter. From primary metastases there is then spread to tumor-specific organs which in the case of head and neck tumors appears to be the lymphatic system of the neck.

CURRENT CONCEPTS IN TREATMENT

Despite impressive improvements in local control with current treatment modalities, 5-year survival rates in patients with advanced head and neck malignancies remain essentially unchanged over the past three decades (1). Palliative chemotherapy is often employed in those individuals who are considered beyond curative treatment or no longer curable. Although chemotherapy now plays an integral role in the treatment of locoregionally advanced disease, it has made little impact on survival in patients with metastatic disease.

Palliative care is defined as the active care of patients whose disease is not responsive to curative treatment. Control of pain, of other symptoms, and of psychological, social, and spiritual problems is paramount. The goal of palliative care is achievement of the best possible quality of life for patients and their families. Radiotherapy, chemotherapy and surgery all have a place in palliative care, provided that the symptomatic benefits of treatment clearly outweigh the disadvantages. Generally speaking, investigative procedures are kept to a minimum.

In keeping with the traditionally expressed role of treatment in recurrent or metastatic head and neck cancer most physicians believe that treatment should be palliative. Therefore, the most important outcomes are related to improvement of disease-related symptoms, such as pain, difficulty in swallowing, asthenia, anorexia and weight loss. Faced with treatment that can improve survival at the cost of severe and/or protracted toxicity, the practitioner must weigh survival benefit against treatment-induced adverse effects. In this kind of disease the quality of survival may be an even more important objective than the duration. If significant progress can be achieved with new therapeutic options, prolongation of survival might outweigh the toxicities of treatment.

INDICATORS PREDICTIVE OF CERVICAL METASTASES

Invasive squamous cell carcinoma of the upper aerodigestive tract has a strong predilection for metastatic spread to the cervical lymphatics. The status of the cervical lymph nodes is perhaps the single most important prognosticator in head and neck cancer, as the presence of metastatic disease significantly decreases chances for survival (7,8,9). Several factors have been shown to increase the risk for cervical metastases. These include the site of the primary tumor, tumor thickness, DNA ploidy, the status of margins, the presence or absence of perineural infiltration, and the presence of angioinvasion (10-12). A recent report by Martin-Villare et al. (13,) includes additional factors such as degree of differentiation and pre-epiglottic space involvement. Using a multiple regression analysis Jones et al. (14) determined that the two most significant variables as regards recurrence were the status of the margins and the depth of the primary tumor

IDENTIFICATION OF CERVICAL METASTASES

It is well established that specific primary sites will metastasize in a predictable manner to specific nodal regions within the neck. For nearly forty years, the classification used to define lymph node groups was that developed by Rouviere (7) in 1938 based on earlier classifications proposed by Trotter and Poirer and Charpy. Shah et al., (15) proposed a system based on levels rather than on triangles of the neck. Using this system we are able to anticipate the most probable sites of metastases for any given primary tumor as well as the most anticipated location of recurrent loco-regional disease. The presence or absence of nodal spread is critical in head and neck cancers as survival is impacted by this variable. Survival rates decrease by approximately 50% when nodal metastases are present with the rate of distant spread seeming to increase as well (16,17).

Given the importance of identifying loco-regional disease, what are the means available to the clinician to help detect or even to prevent the spread of disease to the cervical lymphatics? The most basic tool available is that of physical examination. Yet, it appears that clinical palpation of the neck is not a very accurate diagnostic modality. In fact, the accuracy of palpation for detecting metastatic lymph nodes ranges between 59% and 84%, depending on the site of the primary tumor (18).

Current imaging techniques include ultrasound, FNA-ultrasound, color Doppler ultrasound, CT, MR, and positron emission tomography (PET). Which is accurate, which is reliable and which is indicated to assist the clinician in the diagnostic algorithm? Kau et al., (19) discussing the available diagnostic modalities, determined that based on their data and reported literature, the accuracy of CT scanning (84.9%) and MR imaging (85%) was superior to that if palpation (67.9%) and ultrasound (72.7%). Ultrasound-guided fine needle aspiration cytology, a commonly employed diagnostic modality in Europe, was evaluated in an objective manner with 56 consecutive patients undergoing neck dissections following a US-FNA (20). The results yielded a sensitivity of 89.2%, a specificity of 98.1%, and an accuracy of 94.5%. Additionally, it correctly staged nodal disease in 93% of cases as compared with palpation which correctly diagnosed 61% of patients. This compares favorably with reported rates for positive emission tomography.

Yuasa et al., (21) reported on the use of ultrasonography alone without FNA for the early detection of cervical metastases. These authors accurately identified cervical metastases in 94.1% of patients.

Although generally accurate for soft tissue interpretation, CT scans for recurrent metastatic disease remain replete with diagnostic pitfalls. Three-dimensional spiral computed tomography imaging, however, appears to be a method that is suited to view spatial relationships between tumor, fascial spaces, adjacent soft tissues, and other structures (22). Using reconstructions performed in sagittal, coronal, and oblique planes 3D VR appears to be clearly advantageous over standard CT techniques.

MR imaging with its excellent soft tissue resolution, has been reported to be superior to CT for diagnostic accuracy (23). Limited references exist regarding its efficacy in detecting cervical nodal disease. By comparison with palpation in a prospective study MR demonstrated similar sensitivities and specificities (24). The authors of this study concluded that neither clinical examination nor MR alone can be relied upon to make decisions regarding the status of the neck.

Functional MR is a technique that uses ultra-small super-paramagnetic iron oxide particles known as Combidex MR. Nodes with tumor cells do not have the ability to concentrate iron particles. Hoffman and his colleagues (25) prospectively analyzed patients undergoing functional MR with subsequent neck dissections. This technique demonstrated a sensitivity of 95% and a specificity of 99%. These values were clearly higher than those for standard MR in any prior published study. This technique is limited however by its inability to identify small nodes.

2-fluoro-2-deoxy-D-glucose positron emission tomography (FDG-PET) is felt to be a sensitive tool for detecting primary malignant lesions as well as metastatic spread. Jungehulsing, et al. (26) prospectively investigated the sensitivity of FDG-PET in detecting occult primary carcinomas with manifestation in the head and neck lymph nodes. Only 26% of patients were found to have a primary tumor when thought to have an occult primary that went undiagnosed with conventional workup. Stoeckli et al., (27) found that FDG-PET was not as sensitive or as specific as sentinel node biopsy in diagnosing metastatic tumor in clinically negative nodes.

So where, if at all, is FDG-PET applicable? It may be that its role is more appropriate in identifying recurrent disease. Anzai et al., (28) compared FDG-PET to MR and/or CT in recurrent head and neck cancer. Recurrence was identified in 8 of 12 patients with FDG-PET yielding a sensitivity and specificity of 88% and 100%, respectively. These data were superior to either MR or CT in identifying recurrent disease. Sensitivity and specificity were very similar in work done by Lapela and colleagues (29). Complementary findings were reported by Lowe, (30), DiMartino, (31) Stokkel, (32) and Farber. (33). Lonneux and colleagues (34) studied the role of FDG-PET in symptomatic patients with suspected recurrent disease. In this prospective and consecutive inclusion study sensitivity and specificity of FDG-PET clearly exceeded that of either CT or MR confirming the earlier data of Anzai et al., (28).

Lymphatic mapping is designed to determine the nodal status of a region without the morbidity associated with an elective nodal dissection. In the treatment of regional lymphatics in malignant cutaneous melanoma several authors have shown that if the first drainage echelon (sentinel node) is free of micrometastases on histological examination then the chance of spread to the remaining lymphatics is very small (35-37). Lymphadenectomy in this situation and in breast cancer as well is carried out only when the biopsied sentinel node is positive for micrometastatic disease.

Successful radio-localization of the sentinel node in the upper aerodigestive tract was first described by Alex and Krag (38). Since this initial report these (39) and others have shown that the peritumoral injection of radionuclide/sulfur ^{99m}Tc can be measured in the cervical lymphatic basin with a gamma probe allowing for transcutaneous identification of nodal involvement. In fact, a clinical trial to test the role of selective nodal dissection in the setting of a cervical sentinel node radio-localization is currently ongoing in the American College of Surgeons Oncology Group (ACOSOG).

FACTORS RELATED TO OUTCOME OF SALVAGE THERAPY

The development of a recurrence in the neck following treatment for head and neck squamous cell carcinoma has been associated with a worsened prognosis (40-44). Isolated cervical recurrences occur in less than 5% of all patients with SCC of the head and neck as opposed to the vast majority of recurrences that appear also either at the primary site or in sites distant to the neck. Unfortunately, recurrence in a previously dissected neck carries with it a survival rate of approximately 5%.

Several treatment options have been proposed for recurrent cervical disease. Yet the question remains, what are the clinical factors that are associated with the outcome of salvage therapy? Krol et al., (45) in a retrospective, multi-institutional review of patient records with an isolated cervical recurrence in a previously treated neck, found a median survival for the entire study group of 11 months with a three year disease-free survival of 33%. Better survival appears to be present in the following groups: those with initially negative surgical resection margins, those with a non-surgical initial neck treatment, those with no history of prior recurrence, those with an ipsilateral location of the recurrence relative to the primary, and those undergoing surgical salvage as treatment for the recurrence. This latter point was confirmed by Schwartz et al. (46) in a study comparing treatment modalities for the treatment of recurrent oral cavity tumors.

Pivot and colleagues (47) performed a retrospective analysis of nearly 500 patients with recurrent squamous cell carcinomas of the head and neck. These authors found that statistically significantly favorable prognostic factors include: initially negative nodes, no initial chemotherapy exposure, induction chemotherapy response, long duration of disease-free survival, good performance status and lack of locoregional recurrence. Following a multivariate analysis of these data the authors concluded that loco-regional recurrence, performance status, and no initial chemotherapy exposure remain significant prognostic factors for overall survival following recurrent disease.

Jones et al. (14) retrospectively studied the treatment of recurrent Stage I and Stage II carcinomas of the oral cavity. A multivariate regression analysis revealed that following control for variables the only factors that were deemed significant for recurrence were the presence of a surgically positive margin or a tumor depth greater than 5 mm. The authors concluded that more extensive surgery as an initial therapy is not indicated and would not favorably impact on the recurrence rate.

CLINICAL PRESENTATION OF RECURRENT DISEASE

The most obvious presentations of recurrence include a visible or palpable mass present at the previously treated primary site or in the treated neck, or new onset (or worsening of chronic) dysphagia, odynophagia, dyspnea or swallowing difficultiies. Unusual presentations are often overlooked and factor into the early identification of the recurrence and subsequently the ability to successfully treat the recurrence.

The role of pain as a presenting sign of recurrent head and neck cancer is less often recognized in head and neck cancer is seldom addressed. Smit et al., (48) retrospectively studied the role of pain as a first sign of recurrence in 195 patients with 95 being the treatment group and 100 acting as a control group. Of the patients with proven recurrent disease, 70% reported pain as the primary symptom. The pain was referred in 35% of cases and localized in the remaining 65%. Wong and colleagues (49) evaluated 12 patients who developed head and neck recurrences that were all preceded by severe oro-facial pain. No clear indication of malignant disease was detected in any of these patients despite an extensive work-up. Clearly, pain as a symptom in patients with a history of SCC of the upper aero-digestive tract necessitates identification and treatment of a suspected recurrence with the utmost dispatch.

TREATMENT OPTIONS IN RECURRENT SCC OF THE HEAD AND NECK

Chemotherapy

Concomitant, or in some cases, induction chemotherapy, is appropriate for the treatment of locally advanced SCC of the head and neck because it allows organ preservation without compromising survival and it improves survival in unresectable disease. The choice of palliative chemotherapy treatment in recurrent or metastatic head and neck cancer continues to be controversial as long-term prognosis is poor and quality of life with chemotherapy is not always improved. The topic of chemotherapy for recurrent and metastatic head and neck cancer is covered in a previous chapter.

Re-Irradiation Therapy

Although previously considered "taboo", more and more clinicians today are re-considering the role of re-irradiation in the environment of recurrent head and neck tumors. Levendag, Meeuwis and Visser (44) reviewed their experience with both external beam therapy (EBRT) alone and external beam combined with interstitial radiation therapy (EBRT+IRT). Although improvement in local control was seen this did not translate into improved overall survival. Stevens, Britsch and Moss (50) treated 15 patients with recurrent disease using high-dose re-irradiation with EBRT. Five-year data showed a 17% survival rate with loco-regional control in 27% of patients. This study demonstrated successful curative treatment in a significant proportion of patients.

Brachytherapy alone has been reported in a number of different series. Senan and Levendag (51) utilized endoscopically-controlled IRT on 22 patients describing good results with acceptable complications. Krull et al., (52) retrospectively studied 19 patients all previously treated with ERT who received IRT. CR was achieved in 5 patients while 10 achieved a PR with a survival rate of 49% at 12 months and 35% at 24 months.

Concomitant chemotherapy plus re-irradiation

Multiple studies have begun to appear in the literature exploring the use of combined chemo-radiation in the previously treated patient population.

These studies attempt to replicate the results of those such as Brockstein et al., (53) who employed this type of treatment regimen in a primary treatment setting. Weppelmann and colleagues (54) reported a Phase I/II study of 21 patients treated with recurrent disease. 9 achieved a CR and 6 a PR with a 1-year actuarial survival of 56%. Gasparini et al. (55), treated 51 patients in a Phase II study with 5 having recurrent disease. Only one of these achieved an objective CR. Haraf and colleagues (56,57) reported on the use of continuous infusion 5-FU and hydroxyurea, both with and without paclitaxel, and concomitant RT, demonstrating overall survival, progression-free survival, and local/regional control at 5 years of 14.6%, 13.5%, and 20%, respectively. Spencer et al. (58), treated 35 patients with inoperable recurrent head and neck cancer using RT and 5-FU with hydroxyurea. Fifteen of 35 achieved a CR while 11 of 35 achieved a PR. The median survival rate was 10.5 months. Acceptable acute toxicity and minimal late effects resulted in encouraging response and survival rates.

Surgery

Salvage surgery appears to be a "double-edged sword" in that it may be the best option for many patients with recurrent tumor yet the benefit that it provides may come at an extremely high personal cost to the patient. Goodwin (59) performed a meta-analysis of 32 published reports to obtain an estimate of the average treatment effect for salvage surgery with regard to survival, disease-free survival, surgical complications, and operative mortality. The weighted average of 5-year survival was 39% of 1,080 patients. In the prospective study of 109 patients who underwent salvage surgery the median disease-free survival was 17.9 months correlating strongly with recurrent stage, weakly with recurrent site, and not at all with time to pre-salvage recurrence. Goodwin believed that the decision to undergo salvage surgery should be a personal choice made by the patient after an honest and compassionate discussion with the surgeon. Questions that need to be asked prior to deciding include:

Is the recurrence limited in scope and amenable to local therapy with curative intent?
Is safety altered by previous treatment?
Are function-preserving procedures possible despite prior treatment?
Is the success rate unacceptably low?
Is surgical decision making hindered by prior treatment?

Experimental Therapies

The goal of gene therapy is to introduce new genetic material into cancer cells that will selectively kill the cancer cells with no toxicity to the surrounding nonmalignant cells. Gene therapy uses a vector that is able to deliver a DNA sequence into cells which, in turn, incorporates itself into the cellular genome and produces proteins that will have a therapeutic effect (60). In vivo gene therapy involves the introduction of the vector directly with the gene into the tissues to be treated. The vector acts as a transport while the desired gene is contained, for example, in a plasmid which is a DNA strand that can result in messenger RNA production and, hence, protein production. Currently, the lack of an ideal vector is one of the major stumbling blocks of gene therapy. Gleich (60) reported on 20 patients who had failed conventional therapy and were treated with human leukocyte antigen (HLA)-B7 using a lipid vector. No adverse effects were seen with 4 patients having had a partial response and 2 with stable disease. The remaining 14 patients all demonstrated disease progression.

Ganly and colleagues (61) reported a Phase I study using Onyx-15, an E1B 55 kDa gene-detected adenovirus, administered by a single intratumoral injection to a total of 22 patients. No objective responses were observed however, MR studies suggested tumor necrosis in 5 patients. An additional 8 had stable disease lasting from 4-8 weeks. Hong et al used ONYX alone (62), and Khuri et al., (63) reporting from multiple centers, used ONYX -015 in combination with cisplatin and 5-FU. This Phase II trial enrolled 37 patients with documented objective shrinkage of tumor in 63% of patients who could be evaluated. Of these, there were 27% with a CR and 36% with a PR. The median survival overall was 11 months with the observation that by six months none of the responding tumors had progressed whereas all non-injected tumors treated with chemotherapy alone had progressed. Finally, Clayman (64), reporting on the current status of gene therapy, noted that several randomized studies of the p53 adenovirus (AdCMVp53) have been initiated to determine its role as a surgical adjuvant in untreated disease and in combination with DNA-damaging agents.

Intratumoral injections also include the possibility of utilizing chemotherapeutic agents delivered directly into recurrent disease. Cisplatin-epinephrine gel has been tested in comparable randomized, prospective, double-blinded studies yielding similar results in North American and European study groups (65). A durable CR was reported in 19% of patients with a PR being seen in an additional 11%. Systemic toxicities were minimal and side effects were generally limited to local pain and swelling. These results were comparable to other, more traditional modalities.

Photodynamic therapy is a treatment modality that combines the use of a photosensitizing injectable dye with specific laser wavelength (energy) resulting in the activation of the dye and the production of a singlet oxygen reaction. This, in turn, produces tumor necrosis and death. Although highly effective, this treatment is currently limited to tumors that are relatively superficial (depth of less than 10mm) as the laser light is delivered in a manner that is described as "front surface" (directed on the tumor) rather than in an implantable manner. Activation of the drug is thereby limited by the thickness or depth of the tumor that will allow only a certain amount of penetration of the laser light. In patients with recurrence on the mucosal surface of the aero-digestive tract rather than in the cervical lymphatics that are not easily accessible, reports indicate excellent, durable responses (66).

CONCLUSIONS

Despite advances in treatment of primary tumors of the head and neck region, recurrent disease signals an ominous outcome for the patient. Recurrent and/or metastatic head and neck squamous cell carcinoma continues to be a significant cause of cancer-related morbidity and mortality. Improved surveillance and surgical reconstruction methods should help to enhance the capability of surgery to salvage tumors resistant to prior chemotherapy and radiation therapy. Several recently introduced chemotherapeutic agents either alone or in combination with other agents or re-irradiation appears to be extremely active and effective in this patient population. The upcoming decade is likely to see many trials of novel agents either alone or in combination with currently available treatment options. The availability of these new therapeutic regimens may expand the options of patients with recurrent disease and hopefully will help improve the outcome in a group of patients who otherwise have little prospect of attaining cure.

REFERENCES

1. Vokes, E.E., Weichselbaum, R.R., Lippman, S.M., Hong, W.K. (1993). Head and Neck Cancer. New Engl J Med 328, 185-194.
2. Suit, H.D., and Westgate, S.J. (1986). Impact of improved local control on survival. Int J Radiat Oncol Biol Phys 12, 453-458.
3. Strong, E.W. (1983). Treatment failure in head and neck cancer. Cancer Treat Symp 2, 5-20.
4. Tomlinson, R.H., and Gray, L.H. (1955). The histological structure of some human lung cancers and the possible implications for radiotherapy. Br J Cancer 9, 539-549.

5.   Folkman, J. (1971). Tumor angiogenesis: Therapeutic implications. N Eng J Med 285, 1182-1186.

6.   Hart, A., and Saini, A. (1992) Biology of Tumor Metastasis. Lancet 339, 1453-1457.

7.   Som, P.M. (1987). Lymph nodes of the neck. Radiology 165, 593-600.

8.   Shah, J.P. (1990). Patterns of cervical lymph node metastasis from squamous cell carcinomas of the upper aerodigestive tract. Am J Surg 160, 405-409.

9.   Shah, J.P., and Tollefsen, H.R. (1974). Epidermoid carcinoma of the supraglottic larynx: role of neck dissection in initial surgical treatment. Am J Surg 128, 494-499.

10.   Ho, C.M., Lam, K.H., Wei, W.I., Lau, S.K., Lam, L.K. (1992). Occult lymph node metastasis in small oral tongue cancers. Head Neck 14, 359-363.

11.   Johnson, J.T. (1990). A surgeon looks at cervical lymph nodes. Radiology 175, 607-610.

12.   Fakih, A.R., Rao, R.S., Borges, A.M., Pate, A.R. (1989). Elective versus therapeutic neck dissection in early carcinoma of the oral tongue. Am J Surg 158, 309-313.

13.   Martin-Villares, C., Poch Broto, J., Ortega Medina, L., Iglesias Moreno, M.C., Gonzalez Gimeno, M.J. (2000). Acta Otorrinolaringol Esp 51, 330-334.

14.   Jones, K.R., Lodge-Rigal, R.D., Reddick, R.L., Tudor, G.E., Shockley, W.W. (1992). Prognostic factors in recurrence of stage I and II squamous cell carcinoma of the oral cavity. Arch Otolaryngol Head Neck Surg 118, 483-485.

15.   Shah, J.P., Strong, E.W., Spiro, R.H., Vikram, B. (1981). Surgical grand rounds: neck dissection: current status and future possibilities. Clin Bull 11, 25-33.

16.   Leemans, C.R., Tiwar, R., Nauta, J.J.P., van der Waal, I., Snow, G.B. (1993). Regional lymph node involvement and its significance in the development of distant metastases in the head and neck carcinoma. Cancer 71, 452-456.

17.   Leemans, C.R., Tiwar, R., Nauta, J.J.P., van der Waal, I., Snow, G.B. (1994). Recurrence at the primary site in head and neck cancer and the significance of neck lymph node metastases as a prognostic factor. Cancer 73, 187-190.

18.   Sako, K., Pradier, R.N., Marchetta, F.C., Pickren, J.W. (1964). Fallibility of palpation in the diagnosis of metastases to cervical nodes. Surg Gynaecol Obstet 118, 989-990.

19.   Kau, R.J., Alexiou C., Stimmer, H., Arnold, W. Diagnostic procedures for detection of lymph node metastases in cancer of the larynx. J Oto Rhino Laryngol 62, 199-203.

20.   Knappe, M., Louw, M., Gregor, R.T. (2000). Ultrasonograpgy-guided fine-needle aspiration for the assessment of cervical metastases. Arch Otolaryngol Head Neck Surg 126, 1091-1096.

21.   Yuasa, K., Kawazu, T., Kunitake, N., Uehara, S., Omagari, J., Yoshiura, K., Nakayama, E., Kanda, S. (2000). Sonography for the detection of cervical lymph node metastases among patients with tongue cancer: criteria for early detection and assessment of follow-up examination intervals. Am J Neuroradiol 21, 1127-1132.

22. Franca, C., Levin-Plotnik, D., Sehgal, V., Chen, R.T., Ramsey, R.G. (2000). Use of three-dimensional spiral computed tomography imaging for staging and surgical planning of head and neck cancer. J Digital Imag 13, 24-32.

23. Lufkin, R.B., and Hanafee, W.N. (1988). Magnetic resonance imaging of the head and neck. Invest Radiol 23, 162-169.

24. Hao, S.P., and Ng, S.H. (2000). Magnetic resonance imaging versus clinical palpation in evaluating cervical metastasis from head and neck cancer. Otolaryngol Head Neck Surg 123, 324-327.

25. Hoffman, H.T., Quets, J., Toshiaki, T., Funk, G.F., McCulloch, T.M., Graham, S.M., Robinson, R.A., Schuster, M.E., Yuh, W.T. (2000). Functional magnetic resonance imaging using iron oxide particles in characterizing head and neck adenopathy. Laryngoscope 110, 1425-1430.

26. Jungehulsing, M., Scheidhauer, K., Damm, M., Pietrzyk, U., Eckel, H., Schicha, H., Stennert, E. (2000). 2(F)-fluro-2-deoxy-D-glucose positron emission tomography is a sensitive tool for the detection of occult primary cancer with head and neck lymph node manifestation. Otolaryngol Head Neck Surg 123, 294-301.

27. Stoeckli, S.J., Steinert, H., Pfaltz, M., Schmid, S. (2002). Is there a role for positron emission tomography with 18-F fluorodeoxyglucose in the initial staging of nodal negative oral and oropharyngeal squamous cell carcinoma. Head Neck 24, 345-349.

28 .Anzai, Y., Carroll, W.R., Quint, D.J., Bradford, C.R., Minoshima, S., Wolf, G.T., Wahl, R.L. (1996). Recurrence of head and neck cancer after surgery or irradiation: prospective comparison of 2-deoxy-2-(F-18) fluoro-D-glucose PET and MR imaging diagnoses. Radiology 200, 135-141.

29. Lapela, M., Grenman, R., Kurki, T., Joensuu, H., Leskinen, S., Lindholm, P., Haarparanta, M., Ruotsalainen, U., Minn, H. (1995). Head and neck cancer: detection of recurrence with PET and 2-(F-18) fluoro-2-deoxy-D-glucose. Radiology 197, 205-211.

30. Lowe, V.J., Boyd, J.H., Dunphy, F.R., Kim, H., Dunleavy, T., Collins, B.T., Martin, D., Stack, B.C. Jr., Hollenbeak, C., Fletcher, J.W. (2000). Surveillance for recurrent head and neck cancer using positron emission tomography. J Clin Oncol 18, 651-658.

31. Westhofen, M. (2000). Diagnosis and staging of head and neck cancer: a comparison of modern imaging modalities with panendoscopic and histopathologic findings. Arch Otolaryngol Head Neck Surg 126, 1457-1461.

32. Stokkel, M.P., Terhaard, C.H., Hordijk, G.J., van Rijk, P.P. (1999). The detection of local recurrent head and neck cancer with fluorine-18 fluorodeoxyglucose dual-head positron emission tomography. Europ J Nucl Med 26, 767-773.

33. Farber, L.A., Benard, F., Machtay, M., Smith, R.J., Weber, R.S., Weinstein, G.S., Chalian, A.A., Alavi, A., Rosenthal, D.I. (1999). Detection of recurrent head and neck squamous cell carcinomas after radiation therapy with 2-18F-fluoro-2-deoxy-D-glucose-positron emission tomography. Laryngoscope 109, 970-975.

34. Lonneux, M., Lawson, G., Ide, C., Bausart, R., Remacle, M., Pauwels, S. (2000). Positron emission tomography with fluorodeoxyglucose for suspected head and neck tumor recurrence in the symptomatic patient. Laryngoscope 110, 1493-1497.

35. Morton, D.L., Duan-Ren, W., Wong, J.H., Economou, J.S., Cagle, L.A., Storm, F.K., Foshag, L.J., Cochran, A.J. (1992). Technical details of intraoperative lymphatic mapping for early stage melanoma. Arch Surg 127, 392-399.

36. Thompson, J.F., McCarthy, W.H., Bosch, C.M.J., O'Brien, C.J., Quinn, M.J., Paramaesvaran, S., Crotty, K., McCarthy, S.W., Uren, R.F., Howman-Giles, R. (1995). Sentinel lymph node status as an indicator of the presence of metastatic melanoma in regional lymph nodes. Melanoma Res 5, 255-260.

37. Albertini, J.J., Cruse, C.W., Rapaport, D., Wells, K., Ross, M., DeConti, R., Berman, C.G., Jared, K., Messina, J., Lyman, G., Glaus, F., Fenske, N., Reintgen, D.S. (1996). Intraoperative radiolymphoscintigraphy improves sentinel lymph node identification for patients with melanoma. Ann Surg 223, 217-224.

38. Alex, J.C., and Krag, D.N. (1993). Gamma-probe-guided localization of lymph nodes. Surg Oncol 2, 137-144.

39. Alex, J.C., Sasaki, C.T., Krag, D.N., Wenig, B.L., Pyle, P.B. (2000). Sentinel lymph node radiolocalization in head and neck squamous cell carcinoma. Laryngoscope 110, 198-203.

40. Pearlman, R.W. (1979). Treatment outcome in recurrent head and neck cancer. Arch Surg 114, 39-42.

41. Khafif, R.A., Gelbfish, G.A., Attie, J.N., Tepper, P., Zingale, R. (1989). Thirty-year experience with 457 radical neck dissections in cancer of the mouth, pharynx, and larynx. Am J Surg 158, 303-307.

42. Sisson, G.A. (1974). The philosophy underlying the treatment of recurrent cancer of the head and neck. Otolaryngol Clin N Am 7, 153-161.

43. Kohal, W.A., Neifeld, J.P., Eisert, D.R., Terz, J.J., Lawrence Jr., W. (1983). Management of locoregional recurrent oropharyngeal carcinoma. Am J Surg 146, 436-438.

44. Levendag, P.C., Meewis, C.A., Visser, A.G. (1992). Reirradiation of recurrent head and neck cancers: external and/or interstitial radiation therapy. Radiotherap Oncol 23, 6-15.

45. Krol, B.J., Righi, P.D., Paydarfar, J.A., Cheng, E.T., Smith, R.M., Lai, D.C., Bhargava, V., Piccirillo, J.F., Hayes, J.T., Lue, A.J., Scher, R.L., Weisberger, E.C., Wilson, K.M., Tran, L.E., Rizk, N., Pellitteri, P.K., Terris, D.J. (2000). Otolaryngol Head Neck Surg 123, 368-376.

46. Schwartz, G.J., Mehta, R.H., Wenig, B.L., Shaligram, C., Portugal, L.G. (2000). Salvage treatment for recurrent squamous cell carcinoma of the oral cavity. Head Neck 22, 34-41.

47. Pivot, X., Niyikiza, C., Poissonnet, G., Dassonville, O., Bensadoun, R.J., Guardiola, E., Foa, C., Benezery, K., Demard, F., Thyss, A., Schneider, M. (2001). Clinical prognostic factors for patients with recurrent head and neck cancer: implications for randomized trials. Oncology 61, 197-204.

48. Smit, M., Balm, A.J., Hilgers, F.J., Tan, I.B. (2001). Pain as a sign of recurrent disease in head and neck squamous cell carcinoma. Head Neck 23, 372-375.

49. Wong, J.K., Wood, R.E., McLean, M. (1998). Pain preceding recurrent head and neck cancer. J Orofacial Pain 12, 52-59.
50. Stevens, K.R. Jr., Bristch, A., Moss, W.T. (1994). High-dose reirradiation of head and neck cancer with curative intent. Int J Rad Oncol Biol Physics 29, 687-698.
51. Senan, S., and Levendag, P.C. Brachytherapy for recurrent head and neck cancer. (1999). Hematol Clin N Am 13, 531-542.
52. Krull, A., Friedrich, R.E., Schwarz, R., Thurmann, H., Schmelzle, R., Alberti, W. (1999). Anticancer Res 19, 2695-2697.
53. Brockstein B. E., Haraf, D.J., Stenson, K., Sulzen, L., Witt, M.E., Weichselbaum, R.W., Vokes, E.E. (2000). A phase I-II study of concomitant chemoradiotherapy with paclitaxel, 5-fluorouracil and hydroxyurea with granulocyte colony stimulating factor support for patients with poor prognosis head and neck cancer. Ann Oncol 11, 721-728.
54. Weppelmann, B., Wheeler, R.H., Peters, G.E., Kim, R.Y., Spencer, S.A., Meredith, R.F., Salter, M.M. (1992). Treatment of recurrent head and neck cancer with 5-fluorouracil, hydroxyurea, and reirradiation. Int J Radiat Oncol Biol Phys 22, 1051-1056.
55. Gasparini, G., Recher, G., Testolin, A., DalFior S., Panizzoni, G.A., Cristoferi, V., Squaquara, R., Pozza, F. (1992) Synchronous radiotherapy and chemotherapy with cisplatin in the management of locally advanced or recurrent head and neck cancer. Am J Clin Oncol 15, 242-249.
56. Haraf, D.J., Weichselbaum, R.R., Vokes, E.E. (1996). Re-irradiation with concomitant chemotherapy of unresectable recurrent head and neck cancer: a potentially curable disease. Ann Oncol 7, 913-918.
57. Haraf, D.J., Stenson, K., List, M., Witt, M.E., Weichselbaum, R.R., Vokes, E.E. (1997). Continuous infusion paclitaxel, 5-fluorouracil, and hydroxyurea with concomitant radiotherapy in patients with advanced or recurrent head and neck cancer. Sem Oncol 24, S2-68-S2-71.
58. Conner, W., Salter, M.M. (1999). Concomitant chemotherapy and reirradiation as management for recurrent cancer of the head and neck. Am J Clin Oncol 22, 1-5.
59. Goodwin, W.J. (2000). Salvage surgery for patients with recurrent squamous cell carcinoma of the upper aerodigestive tract: when do ends justify means? Laryngoscope 110, 1-18.
60. Gleich, L.L. (2000). Gene therapy for head and neck cancer. Laryngoscope 110, 708-726.
61. Ganly, I., Eckhardt, S.G., Rodriguez, G.I., Soutar, D.S., Otto, R., Roberston, A.G., Park, O., Gulley, M.L., Heise, C., Von Hoff, D.D., Kaye, S.B. (2000). A phase I study of Onyx-015, an E1B attenuated adenovirus, administered intratumorally to patients with recurrent head and neck cancer. Clin Cancer Res 6, 798-806.
62. Hong, W.K., Kirn, D.H. (2000). A controlled study of intratumoral ONYX-015, a selectively-replicating adenovirus, in combination with cisplatin and 5-fluorouracil in patients with recurrent head and neck cancer. Nature Med 6, 879-885.

63.   Khuri F.R., Nemunaitis, J, Arseneau, J., Tannock, I.F., Romel, L, Gore, M., Ironside, J., MacDougall, R.H., Heise, C., Randlev, B., Gillenwater, A.M., Bruso, P., Kaye, S.B.,

64.   Clayman, G.L. (2000). The current status of gene therapy. Sem Oncol 27, 39-43.

65.   Wenig, B.L., Werner, J.A., Castro, D.J., Sridhar, K.S., Garewal, H.S., Kehrl, W., Pluzanska, A., Arndt, O., Costantino, P.D., Mills, G.M., Dunphy II, F.R., Orenberg, E.K., Leavitt, R.D. (2002). The role of intratumoral therapy with cisplatin/epinephrine injectable gel in the management of advanced squamous cell carcinoma of the head and neck. Arch Otolaryngol Head Neck Surg 128, 880-885.

66.   Wenig, B.L., Kurtzman, D.M., Grossweiner, L.I. (1990). Photodynamic therapy in the treatment of squamous cell carcinoma of the head and neck. Arch Otolaryngol Head Neck Surg 116, 1267-1270.

Chapter 14

QUALITY OF LIFE AND LATE TOXICITIES IN HEAD AND NECK CANCER

Marcy A. List, PhD and John StracksB.A.
University of Chicago Cancer Research Center, Chicago, IL 60637

INTRODUCTION

Historically, the success or value of a specific cancer treatment was judged by objective tumor response, overall survival and/or disease-free survival. With the increasing use of multi-modality treatment, particularly in HNC, and the growing number of survivors, the need to understand patients' experience, their perceptions of treatment effects and their priorities has become well recognized. Health care interventions must be evaluated not only by their impact on quantity of life, but also on quality of life (QOL). In certain cases or for certain patients, extended survival with poor QOL may not be the outcome of choice; palliative treatment that reduces symptoms or no treatment—an option that spares patients specific toxicities, while not lengthening life—may enhance QOL.

For patients with HNC in particular, appreciation of the full impact of the disease and its treatment is critical. Since many HNC patients present with advanced stage disease,[1] treatment tends to be aggressive with significant acute and long-term effects. Both the disease and the effects of therapy interfere with basic human functions such as eating, speaking and breathing, which can have a drastic influence on day to day activities and QOL.

DEFINITION OF QOL

Health-related quality of life (HRQOL) may be defined as the patient's perception of the impact of illness and/or treatment. It is distinguished from more standard toxicity ratings in that it is from the perspective of and rated by the patient rather than the physician. There are two fundamental premises of HRQOL: multi-dimensionality, that is, it encompasses a broad range of domains; and subjectivity, referring to the fact that two people may have substantially different reactions to a similar disability. While specific definitions vary, QOL is generally considered to include at least three, and often four domains:[2-5]

- Physical/somatic (eg, pain, nausea, and fatigue)
- Functional (eg, energy level, and activities of daily living)
- Social (eg, maintenance of relationships with family and friends)
- Psychological/emotional (eg, mood, anxiety, and depression)

QOL further differs from traditional treatment endpoints such as response rate or survival in its fluidity, as its level for an individual patient can vary widely over time due to a variety of conditions and events.

HISTORY OF HNC QOL

The understanding that non-medical factors can affect patients' health and well-being has been acknowledged as far back as Hippocrates.[6] The study of QOL in HNC is, of course, a more recent development, with the earliest study being published in 1953.[7] That study, like many of the ones that followed it, was a cross-sectional, descriptive look at the psychological outcome of patients undergoing laryngectomy. Until the mid-1980's, most HNC QOL studies focused only on one aspect (either physical or psychological) of one type of disease (cancer of the larynx).[6] Since 1985, the study of HNC QOL has exploded both in scope and in methodology. A number of well-validated, reliable HNC-specific assessment tools having been developed and research has expanded to include the full spectrum of HNC diagnoses (eg oropharynx, nasopharynx) and treatments (surgery, radiation, chemotherapy, and chemoprevention). One of the most important advances has been the use of prospective, longitudinal designs, that is, the collection of pre-treatment data followed by the systematic collection of post-treatment data over time. Only about a quarter of studies published from 1985-1997 were longitudinal in design,[8,9] compared to well over half the studies done in the past three years.

QOL ASSESSMENT

Measures

There are currently a wide range of QOL instruments available to researchers and clinicians and the measure selected for use in a given study should be based on the purpose of the assessment. General measures, such as the Medical Outcomes Study 36-Item Short Form (MOS SF-36)[10] or the Psychosocial Adjustment to Illness Scale-Self Report (PAIS-SR)[11] can be used to evaluate a patient's overall adjustment to one's illness. With questions such as "has your overall health significantly increased or decreased over the past month," and "can you walk up a flight of stairs" the use of a general health measure can capture the patient's opinion of whether the disease has had a substantial affect on one's overall physical and emotional health.

A second level of information can be obtained using measures that are specific to cancer such as The Functional Assessment of Cancer Therapy (FACT-G)[2,12] and the European Organization for Research and Treatment of Cancer Quality of Life Questionnaire Core 30 Items (EORTC QLQ-30).[13,14] These instruments address global QOL as well as the multitude of ways in which cancer and cancer treatments can affect patients. For example, they include items related to symptoms such as nausea and vomiting, fatigue, relationships with family and friends, and the ability to work and do normal activities. In general, individual items are collapsed and summarized as domain scores including but not limited to physical, emotional, functional, and social well-being or function. These cancer specific instruments allow for comparison between patients with different types of cancers.

Most cancers and cancer treatments have side effects, symptoms and/or residual effects that are disease specific (e.g., swallowing related to HNC or lymphedema related to breast cancer). The FACT and the EORTC have HNC specific modules which are added to the general measure (FACT Head and Neck subscale (FACT H&N)[15,16] and EORTC QLQ Head and Neck (H&N-35)[17-19]). Other measures such as the Performance Status Scale-Head and Neck (PSS-HN)[20] and the University of Washington Quality of Life Questionnaire (UW-QOL)[21] are available to specifically assess patients' ability to eat, their ability to swallow and communicate, and other symptoms that are more severe in HNC treatment than in other types of cancer treatment. Several studies have suggested that combining general measures with HNC specific measures provide the most complete picture of QOL.[15-17]

Finally there are a number of modality specific measures such as the McMaster Radiotherapy Questionnaire (RTQ),[22] which measures the effect of radiation on skin, swallowing, levels of saliva and other symptoms, and the Quality of Life-Radiation Therapy Instrument (QOL-RTI),[23] a non-site specific measure of the effect of radiation therapy using a visual analog scale. The QOL-RTI also has a companion measure for HNC (H&N module).[24]

In addition, one might assess depression, anxiety or other psychological factors using any number of reliable and valid tools. The Beck Depression Inventory (BDI)[25] or the Centers for Epidemiologic Studies-Depression Scale (CES-D)[26] can quickly screen patients at every assessment point for the prevalence of depressive symptoms.

Choosing Measures

Choice of measure will depend on the question being asked (e.g., comparing the specific effects of different radiation treatment regimens, a comprehensive assessment of the broad range of potential symptoms and side effects of a new treatment) and available resources. For instance, investigators at the University of Chicago have focused, clinically, on the refinement of chemoradiotherapy regimens for locoregionally advanced HNC patients. The purpose of the accompanying QOL research has been to examine both the acute and long-term effects of each of these regimens.[27-29] This goal has necessitated a rather comprehensive assessment with longitudinal follow-up. Patients enrolled on specific protocols are assessment pre-treatment, on-treatment and at several time points post treatment. Assessment includes overall QOL (FACT-G), HNC-specific functional status (PSS-HN eating, speaking, and socializing), HNC-specific symptoms (FACT H&N subscale), overall performance status (Karnofsky performance status scale),[30] the specific effects of radiation therapy (RTQ), and depression screen (CES-D). The entire assessment takes 10-20 minutes per assessment point.

Schedule of assessments

The schedule of assessments is also dependent on the research question of interest. Because HNC patients may present with co-morbidities related to tobacco and alcohol abuse and because studies have shown that pre-treatment QOL is the best predictor of post-treatment QOL,[29,31,32] the collection of baseline data is imperative. Post-treatment, the question of how often to assess patients requires a balance between the desire to closely track changes in patients' QOL over time and the financial, personnel, and analytic burdens of assessing patients too frequently. Studies often assess patients at baseline and the end of treatment, and then 1, 6, 12, and 24 months following treatment. Figure 1 below presents a schematic example of how the longitudinal collection of QOL data can be vital to truly differentiating the effect of two different types of treatments.

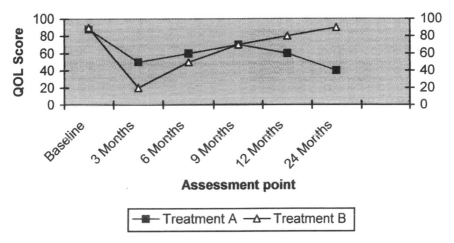

Figure 1. **QOL Assessment Schedule**

In this illustration, the different lines represent different treatment arms. The QOL scores are shown on the Y-axis while the time since treatment is shown on the X-axis. At baseline groups have similar QOL scores; during treatment patients receiving treatment B show a more profound decline in QOL and by 6 months both groups have returned to about 50% of pre-treatment levels. If one had stopped following patients at 3 months, however, one might have concluded that treatment B had more residual toxicity. If stopped at 6 months, treatments would have been considered equivalent. At 12 months it is beginning to appear that treatment B patients are doing better and at 24 months, treatment B patients have returned to their pre-treatment levels while those receiving treatment A are declining.

CURRENT RESEARCH

As described above, there has been both a broadening of the spectrum of HNC research as well as a more focused approach to specific issues and questions. Recent studies have included examinations of: the effects of different treatments on QOL, disease site and stage as related to QOL, the QOL of long-term survivors, specific symptoms of HNC, patients' priorities and preferences in regard to treatment, substance use, the relationship between function and QOL, QOL predictors of disease survival or progression, and, ever increasingly, interventions aimed at maximizing patient QOL during and following treatment. The remainder of this chapter will explore the research done in this area over the past several years.

Effect of treatment on QOL

Impact of surgery

Some of the possible results of surgical resection include disfigurement, voice loss, and difficulty with chewing and/or swallowing (see Table 2 for a complete list). These dysfunctions have been associated with moderate to severe distress, negative self image, and disturbed interpersonal relationships.[33-36] Feelings of shame while eating in the presence of others, a decrease in social and sexual activity, diminished social acceptance, and related financial repercussions have also been reported.[33,34,37]

Over the past decade there has been an emphasis on less extensive surgeries with greater attempts at organ preservation.[1,38] In contrast to earlier cross-sectional studies assessing QOL outcomes in post-laryngectomy patients,[6] recent studies have been longitudinal in design and thus able to provide some data on the effects of different types of surgery on QOL[39-42]. Results suggest that advances in surgical techniques have decreased the long-term morbidity of some procedures. In addition, while significant deficits may be seen during and shortly after treatment, recent data indicate that the overall QOL of many patients returns to pre-treatment levels or beyond with pre-treatment QOL proving to be a good predictor of post treatment QOL. For example, Rogers, et al classified 130 primary surgery patients at baseline into three distinct groups based on their QOL scores at baseline. All groups deteriorated on treatment and recovered post-treatment, but the groups remained distinct over the course of the study.[42]

Researchers have also examined the effects of different types of neck dissections on QOL. For example, surgeries sparing the spinal accessory nerve (CN XI) have been associated with significantly less pain at comparable lengths of time post-treatment.[43] Furthermore, when CN XI was spared, patients with no level V dissection scored better on pain and eating scales than patients with level V dissection. The authors caution however, that while such data may assist in decision making, survival and eradication of cancer should be the primary determining factors in decisions about type of neck dissection. Results from a second study found that, at both 6 and 12 months, radical neck dissection was associated with significantly greater shoulder dysfunction than either selective neck or modified radical neck dissections.[44] Comparing the latter two procedures, modified radical neck dissection was associated with greater shoulder disability at 6 months, but by 12 months these patients were comparable to those treated with selective neck dissection.

Impact of radiation therapy

Given the severity of radiation toxicities and the fact that radiation therapy has long been considered an alternative to invasive surgery, there has been considerable exploration of the effects of radiation therapy on QOL. [46-49] While these sequalae generally do not include physical disfigurement or voice loss, the impact on swallowing, chewing, taste and other symptoms (see table 2) may be as bad or worse than those of surgery.

Table 2. **Common Treatment Effects**[27,33,45]

Surgery	Radiation therapy
Impaired speech and/or changes in voice quality	Problems eating – chewing, swallowing
Problems eating and drinking – drooling; choking	Xerostomia (dry mouth)
Disfigurement	Decreased sense of taste/smell
Decreased sense of taste/smell	Esophageal stricture
Respiratory problems	Osteoradionecrosis
	Dental problems: trismus, tooth decay
	Voice hoarseness

Several recent studies have explored the impact of different radiation schedules on HNC patient QOL. In a long- term (7 to 11 years post treatment) follow-up of a randomized study, hypofractionated radiation (2.35 Gy daily, four days per week) was associated with similar or better QOL when compared to conventionally fractionated RT (2 Gy daily, five days per week),[50] though there was considerable psychological distress in all patients. Another study examined laryngeal cancer patients receiving either continuous hyperfractionated accelerated radiation therapy (CHART) (primarily stage II disease) or conventional fractionation (primarily stage I disease). While target volumes and initial QOL scores were similar across groups, those receiving CHART showed greater improvement in QOL at one year despite more severe initial toxicity.[51] In a large randomized trial of 615 patients with advanced HNC, more severe physical and emotional acute effects accompanied CHART, compared to conventional radiotherapy. In contrast, symptoms were more persistent in the conventionally treated group.[52] Finally, A study comparing patients treated with conventional therapy to those treated with concomitant boost RT found no differences between the groups. The researchers did find that xerostomia was a major contributor to poorer QOL.[53]

Impact of surgery vs radiation therapy

With ever greater numbers of patients being treated with radiation therapy with or without surgery, several researchers have attempted to compare QOL in patients treated with radiation alone to those treated with surgery with or without radiotherapy. Results have generally suggested better QOL and functional results in the radiation only group. For example, in a retrospective study of 40 patients with base of tongue tumors, PSS-HN scores for patients treated with primary radiation (n=30) were compared to those in patients treated with initial resection (n =10).[54] Survival and local control rates were similar, but the radiated patients had better scores in all three areas of the PSS-HN even when T-stage was taken into account. In a long-term (median 5-year) follow-up study, the radiation patients reported fairly good QOL, as three-quarters of the group had returned to pre-treatment employment status and their FACT scores were higher than published norms for mixed cancer patients. They did, however, report numerous residual symptoms including xerostomia, difficulty swallowing, decreased energy, worry, change in taste and pain.[47] Another small study of 13 relapse-free survivors of advanced stage (III or IV) oropharyngeal cancer similarly suggested that, at 12 months, the surgically treated patients had more difficulties with appearance and speech although all patients had problems swallowing and chewing.[55] The surgical patients did report less pain. It is important to note that the data presented above derives from small non-randomized studies and thus are subject to selection bias.

Chemoradiotherapy

In the past decade, HNC has been more frequently treated with organ preserving, neo-adjuvant or concomitant chemoradiotherapy. While generally successful in minimizing the disfigurements of surgery, these regimens still have major effects on QOL. In a longitudinal study of 64 patients with advanced HNC treated with curative-intent concomitant chemoradiotherapy, acute treatment toxicities were severe, with initial significant declines in virtually all QOL domains.[29] However, by 12 months, general functional and physical measures had returned to baseline levels (good to excellent). Although up to one-third of patients continued to report difficulties at one year such as swallowing problems, hoarseness, and mouth pain, these were similar to baseline frequencies. Adverse effects that were more prevalent at 12 months post treatment compared to pre-treatment included dry mouth (58% versus 17%), difficulty with taste (32% versus 8%), and diet restricted to soft foods (82% versus 42%). Similar acute declines followed by rebounds in swallowing and overall QOL were reported in a study of intraarterial chemotherapy and radiation.[56] At six months post completion of therapy, mean QOL surpassed pretreatment levels.

Of particular interest in the evaluation of chemoradiotherapy protocols are the follow-up QOL data from the VA Larynx Trial in which patients with stage III or IV laryngeal cancer were randomized to sequential chemotherapy followed by radiotherapy or standard laryngectomy and postoperative radiation. In a report of 46 (25 assigned to surgery plus radiation and 21 to chemotherapy plus radiation) long-term survivors 8-13 years post treatment, significantly better QOL scores and less head and neck pain were found in the chemotherapy plus radiation group.[57] Compared to patients undergoing laryngectomy, those who maintained a functioning larynx had less body pain, better mental health, better emotional scores and less depression. Interestingly, there were no significant differences in speech and communication scores between the two groups. The differences in QOL appear to suggest that the differences are due to the surgery, not the type of surgery (i.e., removal of the larynx), and the differences show up in physical and mental domains, not functional domains as would have been initially postulated.

Combination therapies

QOL research in HNC has clearly demonstrated the toxicity inherent in combination treatment. In addition to the late effects shown in combined chemoradiotherapy protocols, surgery plus radiotherapy has been associated with greater physical morbidity than either one alone,[8,58-60] even in patients more than three years out of treatment.[61]

QOL research by symptom

Pain

There has been considerable variability in the frequency and severity of pain reported by HNC patients. These discrepancies may be attributable, at least in part, to differences in time since treatment as well as how pain was measured. For example, data from several investigations suggest that head and neck pain may increase during or shortly post treatment[62] and then decrease over time.[58,63] Similarly, while long-term head and neck pain or discomfort has been cited in close to 60% of patients,[60,64] considerably fewer patients (2% - 25%) report moderate or severe pain.[60,63-65] Reports of the amount of pain associated with neck dissection have also been variable. While Chaplin[63] noted increased pain over time and no association with type of neck dissection, Kuntz and Weymuller[44] observed improvements in patients who had undergone selective or modified radical neck dissection, but not for those with radical neck dissection. This latter group also had persistent shoulder dysfunction. Terrell found less shoulder pain in a group who had selective neck dissections as compared to modified radical neck dissections, and both groups had less pain than patients who received a radical neck dissection.[43]

Mood disorders

Mood disorders such as depression, anxiety, worry, and fatigue can be serious side effects of HNC treatment.[66-68] Most QOL instruments include several questions on emotional issues, and more recently, studies have used a variety of specific anxiety and depression measures. Studies of mood disorder have consistently reported up to a third of all patients exhibit some depressive symptomotology in the first year following treatment.[58,69,70]

Females have been found to be more anxious than males at diagnosis and patients under 65 years of age were more depressed than those over 65. Patients with lower performance status, those with more advanced disease, and those who lived alone tended to display higher emotional distress as well.[70,71] Like other HNC symptoms, mood disorders tend to dissipate over time, and there appears to be gradual improvement of psychological functioning and global quality of life.[32] Additionally, recent studies have suggested that post-treatment depressive symptoms might be predicted by a few pre-treatment variables including pre-treatment depressive or physical symptoms.[70,72] Because depression and anxiety can be associated with alcohol abuse,[73,74] a known contributor to HNC, care must be taken to separate mood disorders caused by disease and treatment from disorders existing before the development of HNC, although both should be treated.

Xerostomia

Xerostomia has long been known as one of the most prevalent and long- term side effects of radiation and/or chemotherapy treatment for HNC. Not only is dry mouth aggravating in and of itself, but it can also lead to other severe conditions such as anorexia and multiple dental and gum related problems, all of which can affect patient QOL. A recently published study found xerostomia to be the symptom most frequently associated with poorer QOL on EORTC QLQ-30 domain scores and symptom scales in HNC.[53] In response to the prevalence and severity of xerostomia, has been the development and testing of an increasing number of new strategies for minimizing this troublesome sequalae. While the use of oral care products (e.g., Biotene and Salagen) during treatment[75,76] appears to lessen patients' discomfort and increase QOL, these data are from non-randomized trials and may, in part, reflect a placebo effect.[77] Phase III randomized studies are warranted. Studies of the relationship between radiation field and dry mouth suggest that sparing the parotid gland led to significant recovery of salivary flow at one year post-treatment.[78] In contrast, patients whose parotid glands were included in the radiation field did not recover their salivary flow.

More extensive research has been done on the cytoprotective agent amifostine. Phase III placebo controlled trials have documented that amifostine protects against xerostomia[79,80] and dental caries.[81] Amifostine's ability to protect against mucositis is less clear. While some early studies have suggested lower levels of mucositis in patients receiving subcutaneously administered amifostine as compared to those receiving radiotherapy alone,[82] other studies have found no such protective effect.[79]

Patient Priorities and Preferences

There are data to suggest that patients' attitudes towards potential treatment outcomes may differ from those of their health care providers, relatives or the public.[83,84] Yet, the majority of QOL instruments do not measure which treatment outcomes are most important to patients (i.e., whether patients would rather have a moister mouth or a clearer voice). There has been growing interest in this question and it has been approached in variety of ways. For instance, Terrell asked patients for an "overall bother" score and then examined the degree to which this score correlated with individual QOL domain scores (communication, eating, pain, emotion).[85] Another strategy involves patient ranking of potential treatment outcomes.[86,87] Still others used logistic regression to determine the domains that most highly correlated with overall QOL score,[88] or the derivation of utility ratings towards particular health states.[89] Determining which domains and/or parameters most influence QOL or are most important to patients has implications for education, treatment development, and intervention.

Since early studies in HNC QOL targeted laryngectomy, initial investigations of attitudes and preferences focused on speech function,[90] with somewhat surprising results. For example, patients often rate other problems, such as interference with social activities, as more significant or bothersome than speech disturbance, [57,83,84,87,91-93] although Karnell did find that speech problems are correlated with negative well-being.[88] The VA Larynx study[57] found that although there were QOL differences between the laryngectomy and organ preservation groups, those differences were not correlated with speech function. These results may be partly explained by the enhanced ability of patients to recover their speech after laryngectomy due to new technology, better therapy, and advances in the field.[84]

Smoking and Drinking

Tobacco and alcohol are well known risk factors for HNC and continued smoking has been associated with decreased response to treatment and lower rates of survival.[94] Yet, studies have shown that between 25 and 50% of patients continue to smoke both during and after their treatment.[95,96]

Similar smoking relapse rates were seen by Gritz and colleagues whose findings also indicated that relapse was best predicted by treatment (radiation vs surgery), readiness to quit (precontemplators), age at initiation (younger) and greater addiction.[97] Additionally, Ostroff found that patients with less severe disease were more likely to continue smoking. These findings are obviously concerning and highlight the need for increasing attention to these issues. Although cessation programs are numerous for the general public, programs for HNC patients are lacking, and a recent literature search found that the last published report of a cessation program with this population was published in 1993,[98,99] and its findings were positive although non-significant.

INTERACTION AMONG ASPECTS OF QOL

Studies of function and QOL

Early assumptions were that functional (speech, swallowing, etc) deficits translated into poor overall QOL or increased risk of depression. There are considerable recent data, however, that challenge these common expectations. In spite of residual functional deficits, many HNC patients appear to recover to pre-treatment QOL levels, perhaps by adapting to their deficits.

Data challenging the notion that there is a direct correlation between functional deficits derive from studies of both long-term survivors and newly treated patients. In a study of 47 relapse-free patients (12 to 60 months following chemotherapy and radiation), about 50% reported an inability to eat a normal solid food diet.[28] However, this deficit did not correlate with either global QOL or specific QOL dimensions. Similarly, others have reported that performance parameters (eating in public, speech, normalcy of diet) showed little relationship to depression, global QOL or emotional well-being.[100] They also found that more than 5 years post radiation, patients with nasopharyngeal cancer, although reporting higher rates of residual problems (e.g., dry mouth, sticky saliva and trouble eating), indicated better overall QOL than other advanced disease patients.[65]

Parallel results have been found in larynx cancer patients, who, as noted above, have long been presumed to have poor QOL if they had severe speech deficits. In a series of very small studies of laryngectomy patients, neither stoma nor alaryngeal voice was associated with differences in QOL,[84,101] nor was functional disability significantly correlated with its importance.[92] In the larger VA larynx study, the better QOL scores in the group treated with chemotherapy and radiation appeared to be related not to speech function, but rather to freedom from pain, better emotional well-being and lower levels of depression.[57]

Differences in pattern of recovery over time

In many longitudinal studies, investigators have detected some decline, on treatment, in general QOL measures (global and subscale scores), but recovery to pre-treatment or near pre-treatment levels by 12 months.[102] This recovery occurs in spite of the persistence of many symptoms or functional deficits (e.g., inability to eat a normal diet), with post-treatment QOL showing little relationship at all to residual side effects. Rather post-treatment QOL was best predicted by pre-treatment QOL.[29] Still others have noted little or no decline in emotional well being, or increase in depression, even in the presence of physical deterioration.[58,69] Finally, the most recent longitudinal studies have also shown a return to baseline levels in many domains and especially in overall QOL by long-term (greater than three years) surviving HNC patients.[31,32]

Predictors of 12 month QOL

Observations such as those described above have stimulated the search for predictors or correlates of long-term QOL. A number of disease or patient characteristics (e.g., age, gender, advanced disease, lower performance status, type of reconstruction) have been associated with mental distress or lower QOL.[58,59,69,70,72,103,104] Research on these interactions has emerged in the last few years and results have been mostly inconclusive, although one consistent interaction has emerged. That is, patients with more advanced disease and more physical deficits pre-treatment have been shown to have increased physical and depressive symptoms post-treatment. [58,59,69,70,72,103] A study examining correlations between QOL parameters and survival noted longer survival and fewer recurrences in patients with higher perceived physical abilities.[105]

Determination of the relationship between functioning or symptoms and overall QOL as well as identification of predictors of outcome are questions for continued inquiry. At the same time, however, the fact that many patients appear to adapt in spite of persistent functional deficits and symptoms should not lead to complacency on the part of clinicians or researchers. Identifying which symptoms are most troublesome and important to patients and developing strategies for minimizing these negative sequelae must remain a high priority.

CONCLUSION

While the past fifteen years have shown many advances in the field of HNC QOL research, there are still a number of continued challenges that command attention. Little QOL research has been included in randomized trials. As survival rates continue to improve and methods of treatment become potentially more toxic, the inclusion of QOL data in randomized trials can be invaluable in interpreting the results of those studies. On the other hand, while mean QOL scores, (i.e., group averages) are necessary for these types of comparisons, how that same data might be useful clinically for an individual patient is a relatively uncharted area of investigation. The end result of QOL research should be to make treatment decisions easier and better for individual patients. How that can be done remains to be seen. Additionally, a review of all the HNC QOL literature published in 1999 and 2000 included only one study devoted to interventional research with HNC patients.[106] While difficult to evaluate with traditional methods of statistical analysis, continued and expanded application of QOL data to the design of psychosocial or other interventions is now necessary and warranted.

REFERENCES

1. Vokes EE, Weichselbaum RR, Lippman SM, et al. Head and neck cancer. N Engl J Med. 1993;328:184-94.
2. Cella D. F.A.C.I.T. MANUAL: Manual of the Functional Assessment of Chronic Illness Therapy (FACIT) Scales - Version 4. In:. Chicago: Center on Outcomes, Research and Education; Evanston Hospital Healthcare And Northwestern University; 1997.
3. Schipper H, Levitt M. Measuring quality of life: risks and benefits. Cancer Treat Rep. 1985;69:1115.
4. Cella D. Instruments and assessments methods in psycho-oncology quality of life. In: Holland J, al. e, eds. Textbook of Psycho-Oncology. New York: Oxford University Press; In press.

5. Schipper H, Clinch JJ, Olweny CLM. Quality of Life Studies: Definitions and Conceptual Issues. In: Spilker B, ed. Quality of Life and Pharmacoeconomics in Clinical Trials. Second ed. Philadelphia: Lippincott-Raven; 1996:11-23.
6. Morton RP. Evolution of quality of life assessment in head and neck cancer. J Laryngol Otol. 1995;109:1029-35.
7. Pitkin YN. Factors affecting psycholgic adjustment in the laryngectomised patient. Arch Otolaryngol. 1953;58.
8. De Boer MF, McCormick LK, Pruyn JF, et al. Physical and psychosocial correlates of head and neck cancer: a review of the literature. Otolaryngol Head Neck Surg. 1999;120:427-36.
9. Terrell J. Quality of life assessment in head and neck cancer patients. Hem/Onc Clinics of North America. 1999;13:849-865.
10. Ware JE, Jr., Sherbourne CD. The MOS 36-item short-form health survey (SF-36). I. Conceptual framework and item selection. Med Care. 1992;30:473-83.
11. Derogatis LR. The psychosocial adjustment to illness scale (PAIS). J Psychosom Res. 1986;30:77-91.
12. Cella DF, Tulsky DS, Gray G, et al. The Functional Assessment of Cancer Therapy scale: development and validation of the general measure. J Clin Oncol. 1993;11:570-9.
13. Aaronson NK, Ahmedzai S, Bergman B, et al. The European Organization for Research and Treatment of Cancer QLQ-C30: a quality-of-life instrument for use in international clinical trials in oncology. J Natl Cancer Inst. 1993;85:365-76.
14. Bjordal K, Kaasa S. Psychometric validation of the EORTC Core Quality of Life Questionnaire, 30-item version and a diagnosis-specific module for head and neck cancer patients. Acta Oncol. 1992;31:311-21.
15. D'Antonio LL, Zimmerman GJ, Cella DF, et al. Quality of life and functional status measures in patients with head and neck cancer. Arch Otolaryngol Head Neck Surg. 1996;122:482-7.
16. List MA, D'Antonio LL, Cella DF, et al. The Performance Status Scale for Head and Neck Cancer Patients and the Functional Assessment of Cancer Therapy-Head and Neck Scale. A study of utility and validity. Cancer. 1996;77:2294-301.
17. Sherman AC, Simonton S, Adams DC, et al. Assessing quality of life in patients with head and neck cancer: cross- validation of the European Organization for Research and Treatment of Cancer (EORTC) Quality of Life Head and Neck module (QLQ-H&N35). Arch Otolaryngol Head Neck Surg. 2000;126:459-67.
18. Bjordal K, Ahlner-Elmqvist M, Tollesson E, et al. Development of a European Organization for Research and Treatment of Cancer (EORTC) questionnaire module to be used in quality of life assessments in head and neck cancer patients. EORTC Quality of Life Study Group. Acta Oncol. 1994;33:879-85.
19. Bjordal K, Hammerlid E, Ahlner-Elmqvist M, et al. Quality of life in head and neck cancer patients: validation of the European Organization for Research and Treatment of Cancer Quality of Life Questionnaire-H&N35. J Clin Oncol. 1999;17:1008-19.
20. List MA, Ritter-Sterr C, Lansky SB. A performance status scale for head and neck cancer patients. Cancer. 1990;66:564-9.
21. Hassan SJ, Weymuller EA, Jr. Assessment of quality of life in head and neck cancer patients. Head Neck. 1993;15:485-96.
22. Browman GP, Levine MN, Hodson DI, et al. The head and neck cancer radiotherapy questionnaire: a morbidity/quality of life instrument for clinical trials of radiation therapy in locally advanced head and neck cancer. J Clin Oncol. 1993;11:863-72.
23. Johnson DJ, Casey L, Noriega B. A pilot study of patient quality of life during radiation therapy treatment. Qual Life Res. 1994;3:267-72.

24. Trotti A, Johnson DJ, Gwede C, et al. Development of a head and neck companion module for the quality of life- radiation therapy instrument (QOL-RTI). Int J Radiat Oncol Biol Phys. 1998;42:257-61.

25. Beck AT, Ward CH, Mendelson M, et al. An inventory for measuring depression. Arch Gen Psychiatry. 1961;4:561-567.

26. Radloff LG. The CES-D scale: A self-report depression scale for research in the general population. Appl Psychol Meas. 1977;3:385-401.

27. List MA, Ritter-Sterr CA, Baker TM, et al. Longitudinal assessment of quality of life in laryngeal cancer patients. Head Neck. 1996;18:1-10.

28. List MA, Mumby P, Haraf D, et al. Performance and quality of life outcome in patients completing concomitant chemoradiotherapy protocols for head and neck cancer. Qual Life Res. 1997;6:274-84.

29. List MA, Siston A, Haraf D, et al. Quality of life and performance in advanced head and neck cancer patients on concomitant chemoradiotherapy: a prospective examination. J Clin Oncol. 1999;17:1020-8.

30. Karnofsky DA, Burchenal JH. The clinical evaluation of chemotherapeutics in cancer. In: MacLeod CM, ed. Evaluation of Chemotherapeutic Agents. New York: Columbia University; 1949.

31. Hammerlid E, Taft C. Health-related quality of life in long-term head and neck cancer survivors: a comparison with general population norms. Br J Cancer. 2001;84:149-56.

32. de Graeff A, de Leeuw JR, Ros WJ, et al. Long-term quality of life of patients with head and neck cancer. Laryngoscope. 2000;110:98-106.

33. De Boer MF, Pruyn JFA, Van den Borne HW, et al. Rehabilitation outcomes of long-term survivors treated for head and neck cancer. Head Neck. 1995;17:503-515.

34. Deshmane VH, Parikh HK, Pinni S, et al. Laryngectomy: a quality of life assessment. Indian J Cancer. 1995;32:121-30.

35. Gamba A, Romano M, Grosso IM, et al. Psychosocial adjustment of patients surgically treated for head and neck cancer. Head Neck. 1992;14:218-23.

36. Langius A, Bjorvell H, Lind MG. Functional status and coping in patients with oral and pharyngeal cancer before and after surgery. Head Neck. 1994;16:559-68.

37. Siston AK, List MA, Schleser R, et al. Sexual functioning in head and neck cancer. J Psychosoc Oncol. 1997;15:107-122.

38. Lefebvre JL, Chevalier D, Luboinski B, et al. Larynx preservation in pyriform sinus cancer: preliminary results of a European Organization for Research and Treatment of Cancer phase III trial. EORTC Head and Neck Cancer Cooperative Group. J Natl Cancer Inst. 1996;88:890-9.

39. Schliephake H, Ruffert K, Schneller T. Prospective study of the quality of life of cancer patients after intraoral tumor surgery. J Oral Maxillofac Surg. 1996;54:664-9; discussion 669-70.

40. Rogers SN, Humphris G, Lowe D, et al. The impact of surgery for oral cancer on quality of life as measured by the Medical Outcomes Short Form 36. Oral Oncol. 1998;34:171-9.

41. Netscher DT, Meade RA, Goodman CM, et al. Quality of life and disease-specific functional status following microvascular reconstruction for advanced (T3 and T4) oropharyngeal cancers. Plast Reconstr Surg. 2000;105:1628-34.

42. Rogers SN, Lowe D, Humphris G. Distinct patient groups in oral cancer: a prospective study of perceived health status following primary surgery. Oral Oncol. 2000;36:529-38.

43. Terrell JE, Welsh DE, Bradford CR, et al. Pain, quality of life, and spinal accessory nerve status after neck dissection. Laryngoscope. 2000;110:620-6.

44.   Kuntz AL, Weymuller EA, Jr. Impact of neck dissection on quality of life. Laryngoscope. 1999;109:1334-8.

45.   Beumer Jr, Curtis T, Harrison R. Radiation therapy of the oral cavity: sequelae and management, part 1. Head Neck Surg. 1979;1:301-312.

46.   Bundgaard T, Tandrup O, Elbrond O. A functional evaluation of patients treated for oral cancer. A prospective study. Int J Oral Maxillofac Surg. 1993;22:28-34.

47.   Harrison LB, Zelefsky MJ, Pfister DG, et al. Detailed quality of life assessment in patients treated with primary radiotherapy for squamous cell cancer of the base of the tongue. Head Neck. 1997;19:169-75.

48.   Cooper JS, Fu K, Marks J, et al. Late effects of radiation therapy in the head and neck region. Int J Radiat Oncol Biol Phys. 1995;31:1141-64.

49.   Constine LS. What else don't we know about the late effects of radiation in patients treated for head and neck cancer? Int J Radiat Oncol Biol Phys. 1995;31:427-9.

50.   Bjordal K, Kaasa S, Mastekaasa A. Quality of life in patients treated for head and neck cancer: a follow- up study 7 to 11 years after radiotherapy. Int J Radiat Oncol Biol Phys. 1994;28:847-56.

51.   Hammerlid E, Mercke C, Sullivan M, et al. A prospective quality of life study of patients with laryngeal carcinoma by tumor stage and different radiation therapy schedules. Laryngoscope. 1998;108:747-59.

52.   Griffiths GO, Parmar MK, Bailey AJ. Physical and psychological symptoms of quality of life in the CHART randomized trial in head and neck cancer: short-term and long-term patient reported symptoms. CHART Steering Committee. Continuous hyperfractionated accelerated radiotherapy. Br J Cancer. 1999;81:1196-205.

53.   Allal AS, Dulguerov P, Bieri S, et al. Assessment of quality of life in patients treated with accelerated radiotherapy for laryngeal and hypopharyngeal carcinomas. Head Neck. 2000;22:288-93.

54.   Harrison LB, Zelefsky MJ, Armstrong JG, et al. Performance status after treatment for squamous cell cancer of the base of tongue--a comparison of primary radiation therapy versus primary surgery. Int J Radiat Oncol Biol Phys. 1994;30:953-7.

55.   Deleyiannis FW, Weymuller EA, Jr., Coltrera MD. Quality of life of disease-free survivors of advanced (stage III or IV) oropharyngeal cancer. Head Neck. 1997;19:466-73.

56.   Murry T, Madasu R, Martin A, et al. Acute and chronic changes in swallowing and quality of life following intraarterial chemoradiation for organ preservation in patients with advanced head and neck cancer. Head Neck. 1998;20:31-7.

57.   Terrell JE, Fisher SG, Wolf GT. Long-term quality of life after treatment of laryngeal cancer. The Veterans Affairs Laryngeal Cancer Study Group. Arch Otolaryngol Head Neck Surg. 1998;124:964-71.

58.   de Graeff A, de Leeuw JR, Ros WJ, et al. A prospective study on quality of life of patients with cancer of the oral cavity or oropharynx treated with surgery with or without radiotherapy. Oral Oncol. 1999;35:27-32.

59.   de Graeff A, de Leeuw JR, Ros WJ, et al. Pretreatment factors predicting quality of life after treatment for head and neck cancer. Head Neck. 2000;22:398-407.

60.   Epstein JB, Emerton S, Kolbinson DA, et al. Quality of life and oral function following radiotherapy for head and neck cancer. Head Neck. 1999;21:1-11.

61.   Campbell BH, Marbella A, Layde PM. Quality of life and recurrence concern in survivors of head and neck cancer. Laryngoscope. 2000;110:895-906.

62.   Trotti A, Johnson DJ, Gwede C, et al. Development of a head and neck companion module for the quality of life- radiation therapy instrument (QOL-RTI) [published erratum appears in Int J Radiat Oncol Biol Phys 1998 Dec 1;42(5):1181-2]. Int J Radiat Oncol Biol Phys. 1998;42:257-61.

63. Chaplin JM, Morton RP. A prospective, longitudinal study of pain in head and neck cancer patients. Head Neck. 1999;21:531-7.

64. Rogers SN, Hannah L, Lowe D, et al. Quality of life 5-10 years after primary surgery for oral and oro- pharyngeal cancer. J Craniomaxillofac Surg. 1999;27:187-91.

65. Huguenin PU, Taussky D, Moe K, et al. Quality of life in patients cured from a carcinoma of the head and neck by radiotherapy: the importance of the target volume. Int J Radiat Oncol Biol Phys. 1999;45:47-52.

66. Breitbart W, Holland J. Psychosocial aspects of head and neck cancer. Semin Oncol. 1988;15:61-9.

67. Breitbart W. Identifying patients at risk for, and treatment of major psychiatric complications of cancer. Support Care Cancer. 1995;3:45-60.

68. Espie CA, Freedlander E, Campsie LM, et al. Psychological distress at follow-up after major surgery for intraoral cancer. J Psychosom Res. 1989;33:441-448.

69. de Graeff A, de Leeuw RJ, Ros WJ, et al. A prospective study on quality of life of laryngeal cancer patients treated with radiotherapy. Head Neck. 1999;21:291-6.

70. Hammerlid E, Ahlner-Elmqvist M, Bjordal K, et al. A prospective multicentre study in Sweden and Norway of mental distress and psychiatric morbidity in head and neck cancer patients. Br J Cancer. 1999;80:766-74.

71. Kugaya A, Akechi T, Okuyama T, et al. Prevalence, predictive factors, and screening for psychologic distress in patients with newly diagnosed head and neck cancer. Cancer. 2000;88:2817-23.

72. de Leeuw JR, de Graeff A, Ros WJ, et al. Prediction of depressive symptomatology after treatment of head and neck cancer: the influence of pre-treatment physical and depressive symptoms, coping, and social support. Head Neck. 2000;22:799-807.

73. Brietbart W, Holland JC. Head and neck cancer. In: Holland JC, Rowland JII, eds. Handbook of Psychooncology. New York: Oxford; 1989:233-239.

74. Windle M, Miller BA. Alcoholism and depression symptomatology among convicted DWI men and women. J Stud Alcohol. 1989;50:406-413.

75. Warde P, Kroll B, O'Sullivan B, et al. A phase II study of Biotene in the treatment of postradiation xerostomia in patients with head and neck cancer. Support Care Cancer. 2000;8:203-8.

76. Horiot JC, Lipinski F, Schraub S, et al. Post-radiation severe xerostomia relieved by pilocarpine: a prospective French cooperative study. Radiother Oncol. 2000;55:233-9.

77. Rieke JW, Hafermann MD, Johnson JT, et al. Oral pilocarpine for radiation-induced xerostomia: integrated efficacy and safety results from two prospective randomized clinical trials. Int J Radiat Oncol Biol Phys. 1995;31:661-9.

78. Henson BS, Inglehart MR, Eisbruch A, et al. Preserved salivary output and xerostomia-related quality of life in head and neck cancer patients receiving parotid-sparing radiotherapy. Oral Oncol. 2001;37:84-93.

79. Brizel DM, Wasserman TH, Henke M, et al. Phase III randomized trial of amifostine as a radioprotector in head and neck cancer. J Clin Oncol. 2000;18:3339-45.

80. Bohuslavizki KH, Klutmann S, Brenner W, et al. Radioprotection of salivary glands by amifostine in high-dose radioiodine treatment. Results of a double-blinded, placebo-controlled study in patients with differentiated thyroid cancer. Strahlenther Onkol. 1999;175 Suppl 4:6-12.

81. Rudat V, Meyer J, Momm F, et al. Protective effect of amifostine on dental health after radiotherapy of the head and neck. Int J Radiat Oncol Biol Phys. 2000;48:1339-43.

82. Koukourakis MI, Kyrias G, Kakolyris S, et al. Subcutaneous administration of amifostine during fractionated radiotherapy: a randomized phase II study. J Clin Oncol. 2000;18:2226-33.

83.   Mohide EA, Archibald SD, Tew M, et al. Postlaryngectomy quality of life dimensions idenfied by patients and health care professionals. Am J Surg. 1992;164:619-622.
84.   Finizia C, Hammerlid E, Westin T, et al. Quality of life and voice in patients with laryngeal carcinoma: a posttreatment comparison of laryngectomy (salvage surgery) versus radiotherapy. Laryngoscope. 1998;108:1566-73.
85.   Terrell J, Nanavati K, Esclamado R, et al. Health impact of head and neck cancer. Otolaryngol Head Neck Surg. 1999;120:852-9.
86.   List MA, Butler P, Vokes EE, et al. Head and neck cancer patients: How do patients prioritize potential treatment outcomes? In: American Society of Clinical Oncology; 1998:382.
87.   Sharp HM, List M, MacCracken E, et al. Patients' priorities among treatment effects in head and neck cancer: evaluation of a new assessment tool. Head Neck. 1999;21:538-46.
88.   Karnell LH, Funk GF, Hoffman HT. Assessing head and neck cancer patient outcome domains. Head Neck. 2000;22:6-11.
89.   Jalukar V, Funk GF, Christensen AJ, et al. Health states following head and neck cancer treatment: patient, health- care professional, and public perspectives. Head Neck. 1998;20:600-8.
90.   Karnell LH, Funk GF, Tomblin JB, et al. Quality of life measurements of speech in the head and neck cancer patient population. Head Neck. 1999;21:229-38.
91.   List MA, Stracks J, Colangelo L, et al. How do head and neck cancer patients prioritize treatment outcomes before initiating treatment? J Clin Oncol. 2000;18:877.
92.   Deleyiannis F, Weymuller E, Coltera M, et al. Quality of life after laryngectomy: Are functional disabilities important? Head Neck. 1999;21:319-324.
93.   DeSanto LW, Olsen KD, Perry WC, et al. Quality of life after surgical treatment of cancer of the larynx. Ann Otol Rhinol Laryngol. 1995;104:763-769.
94.   Browman GP, Wong G, Hodson I, et al. Influence of cigarette smoking on the efficacy of radiation therapy in head and neck cancer [see comments]. N Engl J Med. 1993;328:159-63.
95.   List MA, Haraf D, Hagerman D, et al. Two-four years post chemoradiotherapy (CT/XRT) for stage IV head and neck cancer (HNC): How are our patients doing? In: American Society of Clinical Oncology. Atlanta, GA; 1999:391a.
96.   Ostroff JS, Jacobsen PB, Moadel AB, et al. Prevalence and predictors of continued tobacco use after treatment of patients with head and neck cancer. Cancer. 1995;75:569-76.
97.   Gritz ER, Schacherer C, Koehly L, et al. Smoking withdrawal and relapse in head and neck cancer patients. Head Neck. 1999;21:420-7.
98.   Gritz ER, Carr CR, Rapkin D, et al. Predictors of long-term smoking cessation in head and neck cancer patients. Cancer Epidemiol Biomarkers Prev. 1993;2:261-70.
99.   Gritz ER, Carr CR, Rapkin DA, et al. A smoking cessation intervention for head and neck cancer patients: trial design, patient accrual, and characteristics. Cancer Epidemiol Biomarkers Prev. 1991;1:67-73.
100.   D'Antonio LL, Long SA, Zimmerman GJ, et al. Relationship between quality of life and depression in patients with head and neck cancer. Laryngoscope. 1998;108:806-11.
101.   Herranz J, Gavilan J. Psychosocial adjustment after laryngeal cancer surgery. Ann Otol Rhinol Laryngol. 1999;108:990-997.
102.   Rogers SN, Lowe D, Brown JS, et al. A comparison between the University of Washington Head and Neck Disease- Specific measure and the Medical Short Form 36, EORTC QOQ-C33 and EORTC Head and Neck 35. Oral Oncol. 1998;34:361-72.

103. Rogers SN, Lowe D, Brown JS, et al. The University of Washington head and neck cancer measure as a predictor of outcome following primary surgery for oral cancer. Head Neck. 1999;21:394-401.
104. Wilson KM, Rizk NM, Armstrong SL, et al. Effects of hemimandibulectomy on quality of life. Laryngoscope. 1998;108:1574-7.
105. De Boer MF, Van den Borne B, Pruyn JF, et al. Psychosocial and physical correlates of survival and recurrence in patients with head and neck carcinoma: results of a 6-year longitudinal study. Cancer. 1998;83:2567-79.
106. List MA, Stracks J. Evaluation of quality of life in patients definitively treated for squamous carcinoma of the head and neck. Curr Opin Oncol. 2000;12:215-20.

Chapter 15

ORAL, DENTAL, AND SUPPORTIVE CARE IN THE CANCER PATIENT

Harry Staffileno, Jr. DDS, MS and Leslie Reeder, DDS
Northwestern University Medical School, Chicago, IL 60611
Evanston Northwestern Healthcare, Evanston. IL 60201

INTRODUCTION

The management of oral complications in the cancer patient is very challenging. The responses of the oral mucosa can vary in different locations of the oral structures from one patient to another with the same chemotherapy agents. Additionally, the same patient may not show the same lesions with the same dose of chemotherapy on succeeding series or may have a more severe expression of symptoms and lesions at a different cycle with the same agent and same dose.

The patient physiology both before and during chemotherapy will have an impact on oral problems. This makes a changing baseline. In addition, the dose of chemotherapy administered is dependent on the objective response of the tumor and the general well-being of the patient. Thus, the variables multiply.

Now, introduce into the scenario variables such as surgery, chemotherapy, and/or radiation therapy. As one can surmise, the variables are limitless depending on the type and stage of the tumor, type and dose of chemotherapy, and the site and dose of radiation.

This course of events and probabilities has caused the professional care giving community to yield to a palliative approach in treating these problems using methods such as:

1. chemotherapy interruption and/or
2. "cocktails" coating the lesions and/or
3. topical anesthetic agents

Successful management of the cancer patient necessitates a basic appreciation of the tissues and structures of the oral environment and their normal characteristics. Oral problems occur in cancer patients because:

1. The oral mucosa has a high cellular turnover rate.
2. There is complex and diverse microflora.
3. Saliva quality and quantity is altered.
4. Normal oral function such as chewing and eating can cause soft tissue injury [1].

This chapter will discuss the oral side effects of chemotherapy, head and neck radiation treatment and the management of these side effects as well as the dental and oral care for these patients. This chapter will also discuss a treatment protocol that helps to reduce the adverse oral health changes by considering the biology and physiology of the tissues involved. Our goal is to appreciate the problem, establish a diagnosis and enter a treatment plan that seems most appropriate. Palliation is always a by-product of this treatment.

ASSESSMENT OF ORAL HEALTH

Examination of the Chemotherapy Patient

Ideally, the patient undergoing myelosuppressive chemotherapy is seen for oral health assessment prior to initiating chemotherapy [2]. Realistically, this is not always the case but it is preferred. When this is not possible, the patient will generally be seen early in his oncology therapy. Key to successful management of the oncology patient from the perspective of oral and dental health is to establish an assessment prior to chemotherapy. A complete oral and dental exam should be performed including a panoramic x-ray and supplemental dental x-rays as needed. The examination should evaluate all teeth for infection, active periodontal disease, ill-fitting prosthesis or poor state of repair. The oral mucosa should be examined. Is the oral mucosa prior to chemotherapy compromised from the patient taking medications for hypertension, anxiety, depression, or pain? These conditions are treated with agents that predispose the oral environment to modification such as dry mouth. For instance, there may be decreased salivary flow which in turn affects the ecosystem of the oral environment. Additionally, it is important to know the oral health awareness of the patient.

Initial Dental Care for the Chemotherapy Patient

Any positive findings from the dental exam should be scheduled for treatment. This is always done working in close liaison with the oncologist. A dental prophylaxis or periodontal debridement should be done to eliminate bacterial debris on the teeth. Periapical pathology which requires root canal treatment or extraction should be done prior to beginning chemotherapy. Also, caries control is done on carious teeth. Teeth requiring extraction should be extracted at least 10 days prior to the development of neutropenia. Extraction sites should have primary closure to help in the healing process [2,3]. Obviously, the window of time for treatment may be very short, or non-existent. When appropriate, priority should be given to the most essential needs and the patient directed towards definitive treatment.

Education for the Chemotherapy Patient

The patient is educated on the potential oral side effects of chemotherapy: mucositis, changes in taste, bleeding, infection, and salivary dysfunction. The patient is educated on daily oral hygiene including brushing the teeth after each meal and at bedtime and flossing the teeth at least once a day. Depending on the patient's WBC and platelet counts during chemotherapy, the oncologist may, at times, have the patient stop flossing his teeth for a period of time while the blood counts are low. Patients should avoid peroxide, tooth whitening and tartar control toothpaste since these ingredients can be irritating to the tissue during chemotherapy. The patient is advised on diet: avoid spicy, crispy, rough, acidic, hot types of food because these can irritate and traumatize the thin and delicate intraoral tissues during chemotherapy. Patients are also advised to avoid alcohol including mouthwash containing alcohol which can be drying and irritating to the intraoral tissues. Patients should avoid tobacco products such as cigarettes because they are irritating to the intraoral tissues [4]. Atrophy of the oral mucosa is a significant physiologic change with chemotherapy.

Examination of the Head and Neck Radiation Patient

Prior to beginning head and neck radiation treatment, a comprehensive dental exam including a panoramic x-ray with supplemental periapical and bitewing x-rays as indicated should be done to evaluate for dental caries, periapical pathology, periodontal disease, residual root tips, and third molar pathology [4]. The hard and soft tissues should be examined, the patient's oral hygiene should be assessed, and the existing dental restorations should be evaluated for rough, sharp, or overhanging restorations. The fit of existing dental prosthesis [4,5] including orthodontic appliances should also be assessed [5]. A dental treatment plan should be made in consultation with the radiation oncologist. It is important to know the field of radiation, the dosage of radiation and how soon the radiation treatment will begin as these all will be important factors in determining the final dental treatment plan. The patient's level of motivation also will be important in determining the final dental treatment plan [4].

Initial Dental Care for the Head and Neck Radiation Patient

Initial dental care to prevent and eliminate oral bacterial reservoirs should be done prior to beginning head and neck radiation treatment. Non-surgical periodontal therapy such as a dental prophylaxis(cleaning) or a periodontal debridement to remove plaque and calculus should be done. Carious dental lesions that can be restored and teeth requiring root canal treatment should also be done prior to beginning radiation treatment. Impressions of the teeth should be taken for fabrication of vinyl custom fluoride carriers in order for patients to give themselves lifelong daily fluoride treatment to reduce the risk of dental caries. Extraction of hopeless, non-restorable teeth, should be done prior to beginning radiation treatment. Examples include but are not limited to teeth with advanced periodontal disease, large carious lesions, residual root tips not fully covered by bone and, if periapical pathology exists, impacted or partially impacted teeth not fully covered by bone. Ideally, the extractions should be done 21 days prior to beginning radiation treatment to allow for adequate healing time and reduce the risk of osteoradionecrosis(ORN) [4,5,6]. However, this may not always be possible. The extractions should be done with as little trauma as possible and primary closure should be obtained when possible [4].

Education for the Head and Neck Radiation Patient

The patient should be educated on the potential oral side effects of head and neck radiation treatment: mucositis, candidiasis, xerostomia, loss of taste, trismus, dental caries, and ORN. As with the chemotherapy patient, the head and neck radiation patient is educated on diet, daily oral hygiene, the avoidance of alcohol and tobacco products as well as the avoidance of peroxide, tooth whitening and tartar control toothpaste. In addition, food high in sugar content should be avoided in the xerostomic patient due to increased risk of dental caries. Jaw exercises should be done to reduce the risk of trismus. The importance of excellent daily oral hygiene and the use of daily neutral sodium fluoride applied to the teeth with custom fluoride carriers to reduce the risk of caries should be stressed to the patient [4].

SIDE EFFECTS OF CHEMOTHERAPY AND HEAD AND NECK RADIATION TREATMENT AND THEIR MANAGEMENT

Mucositis

By definition, mucositis presents with varying grades of tissue destruction characterized by pain, erythema, and ulceration, with the potential for fungal and bacterial infection. This definition comes close to being accepted by most observers of this oral morbidity.

It is reported in the literature that earlier stages of mucositis may go unrecognized and untreated. Further, the effect on the quality of life from the standpoint of oral mucositis is not appreciated in its initial stages.

The oral mucosa acts as a barrier by protecting the underlying tissues. When this barrier is broken, the normal oral flora can gain entry into the underlying tissues and cause infection. Chemotherapy and head and neck radiation treatment can cause the mucosa to break down. Chemotherapy affects cells with high mitotic activity such as the oral mucosa [1,7]. Therefore, the oral mucosa will become much thinner in dimension which makes the oral mucosa more delicate and fragile. Thus, patients are advised to avoid spicy, crispy, rough, acidic, hot types of food because of the propensity to injure the thin, delicate oral mucosa. Mucositis is usually seen 7 to 14 days after starting chemotherapy. However, patients may experience a burning sensation prior to this [8]. Since the intraoral tissues become thinner and more delicate with chemotherapy, calculus, plaque, rough or sharp teeth or restorations and even ill-fitting prosthesis can cause the tissue to break down more readily [9]. Patients with good dental health and oral hygiene during chemotherapy tend to develop mucositis less often than patients that have poor dental health and oral hygiene [10].

Mucositis is affected by patient's diagnosis, age, and level of oral health and type, dose and frequency of chemotherapy [10]. Mucositis occurs in approximately 40% of patients undergoing chemotherapy [10, 11, 12] whereas almost all patients undergoing head and neck radiation treatment develop mucositis [12]. Chemotherapy can cause a localized or a generalized mucositis, however, radiation mucositis is site specific. Radiation mucositis is related to dose delivered, site delivered and rate at which radiation is delivered [13]. Radiation mucositis may begin as soon as the second week of head and neck radiation treatment [14]. Examples of such chemotherapy agents such include bleomycin, 5-FU, methotrexate, doxorubicin, paclitaxel, etoposide, and hydroxyurea can cause mucosal thinning, erythema and ulceration of intraoral tissues [8] (Fig. 1).

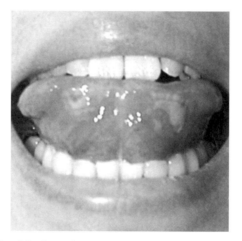

Figure 1. **Mucositis with ulcerations on ventral aspect of tongue.**

The World Health Organization (WHO) criteria for grading mucositis as cited by Raber-Durlacher, et al is submitted so there is a common base of reference (Table 1). Additionally, in an effort to recognize earlier literary contributions to this problem, it is important to mention names such as Peterson, Sonis, Lockhart, Redding, and the Consensus Development Conference of 1989 and the Mucosal Injury Conference of 2000. Early on, Dreizen, Marx, and more recently Raber-Durlacher group and others in the international community contributed diligently in this area.

Table 1. **WHO criteria for grading mucositis [8].**

Grade	Mucositis Description
0	No mucositis
1	Mild tissue changes(focal): white anemic changes; erythematous patches, mucosal thinning; no sensitivity; normal eating
2	Mild tissue changes (focal): erythematous/thinning mucosa; small ulceration<2mm; slight sensitivity; normal eating
3	Moderate tissue changes (focal-diffuse): erythematous/denuded/ ulcerated mucosa; $\leq \frac{1}{2}$ mucosal area involved; blood clots- no active bleeding; moderate sensitivity, difficulty with eating and drinking
4	Marked tissue changes(diffuse): erythematous/denuded/ ulcerated mucosa; $\geq\frac{1}{2}$ mucosal area involved; active oozing/bleeding marked pain; no eating possible

The authors have over 10 years of clinical experience in dealing with oral mucositis and have found the outcomes of their approach to be the most effective to date in treating very refractory problems. It should be noted that treatment of mucositis from the most successful (rapid resolution with the least morbidity) to the most resistant (slowest to resolve with the most morbidity), occurs in the following ordered settings:

1. Solid tumors with chemotherapy - very successful.
2. Solid tumors in the head and neck treated with chemotherapy - successful.
3. Hematological malignancies treated with chemotherapy - moderately successful.
4. Hematological malignancies with chemotherapy and radiation therapy -moderately successful.
5. Solid tumors in the head and neck area receiving radiation therapy - mildly to moderately successful with the final weeks of radiation being difficult for most patients.
6. Solid tumors in the head and neck area treated with radiation therapy and chemotherapy concurrently - mildly successful, but reasonable success in the palliation aspect.
7. Hematological malignancies treated with stem-cell transplants-mildly successful.

With the above stated observations, it becomes evident that management beyond palliation is realistic. However, many oral care practitioners enter into the management of oral mucositis problems with two biases. First, the posture is taken that nothing preventative or therapeutic can be done for patients other than palliation. Secondly, if one is getting results by one measure or another, it must be submitted to double blind, randomized study to prove its value before it can be advocated to the community. This second notion is a very sound premise. However, oncology protocols, dosages, and sequences of management are frequently changed, making it difficult to run controlled studies.

Management of Mucositis

Typically patients with mucositis are treated with:

1. An antimicrobial rinse such as aqueous chlorhexidine 0.2% rinse bid. Chlorhexidine can stain teeth and dental restorations.

2. A cleansing agent such as bicarbonate rinses 2-3x/day. Dissolve ½ teaspoon baking soda in 4 ounces of water and rinse. Follow with clear water rinse.

3. Cephalexin 500mg tid if patient has diffuse mucositis or if patient is neutropenic. If patient has an allergy to cephalosporins or penicillins, doxycycline 100mg qd or clindamycin 150mg tid can be used instead. There may be instances when the oncologist prefers a different antibiotic such as the quinolones.

4. Review of diet with patients. Foods to avoid include acidic, rough, spicy, crispy and hot types of foods since these types of food can irritate and traumatize the intraoral tissues. Patients should choose bland foods such as eggs, puddings, cream of wheat, apple sauce, ice cream, shakes, pasta without tomato sauce.

5. Patients who wear removable dental prosthesis should remove their appliances while they have mucositis.

6. Narcotics are usually not prescribed for pain management of mild mucositis.

For those patients with extreme discomfort and inability to eat, their oral complications are managed much more aggressively and may include:

1.   Cefazolin 1 gm IV. Cefazolin 1 gm can be continued q8 or changed to cephalexin 500mg po tid. If there is an allergy to cephalosporins or penicillin, then Clindamycin 600 to 900mg IV followed by Clindamycin 150mg po tid. There may be instances when the oncologist prefers a different antibiotic.

2.   Dexamethasone 8mg qd for 1 to 2 days to decrease inflammation and discomfort.

3.   Topical analgesics such as viscous lidocaine are not advised because they may be conducive to further injury of the intraoral tissues. Viscous lidocaine is drying to the intraoral tissues and can cause a burning sensation. Patients may even choke or aspirate on food if they use viscous lidocaine prior to eating.

4.   Consider a palliative topical combination rinse:
        Nystatin Oral Suspension   120ml
        Tetracycline powder   2000mg
        Benadryl elixir   40ml
        Dexamethasone elixir   40ml
        Quantities may be varied. Swish with 5ml for 3 minutes and expectorate 3-4x/day. Do not eat or drink for 30 minutes afterwards.

5.   Severe mucositis, such as that experienced with concomitant chemoradiotherapy for head and neck cancer patients, often requires narcotic analgesics for palliation of pain.

With treatment, these acute symptoms generally are alleviated in 24 to 48 hours. When not alleviated, the problem needs to be reviewed for compliance, adjustment of dosages and/or reassessment of diagnosis.

Candidiasis

The prevalence of oropharyngeal candidiasis in the cancer patient may be as high as 60% [8]. There are several types of candidiasis seen in patients undergoing chemotherapy and head and neck radiation treatment.

1.   Pseudomembranous candidiasis is the most common. Clinically it
        appears as white creamy plaques which can be removed leaving the
        underlying tissue red (Fig. 2).

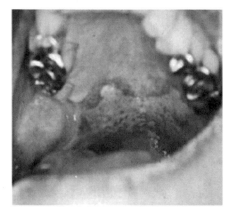

Figure 2. **Pseudomembranous candidiasis on palate. White plaques can be wiped off,
leaving underlying tissue red.**

2.   Erythematous or atrophic candidiasis clinically appears as
        erythematous patches. Usually patients have a burning or painful
        sensation. This form of candidiasis is often overlooked as most
        people think of candidiasis as being white.

3.   Hyperplastic candidiasis clinically appears as white, firm, raised
        plaques that can not be rubbed off.

4.   Angular cheilits clinically appears as red fissured crusts at the corner
        or angle of the mouth which can be covered by white-yellow plaques
        [3].

        Treatment of candidiasis can include topical agents such as nystatin
oral suspension, clotrimazole troches, or systemic agents such as fluconazole.
Nystatin and clotrimazole which contain sugar should be used with caution in
patients who are xerostomic due to the increased risk of caries. Also,
xerostomic patients may find it difficult to dissolve the clotrimazole troche
due to decreased saliva. Patients who develop intraoral candidiasis and wear
removable dental prosthesis, should not only be treated with an antifungal
agent to treat the intraoral tissues but their removable dental prosthesis should
be treated as well. Dentures can be soaked in nystatin oral suspension.
Angular cheilitis can be treated with nystatin/triamcinolone 0.1% ointment
applied to lips tid.

Herpes Simplex Virus(HSV)

HSV is seen more often in patients undergoing chemotherapy rather than head and neck radiation treatment. In the immunocompetent patient, HSV usually only occurs intraorally on the attached gingiva or hard palate as small groups of vesicles arranged in clusters. However, in the immunocompromised patient, these lesions can occur on any of the oral mucosal surfaces such as the dorsum of the tongue, (Fig. 3) ventral and lateral aspects of the tongue, buccal mucosa, soft and hard palate. In the immunocompromised patient, ulcerations, not vesicles, are usually seen. These herpetic lesions are usually larger, more painful and slower to heal than in an immunocompetent patient [15]. In the immunocompetent patient, herpetic lesions usually completely resolve in 7 to 14 days whereas in the immunocompromised patient, herpetic lesions can take much longer to heal [16] and can become secondarily infected.

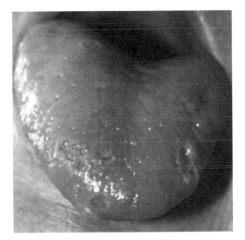

Figure 3 **Herpetic stomatitis on dorsum of tongue in an immunocompromised patient.**

Typically, HSV is treated with acyclovir. If patients have outbreaks of HSV while receiving chemotherapy, acyclovir may be considered prophylactically with future cycles of chemotherapy. The patients level of immunosuppression, creatinine level, and hydration status will all effect the decision of whether to use acyclovir prophylactically.

Salivary Gland Dysfunction

Salivary gland dysfunction is usually milder in the chemotherapy patient than in the head and neck radiation patient. In the cancer patient, medication such as antiemetics, antidepressants, and pain medications, especially the opioids, can cause dry mouth. Modified xerostomia and a change in the quality of saliva is consistent with chemotherapy. These changes make speaking and eating more difficult but with chemotherapy the degree of change is mild. However, with head and neck radiation treatment, xerostomia can be severe. Radiation to the salivary glands causes fibrosis, fatty degeneration, acinar atrophy, and cellular necrosis within the salivary glands [17]. The serous gland acini are affected more than the mucous gland acini [9,17]. Therefore, with radiation treatment the oral secretions become thick and sticky. If the salivary glands are in the field of radiation treatment, permanent damage can be caused to the salivary glands [3]. There may be some regeneration of the salivary glands months after radiation treatment. However, in some patients salivary secretions will never be adequate such as when both the parotid glands are involved in the field of radiation [17].

With xerostomia, the saliva becomes more acidic and there is an increase in the number of cariogenic bacteria. Therefore, head and neck radiation patients are more prone to caries and lifelong daily neutral sodium fluoride should be applied to the teeth to reduce the risk of dental caries. Excellent daily oral hygiene is also extremely important to reduce the risk of dental caries in these patients. An alkaline rinse such as baking soda can be used by the xerostomic patient to help neutralize the acidic environment. Also, baking soda rinse can help dissolve mucous. Pilocarpine tablets (Salagen®) may be usedprophylactically or to treat xerostomia caused by head and neck radiation. It is a cholinergic parasympathomimetic agent increasing secretion not only to salivary glands but to other exocrine glands such as the pancreas, sweat, gastric, intestinal glands and mucous glands of the respiratory tract. It is contraindicated in patients with an allergy to pilocarpine, narrow angle glaucoma, acute iritis, and uncontrolled asthma. Pilocarpine should be used with caution in patients with cardiovascular disease, chronic bronchitis or COPD. Oral Balance® moisturizing gel, Mouth Kote® oral moisturizer or Salivart® synthetic saliva are a few of the over the counter products that can be used to help moisten the intraoral tissues.

SIDE EFFECTS SPECIFIC TO HEAD AND NECK RADIATION TREATMENT AND THEIR MANAGEMENT

Loss of Taste

Patients undergoing head and neck radiation treatment can have partial or complete loss of taste. Radiation damages the cells in the taste buds [17]. Partial taste loss may be noticed two weeks after starting head and neck radiation treatment. Taste is usually partially restored 20 to 60 days after completion of head and neck radiation treatment and usually completely restored within 2 to 4 months after radiation treatment [14,18]. Zinc supplements may improve taste sensation [6,17,19].

Trismus

When the masticatory muscles and/or the TMJ are involved in the field of radiation, trismus can develop due to muscle fibrosis. Trismus is usually noticed 3 to 6 months after radiation treatment [14,18]. Decreased opening of the mouth due to trismus can interfere with oral hygiene, speech and even eating [14]. Therefore, if the muscles of mastication or the TMJ are in the field of radiation, jaw exercises such as basic hinge opening movements should be done several times a day to reduce the risk of trismus [18].

Osteoradionecrosis(ORN)

ORN can be a serious complication of high dose head and neck radiation treatment. Radiation decreases the blood supply to bone and soft tissues by vascular thromboses and fibrosis [7]. Therefore, wound healing is compromised after high dose head and neck radiation treatment. Invasive dental procedures such as extractions in the areas of irradiated bone after high dose head and neck radiation treatment can result in ORN due to the hypovascularity and hypoxia of the bone [3]. It is extremely important that patients undergoing high dose head and neck radiation treatment undergo a thorough dental exam and all the necessary dental treatment including extractions be completed prior to beginning head and neck radiation treatment.

Risk of ORN is lifelong after high dose head and neck radiation treatment [3]. Patients should have frequent dental exams with dental x-rays as needed after high dose head and neck radiation treatment to detect dental problems early e.g. dental caries or periapical pathology, to reduce the risk of ORN. Even ill-fitting prosthesis can cause mucosal injury leading to ORN in the head and neck radiation patient. Dental prosthesis should be evaluated periodically for their fit. ORN is more common in the mandible than the maxilla. ORN may occur even without trauma or infection. Hyperbaric oxygen (HBO), surgical debridement and antibiotics can be used to treat ORN. If patients require extractions after head and neck radiation treatment, prophylactic antibiotics as well as HBO may be required before and after the extractions to reduce the risk of ORN. If patients develop ORN, they should be referred to those who have experience in dealing with ORN [3].

Radiation Caries

Radiation caries may develop rapidly due to radiation induced xerostomia. The decay usually occurs at the cervical area of the teeth and on the cusp tips. If not treated, decay can wrap around the entire tooth which can lead to fracture of the tooth at the gingival margin [9]. Neutral sodium fluoride applied via custom fluoride carriers, excellent daily oral hygiene, a diet low in sugar content, frequent dental exams and prophylaxis can all help to reduce the risk of the head and neck radiation patient developing radiation caries.

Long term effects of head and neck radiation treatment in children

Long term complications of head and neck radiation treatment in children include dental and craniofacial abnormalities. Dental abnormalities include caries, incomplete calcification, premature closure of apices, delayed eruption of teeth, arrested tooth development, altered root development such as shortening or blunting of roots, enamel opacities, enamel grooves and pits, small crowns and small teeth. Craniofacial abnormalities include trismus, malocclusion, and orofacial asymmetry. The location of the tumor, dosage of radiation, and the age of the patient at the time of head and neck radiation are factors in the severity of these abnormalities [5,19,20]. Therefore, children who have received high dose head and neck radiation treatment should be followed closely for the long term complications of radiation treatment.

SUMMARY OF ORAL CARE

Chemotherapy Patient

1.   Since the oral tissues are suppressed in their mitotic activity, they will become much thinner in dimension. This makes the mucosa more delicate and fragile. Thus, the patient is advised to avoid hard, crispy, and spicy foods because of the propensity to injure the oral mucosa.

2.   Another aspect of treating the oral mucosa is to bathe it frequently with an alkaline rinse such as a bicarbonate of soda rinse. Generally, as the patient senses an irritated feeling of the oral mucosa, he/she would begin the bicarbonate of soda rinses consisting of ½ teaspoon of baking soda in 4 ounces of warm water and rinse 2-3x/day. This is to be followed with a clear water rinse.

3.   The patient is advised to discontinue any toothpaste containing peroxide, tooth whitening and tartar control because these ingredients tend to be irritating to a more delicate mucosa.

4.   The patient should avoid alcohol and tobacco products as these are irritating to the intraoral tissues.

5.   The patient should avoid mouthwash containing alcohol as alcohol can be drying and irritating to the intraoral tissues.

6.   Daily oral hygiene consists of brushing teeth with fluoride toothpaste after each meal and at bedtime and flossing daily to reduce plaque. Disclosing tablets may be used to check for plaque to evaluate patients home care.

7.   The patient is advised to brush the dorsum of tongue twice a day with soft toothbrush to remove debris.

8.   The patient should remove dentures at night and soak them in water.

Radiation Treatment

In addition to the recommendations for the chemotherapy patients, the head and neck radiation patients should include the following recommendations:

1. Lifelong, daily neutral sodium fluoride applied to teeth to reduce the risk of dental caries.

2. The head and neck radiation patient must exercise the jaw in an opening and closing exercise twenty times three times a day. This prevents the masticatory muscles from developing stiffness or trismus like condition.

3. Patients are advised to carry a supply of water so he/she may moisten his/her oral tissues frequently.

4. Bicarbonate rinses at least three times a day or more often if possible to help neutralize the acidic environment in the xerostomic patient. Also, the bicarbonate rinse will help loosen debris and dissolve mucus.

5. Saliva substitutes to help moisten the intraoral tissues.

6. Xerostomic patients should avoid food high in sugar content due to their increased risk of caries. Also, patients should moisten their food to help in its digestion.

7. Patients are encouraged not to wear dentures during head and neck radiation treatment.

8. Routine dental exams and x-rays are used to detect dental problems early e.g.. dental caries, and periapical pathology, and to reduce the risk of osteoradionecrosis.

CONCLUSION

Patients undergoing chemotherapy and/or head and neck radiation treatment may have multiple side effects occurring simultaneously such as mucositis, candidiasis, herpetic stomatitis or xerostomia. It is important to make the diagnosis(es) and treat the patient as effectively as possible on the basis of the diagnosis(es). Therapeutic management is generated by the diagnosis (Table 2). The oral and dental care management should be individualized on a case by case basis as there are so many variables involved with the cancer patient.

Table 2. **Treatment Options for Oral Side Effects of Chemotherapy and/or Head and Neck Radiation Treatment**

Name and Typical Dosage of Drug	Indications	Comments
Fluconazole- 200 mg p.o. first day, then 100 mg p.o. for 7-14 days	Oropharyngeal Candidiasis	Numerous drug–drug interactions
Nystatin oral suspension- swish 5 mL for 2 minutes and expectorate/swallow qid for 7-14 days	Oropharyngeal Candidiasis	Use with with caution in xerostomic patient due to sugar content
Clotrimazole- 10 mg troche dissolved slowly in mouth 5x/day for 14 days	Oropharyngeal Candidiasis	May be difficult to dissolve for xerostomic patient Use with with caution in xerostomic patient due to sugar content
Nystatin/Triamcinolone 0.1% oint.- apply to lips t.i.d. with sterile swabs	Angular chelitis due to candidiasis	
Acyclovir- 400 mg tid	Herpetic stomatitis	Modify dose for renal function
Aqueous chlorhexadine 0.2% rinse. Swish with 15 mL for 30 sec and expectorate, b.i.d. (Note: this rinse is not available commercially but can be formulated by a pharmacist)	Antibacterial	Staining of teeth Nystatin and chlorhexidine should be used at least 1 hr apart Need to wait 30 min. before or after use to bruch teeth
Cephalexin- 500 mg p.o. t.i.d. Clindamycin 150 mg p.o. t.i.d.	Diffuse oral ulceras and neutropenia	
Dexamethasone 8 mg p.o. q.d. x 1-2 d	Diffuse painful oral ulcers	Contraindicated if oral herpes present
Flouride "trays"- PreviDent 1.1.% neutral sodium fluoride or Thera-Flur-N neutral sodium fluoride applied via custom fluoride carriers or brushed onto teeth with toothbrush	Xerostomia	As prophylaxis against decay
Sodium bicarbonate rinses- dissolve ½ tsp baking soda in 4 oz water and rinse t.i.d. Follow with clear water rinse.	Xerostomia Post-emesis	Do not swallow bicarbonate rinse Neutralizes oral acid in neutropenic patient, neutralizes stomach acid. Helps dissolve mucus and loosen debris
Salagen- 5 mg p.o. t.i.d	Xerostomia- after head and neck radiation	Contraindicated in narrow angle glaucoma, uncontrolled asthma, acute iritis, pilocarpine allergy
Oral Balance moisturizing gel- apply on tongue- using tongue, apply to oral tissues, prn	xerostomia	.
Mouth Kote oral moisturizer- swish around mouth 8-10 sec. and expectorate, prn	xerostomia	
Salivart synthetic saliva spray- spray into mouth for ½ sec prn	xerostomia	

REFERENCES

1. Peterson DE. Oral problems in supportive care: no longer an orphan topic? Support Care Cancer 2000; 8: 347-348.
2. Peterson DE. Pretreatment Strategies for Infection Prevention in Chemotherapy Patients. NCI Monogr 1990; 9: 61-71.
3. Peterson DE, D'Ambrosio JA. Nonsurgical Management of Head and Neck Cancer Patients. Dent Clin North Am 1994; 38: 425-445.
4. Jansma J, Vissink A, Spijkervet F, et al. Protocol for the Prevention and Treatment of Oral Sequelae Resulting from Head and Neck Radiation Therapy. Cancer 1992; 70: 2171-2180.
5. Consensus Statement: Oral Complications of Cancer Therapies. National Institutes of Health Consensus Development Panel. NCI Monogr 1990; 9: 3-8.
6. Silverman, S Jr. Oral cancer. Oral Surg Oral Med Oral Pathol Oral Radiol Endod 1999; 88(2): 122-126.
7. Silverman S Jr. Oral Defenses and Compromises: An Overview. NCI Monogr 1990; 9: 17-19.
8. Raber-Durlacher JE, Weijl NI, Abu Saris M, et al. Oral mucositis in patients treated with chemotherapy for solid tumors: a retrospective analysis of 150 cases. Support Care Cancer 2000; 8: 366-371.
9. Carl, W. Local Radiation and Systemic Chemotherapy: Preventing and Managing the Oral Complications. JADA 1993; 124: 119-123.
10. Sonis ST. Mucositis as a biological process: a new hypothesis for the development of chemotherapy-induced stomatotoxicity. Oral Oncology 1998; 34: 39-43.
11. Peterson DE. Oral Infection. Support Care Cancer 1999; 7: 217-218.
12. Sonis ST, Eilers JP, Epstein JB, et al. Validation of a New Scoring System for the Assessment of Clinical Trial Research of Oral Mucositis Induced by Radiation or Chemotherapy. Cancer 1999; 85: 2103-2113.
13. Toth B, Martin JW, and Fleming TJ. Oral complications associated with cancer therapy. J Clin Periodontol 1990; 17: 508-515.
14. Meraw SJ. Reeve CM. Dental Considerations and Treatment of the Oncology Patient Receiving Radiation Therapy. JADA 1998; 129: 201-205.
15. Redding SW. Role of Herpes Simplex Virus Reactivation in Chemotherapy-Induced Oral Mucositis. NCI Monogr 1990; 9: 103-105.
16. Epstein JB, Chow AW. Oral Complications Associated with Immunosuppression and Cancer Therapies. Infectious Disease Clin North Am 1999; 13: 901-923.
17. Silverman, S Jr. "Radiation Effects." In Oral Cancer, Sol Silverman, Jr., ed. Atlanta. GA: American Cancer Society, Inc. 1990.
18. Dreizen S. Description and Incidence of Oral Complications. NCI Monogr 1990; 9: 11-15.
19. Majorana A. Schubert MM, Porta F. et al. Oral complications of pediatric hematopoietic cell transplantation: diagnosis and management. Support Care Cancer 2000; 8: 353-365.
20. Jaffe N, Toth BB, Hoar RE, et al. Dental and Maxillofacial Abnormalities in Long-Term Survivors of Childhood Cancer: Effects of Treatment with Chemotherapy and Radiation to the Head and Neck. Pediatrics 1984; 816-823.

INDEX

Acinic cell carcinoma, 159*t*
Acyclovir, 363
Adenoid cystic carcinoma, 159*t*
Adjuvant chemotherapy, 253–54
Aerodigestive tract squamous cell
    carcinoma, 146–58
  etiology of, 147–48
  larynx, 153–58
  medical work-up of, 148
  nasopharyngeal carcinoma (NPC), 149–50
  oral cavity, 151–53
  oropharynx, 150–51
  presentation of, 146–47
  surgical therapy,
    indications/contraindications for, 148
Alcohol, 21–22, 22t, 23–24, 67–68
Alcohol dehydrogenases (ADHs), 34
Alcohol metabolism enzymes, 34
Alpha-tocopherol, 71, 72
Alveolous, cancer of, 90
American Joint Committee on Cancer
    (AJCC), 39–43
Anti-proliferative agents, 70*t*
Auditory canal carcinoma, external, 170–71

Basal cell carcinoma, 177
  surgical treatment for, 177–79, 179*t*
Benadryl elixir, 361
Beta-carotene, 71–72
Betel-nut quid, 25
Brachytherapy, 205–6
Buccal mucosa, cancer of, 90

Cancer
  treatment, nutrients and, 68–70
  head. *See* Head cancer
  neck. *See* Neck cancer
Candidiasis, 361–62, 362*f*
Carbazolin, 361
Carcinoma ex-pleomoprphic adenoma, 159*t*
Cartenoids, 70*t*
Cefazolin, 361
Cervical metastasis
  identification of, 317–20
  predictive indicators for, 317

Chemoradiotherapy, 240–45, 242*t*
  management of neck following, 264–65
  for nasopharyngeal carcinoma, 285–86
  quality of life and, 339
Chemotherapy, 69, 296–97
  adjuvant, 253–54
  combination, 257–59, 297–300, 298*t*,
    299*t*, 300*t*
  concomitant, 256
  dental care and, 355
  education on, 355
  in head and neck cancer, 5–6
  hyperfractionated radiotherapy and,
    260–61
  neoadjuvant, 254–55
  oral hygiene and, 354, 367
  organ preservation-induction
    chemotherapy, 213–29
  radiation therapy and, 6–8, 9
  in recurrent squamous cell carcinoma, 322
  side effects of, 11, 364
  single agent, 256–57
Children
  radiation therapy side effects on, 366
Cigars, 24
Cisplatin, 8, 296*t*, 297
Clear cell carcinoma, 159*t*
Clotrimazole, 362
Color Doppler ultrasound
  cervical metastasis and, 318
Combination chemotherapy, 257–59
Computed tomography (CT), 2, 37
  cervical metastasis and, 318
Concomitant chemotherapy
  radiation therapy and, 256
Cycloxygenase inhibitors, 70*t*
Cytochrome P-450, 33

Dexamethasone, 361
Dexamethasone elixir, 361
Diet, 65–66
DME modulators, 70*t*
Docetaxel, 8, 296*t*
Drinking
  quality of life and, 342–43

Ear, tumors of, 173–75
Epidermal growth factor receptor (EGFR), 8, 301–2
Epithelial carcinoma, 159*t*
Epstein-Barr virus (EBV), 30–31
   head and neck cancer and, 1
Erythroplakia, 63
Ethmoid sinus
   staging of, 42
External auditory canal carcinomas, 170–71

Farnesyl transferase inhibitors, 305–6
Fine needle aspiration (FNA), 36
   ultrasound-guided, 39
   ultrasound-guided, and cervical
      metastasis, 318
Flavonoids, 70*t*
Fluconazole, 362
5-Fluorouracil, 8, 296*t*, 297
Formaldehyde, 26

Gemcitabine, 296*t*
Genetic alterations, testing for
   in head and neck cancer, 2
Glottic larynx carcinoma, 103–7, 104*t*, 105*f*, 107*f*
   carcinoma in situ, 131–32
   classification of, 104*t*
   early vocal cord carcinoma, 132–36, 133*f*, 134*f*, 135*f*
   radiation therapy for, 131–36
   staging of, 41
   treatment of, 3–4
Glutathione S-transferase (GSTs), 33

Hard palate, cancer of, 90
Head and neck cancer
   age and, 20–21
   alcohol and, 21–22, 22*t*, 23–24, 67–68
   chemopreventive agents, 62, 70, 70*t*
   current treatment modalities for, 316–17
   dental care, 355–56
   diagnosis of, 36–39
   diet and, 65–66
   early stage, 3–5
   evaluation in, 36–39
   genetic susceptibility in, 32
   imaging in, 2–3
   late toxicities in, 331–245
   locoregionally advanced, 5–8, 315–25
   lymph node metastasis in, 2
   metastatic, treatment of, 295–309

modified fractionated radiotherapy in, 199–208
   mutagen sensitivity and, 64–65
   oral hygiene in, 9–11, 354–57
   organ preservation for, 235–46
   premalignant lesions, 27
   prevention of, 61–76
   quality of life in, 331–245
   race factors in, 21
   radiation therapy for, 120–21
   radiation therapy in, early stage, 115–41
   recurrent, clinical presentation of, 321
   recurrent, new therapies for, 315–25
   re-irradiation in recurrent, 199–208
   risk factors for, 1–3
   salvage therapy and, 320–21
   screening of, 44–46
   second primary tumors in, 34–36
   side effects of, 357–66
   socioeconomic factors in, 21
   surgery, advanced, 145–87
   surgery, early stage, 85–112
   tobacco and, 21–22, 22*t*, 23, 24, 66–67
   treatment of, 3–9
   United States incidence and mortality in, 17, 17*t*
   unresectable locoregionally advanced, 249–68
      treatment of, 251–52
   viral exposure and, 28–32
   worldwide incidence and mortality in, 16, 17*t*
Health-related quality of life (HRQOL), 331–32
Hemilaryngectomy, vertical, 107*t*
Herpes simplex virus (HSV), 31–32, 363, 363*f*
   head and neck cancer and, 1
Human Papillomavirus (HPV), 28–29
   head and neck cancer and, 1
Hyperfractionated radiotherapy
   chemotherapy and, 260–61
Hypopharyngeal cancer, 98–101
   anatomy of, 98–100, 99*f*, 100*t*
   classification of, 100*t*
   post-cricoid, 100
   posterior pharyngeal wall, 101
   pyriform sinus, 100–101
   radiation therapy for, 136–41, 137*f*, 138*f*, 139*f*, 140*f*, 141*f*
   regional lymph node staging of, 42
   staging of, 40

Ifosfamide, 296*t*
Intratumoral injections, 324

Laryngeal cancer, 102–22
  anatomy of, 102–3
  glottic carcinoma, 103–7, 104*t*, 105*f*, 107*f*
  neck dissection in, 110–12, 111*f*
  regional lymph node staging, 42
  staging of, 40–41
  subglottis, 103, 103*t*
  supraglottic carcinoma, 107–10, 108*f*,
    108*t*, 109*f*
Laryngectomy, supraglottic, 109*f*
Leukoplakia, 63
  tongue cancer with, 92*f*
Lidocaine
  viscous, 361
Lips, cancer of, 88–89
  staging of, 40
Lymph nodes, levels of
  in neck, 111*f*

Magnetic resonance imaging (MRI), 2, 37
  cervical metastasis and, 318–19
Marijuana, 26
Maxillary sinus carcinoma
  staging of, 41
Melanoma, 181–83, 182*t*
  surgical treatment of, 184–86, 186*f*
Meta-analysis, 252–53
Meta-Analysis of Chemotherapy in the Head
  and Neck Cancer (MACH-NC) study,
  253
Metastatic disease, 8–9
  biology of, 315–16
  cervical, identification of, 317–20
  cervical, predictive indicators for, 317
Methotrexate, 8, 296*t*, 297
Middle ear tumor, 173–75
Modified fractionation, 199–203
  conventional radiotherapy and, 200–203
  rational for, 199–200
Molecular staging
  in head and neck cancer, 3
Monoclonal antibodies, 302–4, 303*t*
Mood disorders, quality of life and, 340–41
Mouth, floor of
  cancer of, 90–92
Mucoepidermoid carcinoma, 159*t*
Mucositis, 357–61, 358*f*
  management of, 360–61
  World Health Organization grading of,
    359*t*

Mucositis, acute, 4
Mutagen sensitivity, 64–65
Myoepithelial carcinoma, 159*t*

Nasopharyngeal carcinoma (NPC), 149–50,
  275–90
  chemoradiotherapy, concurrent, 285–86
  combined modality treatment for, 284–86,
    285*t*, 287*f*
  diagnostic work-up of, 278
  distant metastasis treatment in, 288–90,
    289*t*
  epidemiology of, 275
  etiology of, 275–76, 276*f*
  imaging in, 277–80
  incidence and mortality in, 29–30
  molecular monitoring of, 280
  pathology of, 276–77
  presentation of, 277–80
  prognosis of, 280
  radiotherapy for, 280–84, 281*f*
  regional lymph node staging, 42
  salvage of local failure after radiotherapy
    in, 287–88
  staging of, 40, 277–80, 279*t*
  treatment in, 4–5
Navelbine, 296*t*
Neck cancer
  age and, 20–21
  alcohol and, 21–22, 22*t*, 23–24, 67–68
  chemopreventive agents of, 62, 70
  current treatment modalities for, 316–17
  dental care, 355–56
  diagnosis of, 36–39
  diet and, 65–66
  early stage, 3–5
  evaluation in, 36–39
  genetic susceptibility in, 32
  imaging in, 2–3
  late toxicities in, 331–245
  locoregionally advanced, 5–8, 315–25
  lymph node metastasis in, 2
  metastatic, treatment of, 295–309
  modified fractionated radiotherapy in,
    199–208
  mutagen sensitivity and, 64–65
  oral hygiene in, 9–11, 354–57
  organ preservation for, 235–46
  premalignant lesions, 27
  prevention of, 61–76
  quality of life in, 331–245
  race factors in, 21
  radiation therapy for, 120–21, 120*t*, 121*t*

radiation therapy in, early stage, 115–41
recurrent, clinical presentation of, 321
recurrent, new therapies for, 315–25
re-irradiation in recurrent, 199–208
risk factors for, 1–3
salvage therapy and, 320–21
screening of, 44–46
second primary tumors in, 34–36
side effects of, 357–66
socioeconomic factors in, 21
surgery, advanced, 145–87
surgery, early stage, 85–112
tobacco and, 21–22, 22*t*, 23, 24, 66–67
treatment of, 3–9
United States incidence and mortality in,
    17, 17*t*
unresectable locoregionally advanced,
    249–68
    treatment of, 251–52
viral exposure and, 28–32
worldwide incidence and mortality in, 16,
    17*t*
Neck, lymph nodes levels in, 111*f*
Neoadjuvant chemotherapy, 254–55
Nonsmokers, 25–26
Non-steroidal anti-inflammatory drugs
    (NSAIDs), 72–73
Nystatin oral suspension, 361, 362

Oncocytic carcinoma, 159*t*
Oral cavity cancer, 86–92
    alveolous, 90
    anatomy of, 86–88, 87*f*
    buccal mucosa, 90
    floor of mouth, 90–92
    hard palate, 90
    lips, 88–89
    radiation therapy for, 121–25, 122*f*, 123*f*,
        124*f*
    regional lymph node staging of, 42
    staging of, 40
    tongue, 92, 92*f*
    treatment of, 4
Oral hygiene
    in head and neck cancer, 9–11, 354–57
Oral neoplasia, 62–63, 64*t*
Organ preservation-induction chemotherapy,
    213–29
Oropharyngeal cancer, 93–98
    access for, 95*f*
    anatomy of, 93
    base of tongue, 94–96, 95*f*
    posterior pharyngeal wall, 97–98

radiation therapy for, 125–30, 126*f*, 127*f*,
    128*f*, 129*f*
regional lymph node staging of, 42
soft palate tumor, 93–94
staging of, 40
tonsillar pillar, 96–97
tonsils, 96–97
Osteoradionecrosis (ORN), 365–66

Paclitaxel, 8, 296*t*, 299*t*
Pain, quality of life and, 340
Paranasal sinus carcinoma, advanced,
    161–69, 162*t*
    etiology of, 163
    imaging of, 164
    physical examination in, 163
    regional lymph node staging of, 42
    staging of, 41–42
    surgery for, 165–69, 169*f*
    treatment of, 165
Photodynamic therapy, 325
Phytochemicals, 75–76
Pilocarpine, 364
Pipe smoking, 24
Polyphenols, 70*t*
Positron emission tomography (PET), 3, 38
    cervical metastasis and, 318–19
Post-cricoid, cancer of, 100
Potential lethal radiation damage repair
    (PLDR), 239
PPAR-gamma inhibitors, 70*t*
Pro-apoptotic agents, 70*t*
Pyriform sinus, cancer of, 100–101

Quality of life, 331–45
    chemoradiotherapy on, 339
    combination therapies on, 340
    definition of, 331–32
    function studies and, 343–44
    history of, 332
    radiation therapy on, 337–39, 337*t*
    recovery patterns and, 344
    surgery on, 336–37, 338–39
    treatment effect on, 336–40
    twelve month predictors of, 344–45
Quality of life, assessment, 333–35
    measures, choosing, 334
    measures in, 333–34
    schedule of, 334–35, 335*f*
Quality of life, research by symptom, 340–43
    drinking, 342–43
    mood disorders, 340–41
    pain, 340

patient priorities and preferences, 342
smoking, 342–43
xerostomia, 341–42

Radiation caries, 366
Radiation, resistance to, 238–40
mechanisms of, 238–39
overcoming, 239–40
Radiation therapy, 69
concomitant chemotherapy and, 256
data analysis, 119–20
dental care and, 355–56, 368
dose-fractionation consideration in,
118–19, 119*t*
education on, 356–57
modalities, 116, 117*f*, 118*f*
quality of life and, 337–39, 337*t*
results of, 120–31
side effects of, in children, 366
treatment guidelines for, 120–31
Radioresistance, overcoming, 239–40
Radio-surgery, 208
Radiotherapy (RT), 280–84, 281*f*
chemotherapy and, 6–8, 9
in head and neck cancer, 3–5
side effects of, 10
Regional lymph nodes, staging of, 42
Re-irradiation, 204–5
external, 206–8
in recurrent squamous cell carcinoma,
322–23
stereotactic, 208
Retinoids, 70–71

Salivary carcinoma, 158–61
clinical evaluation of, 160
clinical presentation in, 158
etiology of, 158
natural history of, 159, 159*t*
radiographic evaluation of, 160
regional lymph node staging of, 42
staging of, 42
surgery for, 160–61
Salivary gland, dysfunction of, 364
Salted fish, 27
Second primary tumors (SPT), 34–36
Single agent chemotherapy, 256–57
Sinonasal tract malignant tumors, 162*t*
Skin cancer, 176–86
basal cell, 177
excision defect closure of, 179*t*
squamous cell, 179
Smoking

cancer and, 1
quality of life and, 342–43
Snuff, 25
Soft palate tumor, 93–94
Squamous cell carcinoma (SCC)
recurrent, treatment options in, 322–25
chemotherapy in, 322
concomitant chemotherapy plus
re-irradiation in, 322–23
experimental therapies in, 324–25
re-irradiation therapy in, 322
surgery in, 323
surgical treatment for, 179
of vocal cords, 105*f*
Squamous intraepithelial neoplasia (SIN),
63, 64*t*
Stereotactic re-irradiation, 208
Subglottis carcinoma, 103, 103*t*
classification of, 103*t*
staging of, 41
Supraglottic laryngectomy, 109*f*
Supraglottic larynx carcinoma, 107–10,
108*f*, 108*t*, 109*f*
classification of, 108*t*
radiation therapy for, 130–31, 131*f*
staging of, 41
treatment of, 3–4
Surgical therapy
for advanced head cancer, 145–87
for aerodigestive tract squamous cell
carcinoma, 148
for basal cell carcinoma, 177–79
for early stage head cancer, 85–112
for melanoma, 184–86
for neck cancer, 85–112, 145–87
paranasal sinus carcinoma, for advanced,
165–69
quality of life and, 336–37, 338–39
for salivary carcinoma, 160–61
for squamous cell carcinoma, 323
temporal bone carcinoma, for advanced,
172
Surrogate endpoint biomarkers (SEBs), 62
Surveillance Program (SEER) Database
program, 18, 18*f*, 19*f*

Targeting p53, 306–8
Taste, loss of, 365
Temporal bone carcinoma, advanced,
170–75
clinical presentation in, 174–75
diagnostic imaging in, 171
external auditory canal carcinoma, 170–71

middle ear, 173–74
  surgical treatment for, 172, 173*f*
  treatment of, 175
Temporal bone tumor, 173–75
Tetracycline powder, 361
Tobacco, 21–22, 22*t*, 23, 24, 66–67
  nonsmokers, 25–26
  smokeless, 24–25
Tocopherols, 70*t*
Tongue, cancer of, 92, 92*f*
  base of, 94–96, 95*f*
  with leukoplakia, 92*f*
Tonsillar pillar, cancer of, 96–97
Tonsils, cancer of, 96–97
Toxicity
  management of, 265–66
  prevention of, 265–66
Trismus, 365

Tumor node metastasis (TNM) staging
    system, 86
Tyrosine kinase inhibitors, 304–5, 305*t*

United States
  incidence and mortality rate in, 17, 17*t*

Vertical hemilaryngectomy, 107*t*
Viscous lidocaine, 361
Vocal cords
  squamous cell carcinoma of, 105*f*

Wood dust, 26

Xerostomia, 4
  quality of life and, 341–42

Zinc, 74–75